EMERGENCY!
FIRST AID
For Home Recording

Paul White

smt

621.3893

E   CY!

AID

For F   ling

AWN

Also by Paul White and available from Sanctuary Publishing:

Creative Recording Part 1: Effects And Processors (second edition)
Creative Recording Part 2: Microphones, Acoustics, Soundproofing And Monitoring (second edition)
Desktop Digital Studio
Home Recording Made Easy (second edition)
Live Sound For The Performing Musician
MIDI For The Technophobe (second edition)
Recording And Production Techniques (second edition)

The *Basic* series:

Basic Digital Recording
Basic Effects And Processors
Basic Home Studio Design
Basic Live Sound
Basic Mastering
Basic Microphones
Basic MIDI
Basic Mixers
Basic Mixing Techniques
Basic Multitracking
Basic Sampling
Basic VST Effects
Basic VST Instruments

Printed in the United Kingdom by MPG Books, Bodmin

Published by SMT, an imprint of Sanctuary Publishing Limited, Sanctuary House, 45-53 Sinclair Road, London W14 0NS, United Kingdom

www.sanctuarypublishing.com

ISBN: 1-84492-000-3

CONTENTS

INTRODUCTION

This book is written for those people who already have a little experience in recording or using MIDI equipment but who now feel ready to explore different avenues. However, I'm well aware then whenever we enter new territory, we also encounter problems, so the approach is a little different to my other books on recording and MIDI techniques, *Recording And Production Techniques*, *Home Recording Made Easy* and *MIDI For The Technophobe*. In addition to the more usual instruction and explanation, *Emergency! First Aid For Home Recording* specifically concentrates on those areas with which the majority of people have problems. Where possible, it explains how best to avoid those problems, but techniques are also described for improving imperfect existing recordings. The professionals call this 'audio sweetening', but I prefer the rather more pragmatic term 'salvage'!

Emergency! also addresses specific technical issues, such as electrical mains supplies in the studio, ground-loop problems, equipment maintenance, and the cleaning of both analogue and digital tape machines. And of course there's the thorny subject of computer-based audio systems! There's also a discussion on the pros and cons of vintage equipment, and a section on improving your studio acoustics and soundproofing at minimal expense.

Along the way you'll discover new ways of tackling familiar jobs, learn useful techniques to help you with mixing and recording, and find out how to plan and organise a recording session. There's a full section on producing a stereo master tape for CD or tape production, and you even get to learn how to solder and to set up the action on an electric guitar.

Common MIDI problems are discussed, including an extensive section on synchronisation systems and their weaknesses, though there are also plenty of creative suggestions too, such as how to create new synth sounds without extensive editing, or how to add new life to your sequencing. Whichever way your creative nature is trying to take you, this book will help you get there.

1 SESSION PLANNING AND RECORDING

If you've ever spent some time working on a session where the final recordings have been out of tune, or where the instruments have sounded perhaps less than ideal, you're not alone. However, a little preparation can help to eliminate most of the common problems.

It's one thing pottering about with your own material, but when other performers are involved, you need to do a little organisation in advance in order to keep the session flowing smoothly. Musicians are not the most patient of creatures, and if they have to wait around while you clean the tape machines or fix faulty leads, their creativity is likely to suffer.

In order to keep track of what instrument is recorded where, create a track sheet for your studio and then photocopy it. Most computer graphics packages will handle this very easily, but if you don't have access to a computer, a felt pen, a ruler and a steady hand will do just as well. All you need are numbered boxes to represent the recorded tracks, with room inside to write a few notes. If you are using a sequencer on the session, also include a MIDI section on the sheet for your sequencer tracks, showing what patches are used, and which MIDI channels the synths, samplers and drum machines are set to.

Clean Machines

If you're using an analogue tape machine, it's also good practise to clean the heads before every session. This isn't difficult and is best done using cotton buds dipped in isopropyl alcohol. Allow the machine to dry for a minute or so before threading the tape. Make sure all the heads and guides are thoroughly clean (no more brown oxide will come off on the cotton bud when cleaning is complete), and if the rubber pinch roller needs cleaning, use a dilute solution of washing up liquid, not alcohol. If you use alcohol, it will eventually cause the rubber to perish. For further details, see the section in tape-machine maintenance.

Digital tape recorders require less frequent cleaning than analogue machines but be warned that the dry head cleaning tapes often recommended by the manufacturers don't always do a thorough job. If the error readings are significantly higher than normal, and if the numbers don't change when you swap tapes, the machine probably needs a wet clean, though routine wet cleaning doesn't normally need to be carried out more than once every few weeks. If the error figures remain high after cleaning, the machine probably needs a service, and as a rule, digital machines require servicing every 500 hours or so. Most have an inbuilt counter to let you know how long the capstan motor has been running.

Wet cleaning requires a special type of ultra fine, lint free cleaning cloth to apply the cleaning fluid. Isopropyl alcohol is OK, but more effective proprietary fluids are available from studio suppliers. Never, ever use cotton buds on a digital machine. Studio suppliers usually stock ready moistened disposable digital head cleaning wipes in sealed packets, and these are probably the safest bet for the inexperienced user. See the section on tape machine maintenance for further details on cleaning digital machines.

Studio Readiness

Before your performers arrive, you should take the time to get the studio ready for the session, and this includes removing any temporary markings from the mixing console, setting all the channel EQs to neutral, turning down all aux sends and faders, and ensuring all the routing buttons are in their unrouted positions. If you're using a digital mixer or computer system, simply call up your default empty song.

The patch bay should be cleared of all wiring apart from any processors that you know you'll need on the session, and all leads should be neatly stowed ready for use. Tape machines should be cleaned as directed previously, and blank tapes should be to hand. Digital multitrack tapes should be formatted before the musicians arrive.

Reference CDs of material similar to that you'll be working on will help you get the sounds right, and it helps to be able to refer to these as the session progresses, just to make sure you're still going in the right direction. CDs are also invaluable at the mixing stage, as it's very easy for your ears to become accustomed to the sound you're working on, even if it is far too bright or too dull.

The Musician's Part

Part of the musicians' responsibility is to ensure that their instruments are in good working order, and in the case of guitars, that means decent strings should be fitted, the intonation should be correct, and there should be no string buzzes, noisy controls or poor electrical contacts. The same obviously applies to basses. Check tunings before each recording because they have a habit of drifting out as the room warms up. Modern keyboards are generally immune to tuning drift, but old analogue synths should be checked very regularly and be allowed to warm up for as long as possible before recording starts. Keep a can of Deoxit handy for fixing noisy connections.

That Elusive Drum Sound

Drums require special attention, as the only way to record a good drum sound is to start with a good-sounding kit. At the very least, heads should be in good condition and the kit should be properly tuned.

Most contemporary drum sounds rely on the front kick drum head having a hole cut in it, and if the hole is fairly small, you made need to damp the remaining head material with pads of tissue and tape to prevent it ringing. Weak sounding kick drums can often be improved by taping a piece of plastic or an old credit card to the head at the point where the beater impacts. Wooden beaters usually produce a better attack sound for rock sound than cork.

Individual drums may also be damped using small patches of duct tape (gaffa tape), but don't overdamp the drums as small rings and rattles tend to be hidden when everything is playing. As a rule, drums sound best when recorded in a slightly live environment, so if you're working at home on a carpeted floor, you could place a sheet of hardboard beneath the kit when setting up to reflect some of the sound back to the mics. The spurs at the front of the kick drum can rest on the carpet to prevent the drum creeping.

It may help to position additional reflective material around the room if the sound is still too dead, but don't worry about this too much, because if you get a good basic drum sound down, you can do a lot with artificial reverb to add life to the sound. Pay particular attention to siting the drum mics where they won't be in the drummer's way. If getting a drum sound is giving you particular problems, consult the section on recording drums in Chapter 2, 'Vocal And Instrument Recording', which also includes tips on how to rescue substandard drum tracks.

Working Sequence

In most pop or rock sessions, it's best to get the bass and drums down first so that you have a rhythm section to hang the rest of the material on. If you can put down a rough rhythm guitar or keyboard part at the same time, it'll serve as a navigational aid as to whereabouts you are in the song. Vocals, solos and additional instrumentation can be added as overdubs, though it helps to put a guide vocal down early on so that there's no confusion over what part of the song you're working on. This doesn't need to be anything fancy – just give the vocalists a mic, preferably in the control room away from the instruments being recorded 'for real', and record the result onto a spare track. Also make sure the mic is feeding into the musicians' monitor mix so that they know exactly where they are.

When recording vocals, ask the singer which instruments they most need to hear in the headphone mix, and you can also add reverb to the vocals in the cans to make the singer feel more comfortable. Use diplomacy and coaxing to get the best possible performance from all the players, and don't be satisfied with any recording that is out of time, out of tune, or that you know could be done significantly better. The whole beauty of multitrack is that it enables everybody to perform to the best of their abilities, so take advantage of the flexibility it offers.

MDM Slave Reels

When working with multiple modular digital multitrack machines (MDMs), the relatively slow lockup time of the machines can become very frustrating when you move on to doing vocal overdubs and punch ins. To make things easier, do a rough mix of the tracks you've recorded so far onto a spare track on the tape you're using to record the vocals. You can now switch off the other MDMs and just use this 'slave reel' to get the vocals and any other overdubbed parts just right. Once you've got the takes you need, mute or record over the rough guide track, put the other tape machines back on line and mix as usual.

Mixing And Effects

Some engineers like to add effects at the mixing stage – other add them while recording. Leaving effects until the final mix keeps your options open for longer, but more important is capturing a good performance. If playing through effect makes the musicians play better, then it's probably best to work their way. On systems with a limited number of tracks, it may also be necessary to add effect during performance if two or more sounds are to be mixed onto the same track for recording, although this is less of an issue with computer-based systems, where track capacity is less of a problem.

Always try to take a break between recording and mixing to allow your ears to get back to normal, and listen carefully to each track to make sure there are no unwanted noises, wrong notes or unacceptably out of tune bits. If there are sections of recorded background noise between verses or before guitar solos, either erase them or use a gate to keep the track clean. Of course, if you have access to mix automation, you'll be able to do this far more accurately. Only once you are absolutely sure that the recorded tracks are as good as they can be should you move onto mixing. Mixing has problems and pitfalls all of its own, which is why there's a separate chapter dedicated to mixing and balancing. However, don't forget to keep referring to that CD player to maintain your sense of perspective.

After The Mix

When you have a final master mix you are satisfied with, don't reset the desk and unplug everything from the patchbay, because you'll need to listen to copies of your master on other stereo systems, including car stereo cassette systems, to establish how well your mix 'travels'. When making cassette copies, it's usually best to use a Type II or chrome-type tape, but record with the noise reduction switched off. While this will result in more background hiss, it will help to minimise tonal effects due to any misalignment between the deck used to record the tape and those used to play it back.

If your master is intended for commercial release, it will probably be on DAT tape or CD-R, and the company that does your CD mastering should also be able to make final adjustments using EQ and compression. However, don't expect them to work miracles – they can fine-tune a good mix, but they won't be able to salvage a poor balance or a mix where the sounds of the various instruments and voices don't compliment each other.

If the song needs a fade-out ending, don't do this at the mix – instead, make sure you have at least 30 seconds' worth of spare material to cover the fade time and let the company doing your mastering handle the fade. Not only will the fade be smoother, it will also fade into pure silence rather than leaving the background noise from your console exposed. The same is true if you do your own mastering.

That concludes the overview of the recording and mixing session, but not everyone has as much equipment as they'd like. The next part of this chapter deals with using a very basic mixer for multitrack recording n situations where a proper multitrack console may not be available.

Multitracking With A Basic Stereo Mixer

The problem: You have a multitrack session to record, but the only mixer available is a stereo model. It has plenty of inputs, but only two outputs and no tape-monitoring section. How do you use it to do multitrack recording?

Part of the problem is that we're so familiar with the archetypal multitrack mixer, with its fancy monitoring sections and multiple-buss routing, that it's easy to believe it's the only tool for the job, but that's simply not true. In fact, I don't think I know anyone who uses the tape-monitoring section of their console for the intended purpose, anyway. Combine this with the fact that a typical pop session involves a lot of either recording single instruments onto single tracks, or overdubbing, and you soon realise that all the tools you need are there a modest 16 or 24:2 stereo mixer.

Multitrack Paradigm

A studio mixer must serve two functions; during recording, it facilitates signals from microphones and instruments to be routed to specific tracks on a multitrack recorder and along the way it allows you to set the recording levels and EQ. Once you have recorded your first lot of tracks, these need to be monitored somehow so you can play along with what you've already recorded. Being able to hear what you've already recorded is the very essence of multitracking, as it allows your recording to be built up using layers of overdubs.

When all the necessary tracks have been recorded, the mixer assumes its second role – that of providing a means to mix down all the tape tracks

to stereo. This is the conventional way of working, and indeed it is the method most likely explained in your mixer manual, but you still have the means to do all these things using a stereo mixer.

The first problem to solve is that of monitoring, but you'll find most multitrack console owners work the way I'm about to suggest because traditional in-line or split monitoring methods are actually rather cumbersome. All the time you're recording, you're fine-tuning the monitor mix to get a good balance, you're adding effects and tweaking the EQ. When the time comes to do the real mix, however, all this work has to be scrapped if you're using a split console – you have to rebuild your mix from scratch using the mixer's input channels.

In-line monitoring is more flexible, but with the flexibility comes complexity, and a lot of people find it confusing. In fact, most monitor channels seem to be used as spare inputs for synths, samplers and effects returns. The real work is done using perfectly ordinary input channels.

Console Monitoring

A monitor input (whether split or in-line) is just a simplified input channel routed directly to the stereo mix buss; it has no mic amp and usually has less in the way of EQ and aux sends than the main inputs. So, providing you have enough input channels, why not simply use an input channel instead? No reason at all – as I said before, many of us work this way anyway. This is what I call the 'all-input' approach to mixing, and it works like this:

Imagine you have a setup comprising a 16-channel mixer linked to an eight-track recorder. The first thing to do is wire all the tape machine outputs to mixer inputs 1–8 and route all these channels to the left/right stereo mix. In other words, these channels are set up just as they would be for a normal mix-down session. There's no need for monitor channels because we are, in effect, monitoring the output of the recorder at all times via channels 1–8, and most multitrack recorders arrange their internal monitor switching so that the correct signals are always present at the machine's outputs. Because we're using these same channels

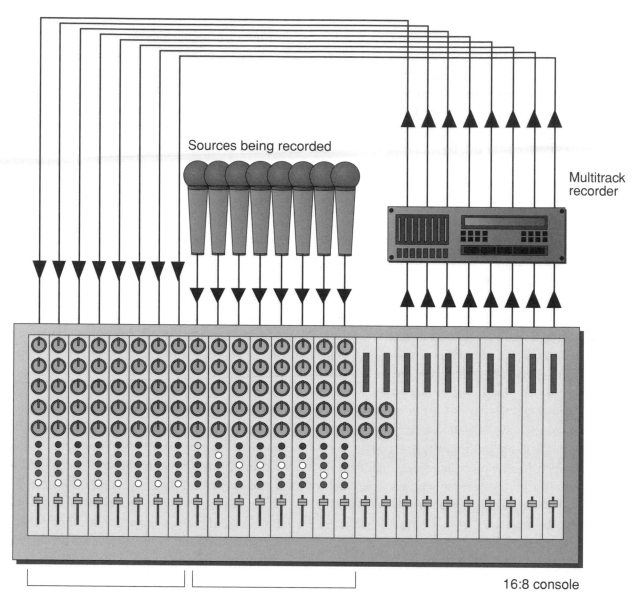

Sources being recorded

Multitrack recorder

16:8 console

Tape returns feed channels 1–8 and are routed to L/R mix

Channels 9–16 are free to feed sources to the multitrack recorder using the usual group-routing buttons. If a simple stereo mixer is to be used, the multitrack recorder may be fed from the channel direct outputs or insert sends, and any spare pre-fade aux sends may be used to create groups

Using this system, the multitrack tape out is always monitored via the mixer's main input channels, so there is no rerouting required between recording and mixing. During mixing, channels 9–16 are free to handle MIDI sources or additional effects returns

Figure 1.1: Console used in all-input mode

to handle the final mix, you can go straight from track-laying to mixing with no repatching at all. And if, during the mix, somebody decides they want to re-record something (as they so often do), there's no need to reset the whole console to make it possible. Figure 1.1 shows how to use a console in 'all-input' mode.

Tracking

That leaves eight spare mixer input channels (9–16) which we can use to handle the mic and line inputs we wish to record. The challenge is to find a way to route these channels to tape without having multiple mix busses to play with.

On the face of it, an eight-track tape machine needs a mixer with eight output groups, otherwise how can you record on all eight tracks at once? Without doubt, multiple output groups make things simple if you do want to record all your tracks at

the same time, but unless you're doing live recording, you'll probably only need to record one or two tracks at a time, especially if most of your backing comes from a MIDI system.

Most mixing consoles have channel-insert points, which can be used to take a signal direct from an input channel to the input of a multitrack recorder. The easiest way to pick up the insert send is to plug in a 'stereo to dual mono' jack adaptor, then use a conventional mono lead to connect the appropriate side of the adaptor to the recorder, as shown in Figure 1.2.

To use the channel for recording, leave the fader fully down, then use the input-gain trim to set the level being fed to your recorder. If the insert point comes post-EQ, then you'll also be able to EQ the signal as you record, but if not, don't worry about it as it's usually best to record flat and EQ during the mix anyway. In addition to enabling you to route

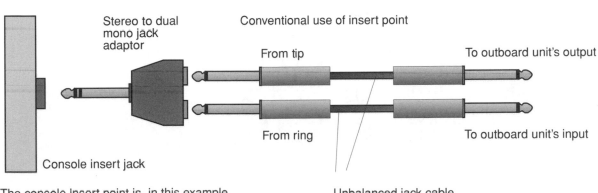

Stereo to dual mono jack adaptor

Conventional use of insert point

From tip

To outboard unit's output

From ring

To outboard unit's input

Console insert jack

Unbalanced jack cable

The console Insert point is, in this example, wired ring send, tip return. Note that some manufacturers use the opposite convention, so always consult your mixer manual

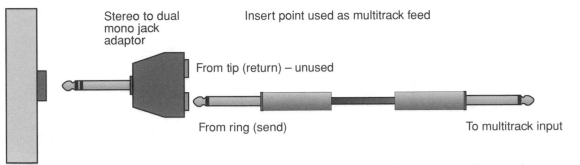

Stereo to dual mono jack adaptor

Insert point used as multitrack feed

From tip (return) – unused

From ring (send)

To multitrack input

Figure 1.2: Picking up insert send from stereo/dual mono jack adaptor

any mixer channel wherever you like, using your insert sends as multitrack feeds gets your signal to the recorder without it having to pass through any unnecessary circuitry. Even the best mixer circuits cause some degradation of the input signal, so if you can avoid the channel pan circuit, the routing switches, the mix busses and the group output amplifiers, then so much the better.

Improvised Grouping

An obvious weakness when working this way is that you have no grouping busses to allow you to mix several mixer channels down to one tape track. However, you do have one or more pre-fade aux sends, and you can use these in exactly the same way as conventional groups. For example, if you want to mix channels 9, 10 and 11 and then send

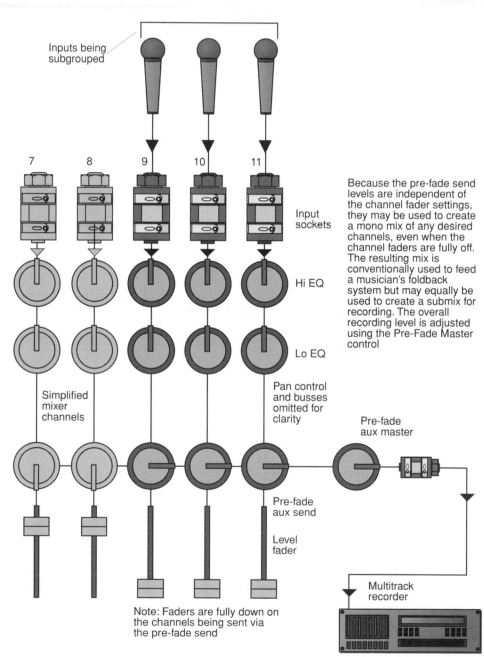

Inputs being subgrouped

7   8   9   10   11

Input sockets

Hi EQ

Lo EQ

Simplified mixer channels

Pan control and busses omitted for clarity

Pre-fade aux master

Pre-fade aux send

Level fader

Note: Faders are fully down on the channels being sent via the pre-fade send

Multitrack recorder

Because the pre-fade send levels are independent of the channel fader settings, they may be used to create a mono mix of any desired channels, even when the channel faders are fully off. The resulting mix is conventionally used to feed a musician's foldback system but may equally be used to create a submix for recording. The overall recording level is adjusted using the Pre-Fade Master control

Figure 1.3: Recording a subgroup via the pre-fade aux send (channels 9, 10 and 11)

the result to multitrack track 1, all you need to do is turn the channel faders down on channels 9, 10 and 11, use the pre-fade aux pots to set the respective levels and use the pre-fade aux master to set the correct recording level. The mixed signal will be monitored at track 1's output via mixer channel 1. Figure 1.3 shows how this may be achieved. Note that the recorder (track 1) is fed from the pre-fade aux send.

Mixers With Groups

While the previously described way of working is fine for set-ups where most of the recording is in the form of overdubs, you can get more flexibility from a mixer with multiple groups. If you're thinking about upgrading your mixer beyond a basic, general-purpose model but you can't justify the expense of an all-singing, all-dancing multitrack desk, a simple 16:4 mixer will provide you with plenty of flexibility for eight-track work.

The limitations are not in the number of tracks you can get onto tape at any one time, because we've seen how the channel-insert sends may be used to accomplish this. Where you are restricted is in the number of submixes you can create, and so far we've only been able to create mono submixes using the pre-fade aux sends.

If you have a four-buss desk (stereo buss plus two additional busses), you'll also be able to set up one stereo submix via the extra busses. This is very useful when you're mixing multiple sources that need to be recorded to two tracks as a stereo submix – for example, drums, backing vocals and so on. Even with relatively complex work, you'll probably have enough flexibility recording individual tracks from insert sends, mono groups from pre-fade aux sends and a single stereo group via your two spare busses. Of course, you may have to do a little patching to get what you want, but that's a small price to pay for getting so much recording flexibility out of such a simple mixer. Given that modern recording systems often offer plenty of tracks, the need to mix signals prior to recording is less pressing than it once was.

The other benefit of having a couple of additional busses is that, when you're mixing, you can create a stereo subgroup to simplify the control of a number of elements that need to maintain their relative levels – for example, the drums in a drum kit.

Making A Choice

The main differences between a general-purpose stereo mixing console and a studio console are the routing, the monitoring and the number of groups provided. Simple general-purpose desks have no monitoring, they usually have more basic routing – and they tend to be a lot cheaper! Even so, many basic general purpose consoles have some provision for playing a two-track recorder back through the desk, but even this can be accomplished using simple patching if the facility is absent.

The very basic 'something into two' live mixer has its shortcomings for multitrack work because of the limited ways in which groups of signals can be routed to the recorder, but a number of inexpensive, general-purpose consoles are available which have routing to either two or four group busses plus the main left/right stereo mix. Providing these consoles have direct channel outputs, or at the very least insert points, it is possible to use them as outlined above for very serious multitrack work, right up to 16- or 24-track.

The Submixer

If using a simpler mixer would leave you short of inputs for your MIDI gear, consider using a separate keyboard mixer for your sequenced instruments and patch this into either two channels of your main mixer or into a pair of aux returns, as shown in Figure 1.4. Because you're not paying for facilities you don't need (such as mic amps and multiple-buss routing), what you get tends to be sensibly priced, compact and with a good audio performance. A rack-mount keyboard mixer can take up just a few U of rack space yet may offer as many as 16 stereo-input channels with EQ and a number of aux sends.

Submixer Limitations

One limitation when adding a separate mixer is that the effects-send systems are also separate. This can

**Figure 1.4: Using a keyboard submixer
(via channels or aux returns)**

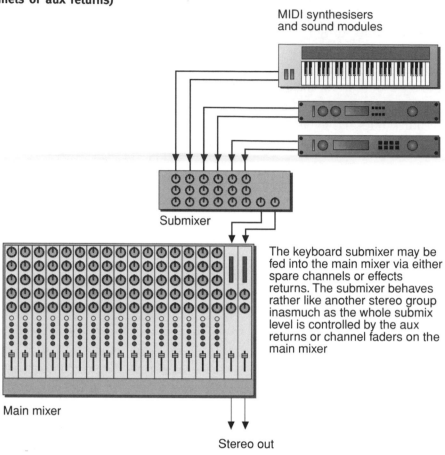

MIDI synthesisers
and sound modules

Submixer

Main mixer

The keyboard submixer may be
fed into the main mixer via either
spare channels or effects
returns. The submixer behaves
rather like another stereo group
inasmuch as the whole submix
level is controlled by the aux
returns or channel faders on the
main mixer

Stereo out

make it difficult to share the same effects units between the two mixer. It is possible to work around this, but the only really simple solution is to use an effects unit with a stereo input, then feed each of the two inputs from each of the two mixers, as shown in Figure 1.5. Alternatively, use a separate effects unit on the keyboard mixer. This may only need to be a quite basic reverb unit, as the majority of modern MIDI instruments come with built in multi-effects capabilities.

Cost Versus Features

By spending your money on a simpler console with more channels, you get full facilities on all channels, a simpler way of working and probably a cleaner signal path. Although you can manage a lot of multitrack work with a general-purpose stereo mixer,

you'll get more flexibility if you have one or two stereo groups available in addition to the main stereo buss.

Adding a separate rack-mount line mixer to handle MIDI instruments and aux returns can also be very cost-effective and saves on studio space. However, it can complicate the way in which effects are shared between the two mixers.

Console-Routing Tricks

Even if you have a multitrack console, you may still find yourself short of facilities, but by applying a little lateral thinking it's possible to make your console's routing system do tricks it was never designed to do.

Mixing consoles are invariably fitted with both pre-fade and post-fade aux sends, with the intention

Figure 1.5: Sharing an effects unit between mixer and submixer (one input from each)

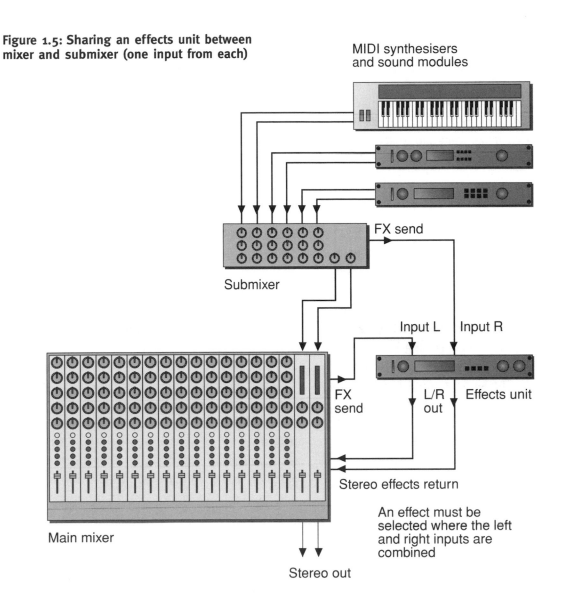

MIDI synthesisers
and sound modules

FX send

Submixer

Input L   Input R

FX
send

L/R
out

Effects unit

Stereo effects return

An effect must be
selected where the left
and right inputs are
combined

Main mixer

Stereo out

of allowing the user to set up foldback mixes or add effects from outboard effects units. These are the applications described in mixer manuals and textbooks, but you can find numerous novel uses for the aux busses that aren't often documented.

Pre-Fade Conventions

During an overdub situation, a cue or foldback mix is generally necessary so that the performers can hear any tracks already recorded. This is routinely set up using a pre-fade send, a control found in the channel strip that feeds some of the channel signal onto a mono mix buss running the length of the

mixer and out via an aux master level control. The output from aux 1, for example, feeds onto the aux 1 buss and then to the aux 1 output socket via the aux 1 master output-level control. Foldback or cue signals are called pre-fade because they're picked up before they reach the channel fader. The significance of this is that, once set, the level of the aux 1 signal doesn't change if the channel-fader setting is varied.

It follows that an independent mono mix of all your channels can be set up using the aux 1 controls, and this will appear at the aux 1 output, where it may be fed to a headphone amplifier or other monitoring system. If you have more than one pre-fade send, you can set up a number of different monitor mixes to satisfy the requirements of each musician, providing you have a multichannel headphone amplifier system. A typical situation is where the backing vocalists want a lot of lead vocal in the cans whereas the drummer and bass player want to hear each other. This is the conventional way to use the pre-fade or foldback sends.

Post-Fade Conventions

Post-fade aux-send controls pick up their signal feeds after the channel fader, so any change to the channel fader also affects the aux-send level. This is exactly what's needed if the aux send is being used to feed an effect such as reverb or echo because, as the channel fader setting is changed during the course of a mix, the amount of effect needs to change by the same amount to maintain the correct proportion of effect to dry signal. By using different settings of the post-fade control on each channel, it is possible to send different amounts of each channel's signal to the same effects unit.

Using the aux-send system has the advantage that different amounts of the same effect can be added to different sounds in a mix. A typical example might be where one reverberation unit is used to provide a rich reverb for the vocals, less reverb for the drums and little or none for the guitars and bass.

Important: an effects unit used in conjunction with a channel aux send should be set up so that it produces only the effected sound and none of the original. This is usually achieved using the mix control, which is either in the form of a physical control or accessed via the effects unit's editing software. In either case, the mix should be set to 100 per cent effect, 0 per cent dry. The amount of effect added to a channel signal is determined by the setting of the pre-fade aux send control.

The output of the effect unit may be fed back into the mixer via spare input channels or via dedicated effects return inputs, also known as *aux returns*. Aux returns are electrically similar to the input channels but usually with far fewer facilities. If a spare input channel (or channels) is used as an effects return, ensure that the aux send on those channels are turned fully down to prevent feedback. To keep the effect in stereo, the two returns or channels must be panned hard left and right.

Also note that, although most stereo reverbs have two input jacks, the reverb itself is generated from a sum of the left and right input signals, so you only need to tie up one aux send. Usually, one of the effect input sockets will have the word 'mono' next to it, indicating that, for mono-in/stereo-out operation, you should send the input to that jack.

These distinctions between pre-fade and post-fade send, and the way in which aux sends are used, also apply to 'virtual' software mixers.

Effects And Insert Points

An insert point is simply a connector that allows the normal signal path to be interrupted and rerouted through an external device. Insert points usually take the form of stereo jacks wired to carry both send and return signals, and if you don't have a patchbay you'll need a Y-lead with a stereo jack on one end and two monos on the other. Inserts are normally fitted to all mixer channels that have mic inputs and often to the groups and main stereo outputs, too.

You can connect either an effects unit or a signal processor to a mixer via an insert point, and in a situation where an effect is required on only a single mixer channel, connecting it via the insert point will provide a cleaner signal path than going via the aux sends, because you'll avoid picking up mix-buss noise from all the other channels connected to the aux-send buss. It will also save tying up aux sends unnecessarily. Note that, when an effect is connected in this way, the dry/effect balance must be set on the effects unit itself. Again, virtual-mixer insert points work on the same principle.

Inserts As Aux Sends

This is where we start to use the mixer less conventionally. For example, if an effect is required on only one channel, a stereo effects processor can be fed from an insert send and the effect outputs brought back into a pair of spare channels or a stereo effect return input as normal. Not only does this conserve your remaining aux sends but it also reduces noise, as the feed to the effects unit doesn't suffer from cumulative mix-buss noise. Figure 1.6 illustrates this method of connection. The effects mix should be set at 100 per cent wet in this case and the effects-return channel controls used to set the effect level.

Note: as the insert point comes before the channel fader, the effect level will remain constant, even if the channel fader is moved. If there is a need to adjust the channel fader during the mix, it helps to return the effects to two adjacent channels so that all three faders can be moved together.

If you don't have your insert points wired to a patchbay, you may have to make up a special lead to allow you to take a feed from the insert point without interrupting the signal flow through the channel. Some mixers allow you to take a direct feed from the insert point by using a mono jack and pushing it into the socket only halfway.

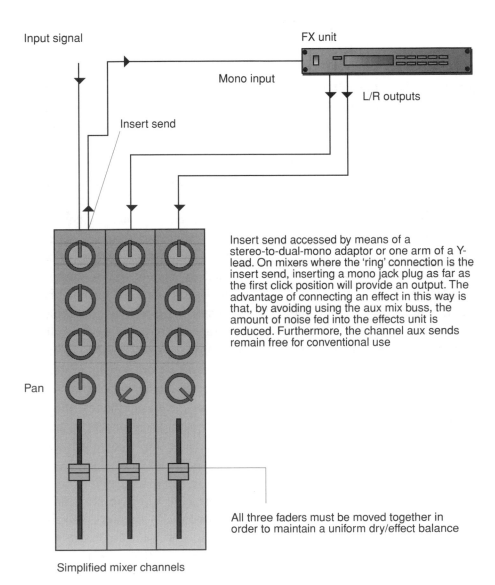

Input signal

FX unit

Mono input

L/R outputs

Insert send

Insert send accessed by means of a stereo-to-dual-mono adaptor or one arm of a Y-lead. On mixers where the 'ring' connection is the insert send, inserting a mono jack plug as far as the first click position will provide an output. The advantage of connecting an effect in this way is that, by avoiding using the aux mix buss, the amount of noise fed into the effects unit is reduced. Furthermore, the channel aux sends remain free for conventional use

Pan

All three faders must be moved together in order to maintain a uniform dry/effect balance

Simplified mixer channels

Figure 1.6: Using an insert send to feed an effects unit (stereo returns into two adjacent spare channels)

You can also use this method for providing a direct channel feed to a multitrack recorder input. In this case, turn the channel fader right down, and/or ensure all routing buttons are in their off positions, then use the input-gain 'trim' control to set the recording level to tape.

Sends As Tape Outs

A pre-fade send is simply an independent mono mix based on the channel pre-fade send control settings, so even if the main channel faders are turned down, you can still create a pre-fade mix. This is potentially useful in a mixer that has fewer output groups than you might like, because you can use any pre-fade send output to feed a multitrack recorder input. In other words, you're using the pre-fade send as an additional output group. You have to control levels using knobs rather than faders, but in all other respects the result is exactly the same. For example, if you have a couple of mics on mixer channels 1 and 2 that you want to mix together and record on tape track 6, all you have to do is turn the channel faders on channels 1 and 2 right down, turn up the pre-fade sends and route the corresponding pre-fade send output to tape-input 6. The send master-level control may then be used to set the correct signal level to tape. The principle here is exactly the same as in Figure 1.3.

Post-fade sends may also be used as tape outs providing your mixer has routing buttons. This is vital, because you don't want the channel signal going anywhere else other than the aux sends, so it's important to make sure any group and 'L,R' routing buttons are off. If you have the facility to do this, then using the post-fade sends instead of the pre-fade sends means you can use the channel faders to adjust the signal level to tape, which may be more convenient.

Sends And Processors

Conventional wisdom tells us not to patch processors via the aux sends, but what if you have a mixer or cassette multitracker with no insert points? In this case, pre-fade aux sends can provide a solution, and the required patching for a compressor is shown in

Figure 1.7. Here, the channel to be compressed is channel 1 and the channel fader must be set fully down. The pre-fade send – on that channel only – is then turned up and the compressor connected to the pre-fade send output, as shown. The output from the compressor can then be fed into a spare mixer channel and the signal routed normally. If you study this patch, you'll see that, because the fader is down on channel 1, the dry signal isn't routed anywhere; the only signal you use is the output from the compressor. In effect, channel 1 has been used as a mic pre-amp and the signal tapped off via the pre-fade send for convenience.

Hidden Flexibility

When I was first introduced to mixers, I found pre- and post-fade send quite confusing, and it's only once I studied the block diagram of the mixer that I realised how simple they really were. Once you realise that the aux-send busses are much like the main group busses, you can use them in any way you wish. Both pre- and post-fade sends may be used to create new tape feeds, and with a four-buss mixer this can make all the difference between four-track and eight-track recording. Cassette-multitracker users can use pre-fade sends as described earlier to patch in compressors or equalisers where there are no insert points, and on more than one occasion I've used the pre-fade or foldback sends on a cassette multitracker to create additional tape outs for remixing. It's often useful to remix a four-track cassette via a more serious mixer, but on cheaper machines you don't have separate tape outputs. In such cases, I've used the left and right outputs to carry a mix of three of the tracks and a pre-fade send to carry the remaining track, and although three sources may not seem like a lot, it's often enough to make a big difference to the final mix. On a machine with two pre-fade sends, you can separate out all four tracks, which is ideal.

The labels associated with mixer inputs and outputs relate to their most common use, but that's not to say you have to use them for that purpose. Quite often, the only way around a sticky problem is to use your mixer in an unorthodox way, and the more you think about it, the more ways there are. I haven't even mentioned the PFL buss, but that provides yet another way out of the a mix – if you PFL-solo one channel while its fader is down, its signal will appear at the headphone and monitor outs while the remaining channels will be routed to the main and output groups as normal. With just a little imagination, a 12:2 mixer can be turned to four-track recording, a 16:4 PA mixer can be used for serious eight-track recording and the limitations you thought your cassette multitracker had can be turned on their heads.

Effects And Processor Patching

Before you can work out the best place to patch in your outboard equipment, you need to know what is an effect and what isn't. I tend to define the various bits of outboard equipment as either effects or processors, according to what they do and how they do it. The main reason for this is that there are certain restrictions on how processors can be connected, while effects enjoy a little more flexibility.

Processors come in the form of boxes or plug-ins and they modify a signal, whereas an effect is a device that leaves the original signal intact and

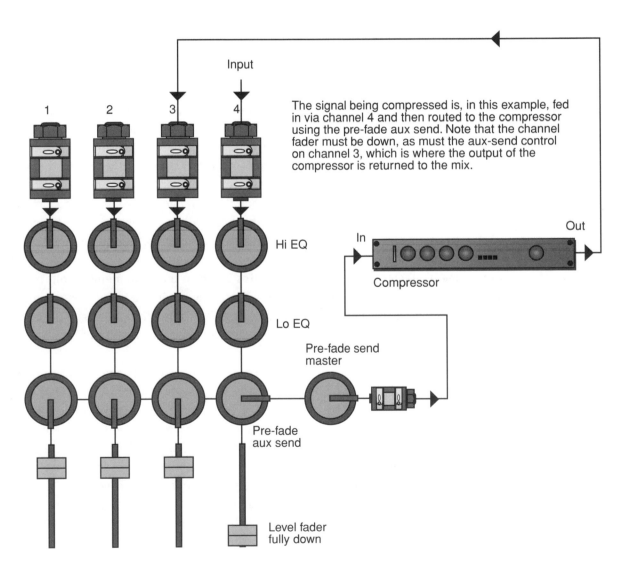

The signal being compressed is, in this example, fed in via channel 4 and then routed to the compressor using the pre-fade aux send. Note that the channel fader must be down, as must the aux-send control on channel 3, which is where the output of the compressor is returned to the mix.

Pan control and busses omitted for clarity

Figure 1.7: Compressing a mic via the pre-fade send (output of compressor fed back into space mixer channel)

adds something else to it. Processors include EQ, compressors, limiters, expander, gates, panners and single-ended noise-reduction units. If you have a box that modifies either the gain of a sound or filters it in some way, it's a reasonably safe bet that it's a processor. Echo units, delay lines, reverbs, chorus/flangers, pitch-shifters, phasers and suchlike are effects, and all effects should have some means of balancing the original and effected signal. Effects may be connected either via console insert points or via the aux sends, but processors can normally be used only at insert points or connected between two pieces of equipment, unless you're using one of the less obvious techniques described here. This also applies to plug-ins and software mixers.

Post-Fade Sends And Subgroups

When you eventually come to mix down, you might create subgroups for things like drums, backing vocals or keyboards so as to reduce the number of faders you have to worry about during the mix. However, if your effects returns come back straight into the main stereo mix, they'll stubbornly refuse to change in level, no matter how far you move the group faders.

The solution is to route the effects used within the subgroup back to the same-numbered groups, so that when each group fader is turned down, the effect level goes down with it. The only time a problem arises is when the same effect is used in two different subgroups, or in both a subgroup and channels routed directly to the stereo mix. There's no easy solution to this, and in extreme cases you might have to patch in a second effects unit to get around the problem.

Metering And Recording Levels

Equipment comes with VU meters, PPM bar-graph meters and peak overload LEDs, but what do these letters mean, and why do these devices all seem to produce different readings for the same signal?

In most cases, meters are designed to tell you when the piece of equipment to which they belong is being fed the correct signal level – all electronic devices have a lower signal limit (where the signal is so small it becomes overpowered by the circuit noise) and an upper limit, where the signal reaches the unit's maximum level, at which time clipping occurs. By using a meter properly, you can choose a signal level that's as high as possible without clipping and which will produce the best possible signal-to-noise ratio. These rules apply similarly to both analogue and digital systems, including computer soundcards.

VU Meters

The first type of meter built specifically for audio use was the VU (Volume Units) meter. The idea was to build a meter that would produce a reading similar to the loudness or volume level perceived by a listener, and the way a human hears sound is that very short-duration sounds appear quieter than longer bursts of sound at the same level. Moving-coil meters can be built to simulate this characteristic pretty well, because the inertia of the mechanism limits the speed at which the meter can respond to transients. Put a drum beat into a VU meter and the meter will barely have begun its climb than the beat will have ended and the meters started back down again. VU meters measure the RMS value of the input voltage; a sine wave that alternates between plus and minus 1 volt, peak to peak, will actually produce a reading on a voltmeter of 0.707 volts, which is what you'd get if the voltage in the sine wave were averaged out into a steady DC voltage.

A conventional mixer designed to operate at a nominal +4dBu should be outputting exactly +4dBu when the VU meters read 0dB, providing the input is a steady sine-wave tone. You might expect the meter to read +4dB, but 0dB simply means the mixer is operating at its optimum level, in this case +4dBu. However, a few manufacturers have decided to make their VU meters read the actual dBu level, so their models will read 0dB for 0dBu and +4dB for a +4dBu signal . They've done this so that you can use the mixer at either +4 or –10, and the meters will always tell you the actual signal level at the output – a practical and sensible option.

VU And Analogue Tape

VU meters work fine with analogue tape because it has quite a lot of headroom above its nominal operating level during which the level of distortion increases progressively, unlike digital systems, which merely clip. For this very reason, when used with digital systems, some engineers claim that VU stands for 'Virtually Useless', because the peak levels produced by something like a drum kit could be driving the digital recorder into clipping while the VU meter is reading around –10dB or less.

And now to dispel the myth that only moving-coil meters are VUs: you can also have bar-graph VU meters, because the characteristics of a bar-graph meter depend entirely on the circuitry or software driving it.

PPM Meters

PPMs (Peak Programme Meters) are more in keeping with the digital age because they are designed to respond fast enough to show any signal peaks that might cause distortion. Some also incorporate a peak hold facility, where the highest peak levels are displayed for several seconds to make sure you don't miss them. However, they still don't read absolute peak values because clipped peaks shorter than a millisecond or so are generally inaudible. Unlike the VU meter, which reads an RMS or average value, the PPM reads the voltage between the negative and positive signal peaks, which explains why you don't see the same reading when a steady sine wave is fed into a VU meter and a PPM. In fact, if you take a typical PPM, it will read 8dB higher than a VU meter monitoring the same signal in the same system.

In real life, you can calibrate a meter to read anything you like, and various professional broadcast institutions around the world have set their own standards. The result is that you can't always expect PPMs to agree. It's also technically possible to build moving-coil PPMs by designing the drive electronics to hold the peak level until the meter has had time to respond. The peaks may register a fraction late, due to the inertia of the meter, but they'll still register. However, such devices are quite esoteric, and in the context of project-studio equipment it's usually safe to assume that all moving-coil meters are VUs and all LED bar-graphs are either PPMs or switchable between VU and PPM functions. Of course, audio software can provide any type of metering of the designer's choosing.

The Peak LED

Simpler pieces of equipment, such as budget effects units, may have only a clip LED to indicate when the input signal is too high. This is less than ideal, but the best way to work in such circumstances is to increase the signal level until the clip LED just flashes on the highest peaks, then back off the level slightly until the peak LED no longer lights. You can consider the peak LED as the top LED on a PPM bar-graph.

Digital Multitrack

A potentially confusing situation arises when using analogue mixers with digital multitrack machines because the meters on the mixer and multitrack don't match up, not even when you put in a steady-state test tone. Even if your mixer has true PPMs, the chances are that the levels still won't match. Why? I've spoken to several different people about this and they all come up with slightly different answers, but as a rule digital multitracks are calibrated so that a 0dB test tone (measured on either a VU or a PPM) coming out of a mixer will read around 12dB below 0dB (clipping) on the digital multitrack. This makes a lot of sense because mixers are designed to be driven 'into the red', and if you have a model with VU meters, you could be a lot further into the red than you imagine. Digital machines won't tolerate any overload unless the period of clipping is so brief that you can't hear it, so calibrating the input electronics in this way is one way of helping the user stay out of trouble. It also means that the mixer can be driven a little further into the red than normal in order to make the most of the available headroom.

Similarly, when the signal comes back from a digital tape recorder, it's often hotter than you expect, for exactly the same reasons. This means that, when you're mixing from ADAT, DA-88 or a professional hard-disk recorder, you might find your mixer once again flicking into the red, even though the meter readings on the multitrack are below 0dB.

Metering Pragmatism

The safest approach when working with either DAT or digital multitrack recorders (including hard-disk-based systems) is to use the meters on the recorders themselves. Pay particular attention to the peak levels, because in digital recording it's the peaks that cause problems. The traditional notion of nominal operating levels isn't really relevant to digital, and whereas with analogue we aimed to get the meters bouncing around the 0dB point, with digital systems the only rule is to record the highest peak level you can without allowing the machine to clip.

When recording to analogue, the meters can give you only a rough guide as to what the right recording level should be, and if they're VU meters, the readings will be different for percussive material and music with more sustained sounds. Add this to the fact that modern tape can often accept a lot more level before saturating than older types and it soon becomes apparent that the only way you can really define the limits is to make a few test recordings at different levels to find at what point distortion becomes audible. After a little experience, you get used to what to expect from a VU meter with different types of input material, but as far as I'm concerned, reading a VU meter is still as much an art as it is a science!

Keeping Creative

Music is an odd kind of art form – its ephemeral nature makes it very hard to quantify. But like most other art forms, there are far more people capable of appreciating it than of creating it. I've often wondered why this should be the case. If you can hear a piece of music and appreciate its intricate harmonies and complex rhythmic structure, then surely you should be able to apply what you like about it to your own work? However, this is obviously not the case, otherwise everyone who liked Mozart would be able to 'imagine' new pieces in Mozart's style.

Some of us have a greater or lesser capacity for original composition, but very few people can be creative all the time. Some have to get in the mood to be creative while others find that ideas simply flash into existence and all too often evaporate again before they can get to a recorder or sequencer. Here are a few tricks and techniques you can use to help stimulate your creativity when your ideas appear to have dried up.

Record Everything

One thing I discovered early on is that it's little use running for the sequencer when a good idea pops into your head because, by the time you have everything up and running, the idea has more often than not been pushed out by the mental demands of loading the software, making any necessary connections, turning that old sampler out of Omni mode and calling up a set of appropriate sounds. A more practical, lower-tech approach is to keep a cheap cassette dictating machine with you at all times so that, if an idea does come along unannounced, you can at least hum it for posterity. This is particularly relevant when you're in the car, as here the creative part of the mind isn't usually too overtaxed, and if a part of the mind isn't currently being used, it's more likely to start making things up.

The same is true when you go into your studio for a workout on your keyboards, guitar or whatever – leave a cassette machine running, because a few worthy bars are quite likely to emerge from half an hour's unfocused rambling. If you have a sequencer, try switching off the metronome, putting it into record and then just playing as if it wasn't on at all. Having a metronome beeping away at you can be very counter-creative when you don't know what you're going to play!

Allow Yourself To Be Uncreative

Part of the problem with composing is that you tend to get annoyed with yourself for not coming up with the goods, and this starts a vicious circle – the more frustrated you get, the less creative you are, and the more frustrated you get. If this sounds familiar, use these times to sort out your patch libraries or rehearse something you already know. The chances are that, by turning your back on your creativity for a while, it will feel left out and try to join in!

You've probably noticed that I've been talking about creativity as is it was in some way separate from the individual, and physiologically this quite clearly isn't the case. But as this is the way it so often behaves, it's often a good way to treat it!

Listen!

Another very worthy non-creative pursuit is sitting down and listening to somebody else's music, especially when you're doing a mechanical task that requires no creative thought – for example, driving, washing up, formatting a box of 100 disks, lying on a sun-soaked beach in the Bahamas and so on. Not only will you soak up ideas (and every musician on the planet has absorbed ideas from other musicians), but your creativity may decide to flex its ego because it thinks it could do better. Any trick to lure it into the open is fair game.

Two's Company

The creative muse is often a gregarious beast by nature and, if forced to work alone, is prone to long bouts of non-productive sulking. That's why composers often work so well in pairs – they can bounce ideas off each other, filter each other's ideas, build on each other's ideas and even compete with each other on a subconscious level.

Another reason why composing teams work so well relates to my introductory comments about how everyone can be a critic, but few can be original. If there are two of you, one person's creativity may come up with the germ of an idea, allowing the other person's critical faculties to focus on what could be done to make it better. In my own experience, it's always easier to spot what's wrong with something, or even to suggest ways to improve it, than it is to come up with something good from scratch. It may be that this symbiotic relationship between the critic and the creator within us is what makes some writing partnerships so successful.

Mechanical Help

If you don't have a composing partner, how about striking up a relationship with a machine? If this sounds like an unlikely source of inspiration, keep in mind that any form of music-composing software is written by human musicians, and if they've done their jobs properly, when you interact with their software, you're interacting with some aspect of them, not with the computer running the program. I know a lot of people scoff at the idea of auto-accompaniment programs, but the better packages are now very sophisticated, and I feel that anybody who writes them off completely is using them the wrong way.

I come from a live-music background, and for more years than I'm prepared to admit I played guitar in what might loosely be described as a rock band. At rehearsals, we'd always put some time aside for jamming, and more often than not we'd decide on a rhythm and a chord progression, then see what evolved. From these jam sessions would come most of our ideas for new songs, and I see compositional or style-based programs as the MIDI equivalent of a band to jam with. It doesn't matter if none of its output makes it into the final composition; if it's helped to provide you with the inspiration to get the tune finished, it's done its job.

One of the great things about style-based auto-accompaniment programs is that, once you've typed in your chord sequence, you can opt to hear it played back in a huge variety of musical styles, and if you're prepared to try some of the less obvious options, you may discover some very fruitful avenues of exploration that you would probably never even have considered had you been working entirely on your own. Because the output from most of these programs can be saved as standard MIDI files, you can load them into your sequencer and then use as much or as little of their contribution as you see fit.

Scales And Keys

Another related example of man/machine symbiosis is evidenced in the scale-transpose facility built into certain sequencer programs. You take something written in, say, C major and then get the program to transpose it into a different key and to move the notes so that they conform to a different scale type. This way you can start out with a trite nursery rhyme type of melody in C major and end up with a Balkan folk melody in E minor! The results aren't always great, but very often something will stimulate your creative muse and prod it back into activity. If you consider compositional software as a catalyst to your own creative ability rather than as a substitute for it, I think you'll find the whole experience more rewarding.

Rhythm Is King

Most pop songs are underpinned by rhythm, but unless you have a lot of experience in playing or programming rhythm parts, the chances are that you'll end up playing along to some well-worn rhythmic cliché that's had all the life quantised out of it. This can be very stifling, as the energy of a rhythm track is quite often what gets your creativity interested in the first place. Give it a four-to-the-bar quantised rock beat and it's likely to pull the metaphorical covers over its head and stay in bed!

A popular way around the rhythm impasse is to use sampled drum loops, and there are literally thousands to choose from on CD or CD-ROM. The great thing about sample CDs is that you get a finished rhythm part complete with good sounds, the right balance and appropriate effects. And because you don't have to worry about these things any more, you can move directly onto the next stage, which is having fun – and having fun is the first step to getting creative. If you feel that this is cheating in some way, you can always replace the drum part using your own ideas at a later stage. Sample loops in REX or Groove Control formats can also be played back over a fairly wide tempo range.

MIDI Loops

The MIDI equivalent of sampled drum loops are now available from a number of companies, and these contain short MIDI files of one- or two-bar rhythm loops in General MIDI (GM) format. Many are recorded by real drummers using drum pads, providing a degree of feel and energy that would

be difficult, if not impossible, for most of us to match at home.

Because the patterns are presented as MIDI files, the tempo can be freely changed, sounds can be substituted at will, and the patterns themselves can be modified in any number of ways. Wading through all the files on a disk can be a long job at first, but I think material of this quality is well worth the small effort required to access it. You'll also find the same companies producing disks containing bass riffs, piano parts, guitar parts, brass licks and little trills and flourishes for more instruments than I could list here, and again these can help to rouse the creative muse from its state of apathy.

Sounds Matter

Read any interview with an A&R man and you'll get the impression that sounds don't count for much – a good tune will shine through on a beat-up old acoustic guitar plus voice recorded on the record company's telephone answering machine. Whether this is actually true isn't the point, but when it comes to actually composing music, I think sounds are very important. It's the sounds you choose that make you feel excited (or not) about the ideas you're trying out, and if I'm trying to write instrumental music that involves the guitar, I'm far more likely to think of something if I've got an effects box plugged in. The same is undoubtedly true for synth sounds and samples.

Of course, today we have so many sounds at our disposal that it's easy to spend all day swapping patches and getting nowhere, so you might try the approach of setting yourself a few limits. For example, you could throw dice to select four or five synth patches, then restrict yourself to working with those and nothing else, at least for the first half an hour or so. Having something limited to focus on certainly helps dispel unwanted distractions, and there's no denying that random chance often pushes you in directions you wouldn't normally go.

The same can be said of my party trick of cleaning the keyboard with a duster while the sequencer is recording, then assigning the result to a drum machine, quantising the data and creating rhythmic loops from the more promising bits. Just occasionally something wonderful pops out and the jaded old creativity sits up and takes notice.

Non-Creative Days

Sometimes, your creativity will decide to stay in bed for the day regardless of what you offer it in the way of temptation. If this happens, try not to fight it – just do something else. Very few people can be creative all the time, and if you try too hard, you risk taking the fun out of music-making. If you enjoy what you're doing, you're much more likely to be good at it than if you're having to force yourself all the time. Treat your creative self as a separate entity and try to get its co-operation by coaxing, not threatening or bullying. Composing music is one area where the carrot invariably produces better results than the stick.

2 VOCAL AND INSTRUMENT RECORDING

This section of the book deals with the problems associated with the recording of the human voice, plus the more common instruments used in contemporary music. A number of recording techniques are discussed, along with possible methods for improving substandard recordings.

Vocal Problems

In theory, getting a great vocal sound should be a matter of simply choosing a good mic, setting it up in front of a competent singer and pressing Record – and sometimes it is, but more often than not some additional treatments and/or precautions are needed. Most vocalists can't control the levels of their performances as precisely as we'd like, especially for pop music, where everything else in the mix probably has very precisely controlled dynamics. Furthermore, the acoustics of the performance space may intrude into the recording, the mic might 'pop' if the singer sings loud B or P sounds, and any tendency towards sibilance on S and T sounds will be exaggerated by a high-quality capacitor studio mic.

Even if all these potential problems are solved, there's still the question of whether or not to use EQ or other processing to enhance the voice, and in a pop-music context some degree of artificial reverberation will almost always be necessary. On top of this, there may be attributes of the performance that are less than perfect, such as pitching or timing, and although re-recording the offending part is usually the quickest and best option, there are technological tricks that can be applied in some circumstances. The aim of this chapter is to explore some of the things that can go wrong during the vocal-recording process and to suggest various measures that can be taken to remedy the problems.

Choice Of Vocal Mic

Sometimes the recording is technically OK but you just don't like the vocal sound you end up with. It's quite common for people not to like recordings of their own voice, because more often than not what you hear is rather different to how you imagine yourself to sound. Having said that, if the sound seems excessively dull, bright, nasal or otherwise coloured, then the choice of microphone or its placement may be the cause.

Not all microphones sound the same, and it isn't always the most highly specified mic that sounds best with a particular vocalist or speaker. Try out whatever vocal mics you have, both dynamic and capacitor, and see how they suit the voice of the performer. For example, a singer with a very bright, almost sibilant voice might be better served by a warm-sounding dynamic mic or a large-diaphragm capacitor model than by a capacitor mic with a pronounced presence boost. A strong presence boost will only further emphasise sibilance, whereas a mic with a warm-sounding low-mid response will help to compensate for the thinness of the original voice.

You may also find that some voices have strong nasal overtones, and in order to minimise these, you need to listen carefully to how different mics sound. For example, dynamic cardioid mics often have a tendency to sound slightly nasal anyway, so if you're noticing problems of this type, try a capacitor or good back-electret mic instead. If you have an omni or figure-of-eight-pattern mic in your collection, try those as well, as they tend to have a more open, natural character than cardioids. Of course, omni mics pick up sound from behind as well as from in front, so you may need to organise an acoustically absorbent surface behind the mic, such as a sheet of acoustic foam or a heavy duvet or blanket draped over a suitable frame.

Vocal Acoustic Considerations

You have a good mic, a singer with a good voice and as far as you know your recording equipment is fine, but every time you record a vocal take, the result sounds boxy. If this sounds familiar, the problem is most likely with the acoustic environment within which you're recording. Even a cardioid-pattern mic picks up some sound from the side, and of course any sound reflected back into the room from a wall behind the singer will also find its way back into the mic, so the solution is to create a relatively dead environment in which to record the performance.

Fortunately, it isn't necessary to treat the whole of the room in which the recording is being made, and if you're using a cardioid mic, it may only be necessary to treat the area behind the singer. The

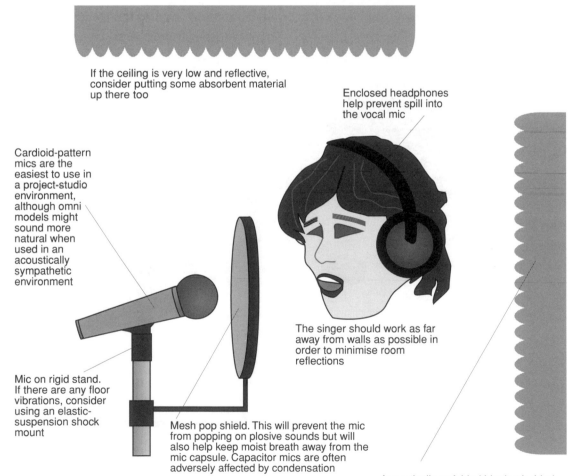

If the ceiling is very low and reflective, consider putting some absorbent material up there too

Enclosed headphones help prevent spill into the vocal mic

Cardioid-pattern mics are the easiest to use in a project-studio environment, although omni models might sound more natural when used in an acoustically sympathetic environment

The singer should work as far away from walls as possible in order to minimise room reflections

Mic on rigid stand. If there are any floor vibrations, consider using an elastic-suspension shock mount

Mesh pop shield. This will prevent the mic from popping on plosive sounds but will also help keep moist breath away from the mic capsule. Capacitor mics are often adversely affected by condensation

Acoustic tile or folded blanket behind the singer to reduce the effect of sound being reflected back into the microphone. If the room is very reflective, hang more blankets around the singing position, especially at the sides, where a cardioid mic is still quite sensitive

Figure 2.1: Mic position and screening used to capture a natural vocal sound

first step is to set up the mic close to the centre of the room, although for technical acoustic reasons it may be advisable to keep away from the exact centre. Setting up away from the walls minimises the amount of reflected sound getting back into the microphone, but you'll probably still need to improvise an absorbent surface behind the singer. A folded blanket, heavy curtain or sheet of foam rubber usually does the trick, and providing the mouth-to-mic distance is kept at between six and nine inches, you should end up with a clean, natural sound. If the room is particularly bad, try introducing more screening at either side of the mic. Figure 2.1 shows the use of mic position and screening to capture a natural vocal sound. In some instances, increasing the mic distance by a few inches, or even lowering the mic so that the singer sings over it, may help to avoid boxiness.

The Proximity Effect

Why does the mic tone seem to keep changing during the performance? All cardioid microphones demonstrate a noticeably increase in bass response when they're used very close to the sound source, and although a skilled vocalist can use this to advantage as a type of real-time tone control, less experienced singers might find it just makes their sound inconsistent. In the studio, both the tonality and level can be made more consistent by keeping the singer at least six inches from the microphone. The closer you get to the mic, the greater the difference in level and bass boost that results from any head movement.

Mic Popping

No matter how good a studio mic is, it will tend to pop if the singer produces a strong B or P sound,

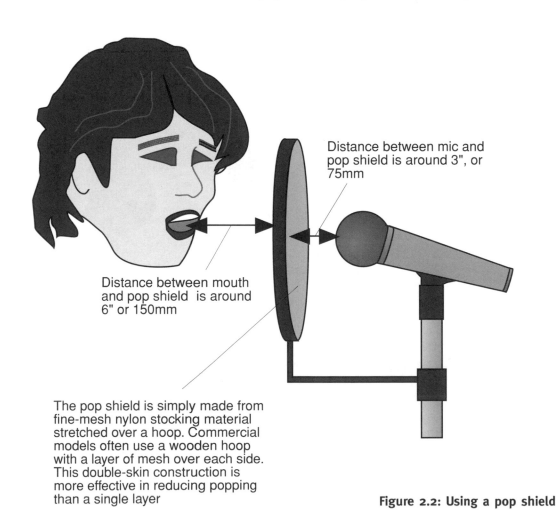

Distance between mic and pop shield is around 3", or 75mm

Distance between mouth and pop shield is around 6" or 150mm

The pop shield is simply made from fine-mesh nylon stocking material stretched over a hoop. Commercial models often use a wooden hoop with a layer of mesh over each side. This double-skin construction is more effective in reducing popping than a single layer

Figure 2.2: Using a pop shield

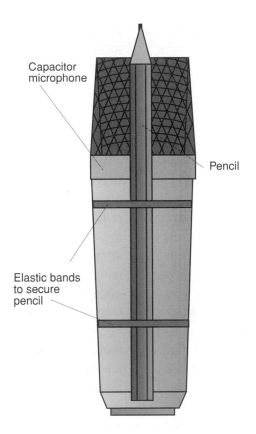

Capacitor
microphone

Pencil

Elastic bands
to secure
pencil

Figure 2.3: The pencil de-esser

and trying to get rid of this after the event using basic EQ is rarely successful. Such pops are caused by blasts of air from the mouth striking the microphone diaphragm, and the worst offenders are the plosive B and P sounds, as holding your hand in front of your mouth while you say different letters will demonstrate. While other sounds produce very little air movement, B and P sounds cause a noticeable gust of air to be expelled from the mouth.

Foam windshields are of little help in reducing popping. The only effective solution is to use a separate pop shield positioned between the microphone and the mouth of the singer. Although commercially made pop shields are available, my own opinion is that they are ridiculously expensive and that you're better off making your own. In effect, a pop shield is simply an area of fine mesh, the purpose of which is to convert blasts of air into harmless turbulence while remaining acoustically transparent to all other sounds. The traditional studio solution is to use a piece of fine nylon stocking material stretched over a hoop made from a wire coathanger, while the commercial models are nearly all made from stocking material fixed to wooden needlepoint hoops (cheaply available from any craft shop). A hoop of between four and six inches in diameter is fine. Figure 2.2 shows how such a pop shield may be constructed, and as you can see, I've suggested putting the material on both sides of the hoop to produce a double-layer filter. Once finished, the pop shield can be supported using a second microphone stand, or you may wish to improvise a stiff wire fitting that allows you to clip the mic to the same stand as the microphone.

Another option, for those who steer clear of the whole subject of DIY, is to buy a kitchen splash guard – a fine wire mesh device designed to be placed over saucepans to prevent splashing when food is being fried. These are very cheap and have the advantage of a built-in handle, which can usually be gripped in a standard mic clip. In my experience, they work every bit as well as the stocking-type pop filter.

Vocal Sibilance

Sibilance is caused by air moving over and between the performer's teeth. In the first instance, try out different mics to see if one produces more acceptable results than the others. Some singers produce virtually no sibilance, whereas others find it extremely problematic. As a rule, mics with presence peaks exaggerate sibilance, although a lot of this also depends on whereabouts in the spectrum the mic designers put the presence boost.

Once you've picked the best-sounding mic, there is a low-tech trick you can try which involves fixing a pencil or pen to the mic so that it shadows the very centre of the mic from the singer. Figure 2.3 shows how the pencil is positioned, and in most cases it can be held in place using thin elastic bands. This technique slightly reduces both sibilance and popping, although I've found that it works better with some mics than with others. Its effect is also

limited, so in very difficult cases you may have to resort to using a dedicated de-esser, either during the recording itself or when mixing.

A dedicated de-esser works in a similar way to a compressor, except that it reacts mainly to sibilant sounds. The simplest de-esser is simply a compressor with an equaliser inserted in the side-chain, as shown in Figure 2.4. The equaliser is set to emphasise signals in the 4–8kHz range, which is generally where sibilance occurs, so that gain reduction occurs only when sibilant sounds are detected. It is necessary to use fast attack and release times in order to keep the processing as unobtrusive as possible, but unless the amount of processing is kept to a minimum, the vocal may take on a lisping quality.

Some dedicated de-essers are better because they produce gain reduction only in those parts of the spectrum where sibilance occurs – the rest of the vocal sound is left untreated. This helps reduce the lisping effect and also enables sibilance to be attenuated more effectively.

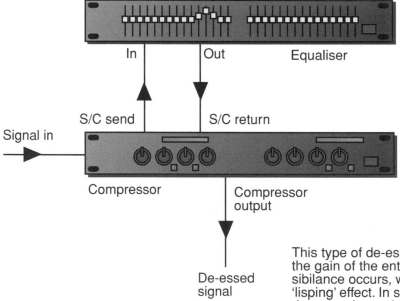

By connecting an equaliser into the side-chain insert points, the compressor can be made more sensitive to whichever frequencies are boosted. By boosting the sibilant part of the spectrum, the compressor will react most strongly to sibilant sounds, reducing their levels

This type of de-esser should be used sparingly as the gain of the entire signal is reduced whenever sibilance occurs, which can produce an audible 'lisping' effect. In serious cases, a dedicated de-esser that reduces the gain of only the high frequencies is preferable, as the resulting side-effects are less obtrusive

Figure 2.4: De-essing with a compressor

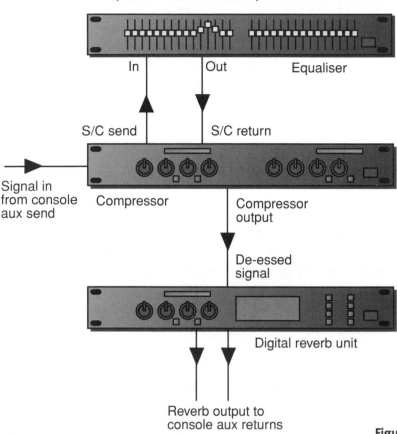

Compressor and EQ set to operate as a de-esser

In   Out   Equaliser

S/C send   S/C return

Signal in
from console
aux send   Compressor   Compressor
output

De-essed
signal

Digital reverb unit

Reverb output to
console aux returns

**Figure 2.5: De-esser in series
with reverb feed**

De-essing the feed to the reverb unit allows brighter reverb
settings to be used without the reverb becoming siblant or
splashy. Very often, slightly sibilant vocals don't become a
problem until reverb is added, so if you can get away with
de-essing only the reverb feed, and not processing the dry
sound, the result is likely to sound more natural

As a general rule, it's usually better to leave any corrective processing to the mixing stage, as an incorrectly set-up processor may ruin what is otherwise a perfectly good take.

Although I know some engineers who work differently, I usually prefer to record vocals with no EQ at all. It's often necessary to use EQ at the mixing stage, but if you've already added EQ when recording, you may never be able to get back to a natural sound if you need to.

Note that even an apparently clean-sounding vocal track can appear sibilant when processed via a bright reverb setting. The obvious alternative is to use a less bright reverb patch, but if the song production calls for a bright sound, then try patching a de-esser in series with the reverb feed, as shown in Figure 2.5. This way, the original vocal sound won't be processed, but the reverb will be fed from a source where sibilant sounds have been suppressed.

Vocal Levels And Compression

Unless the singer is well trained or has had a lot of experience, it's almost certain that some parts of the performance will be too loud, whereas others will be too quiet. It is possible to compensate for this to some extent while mixing by constantly moving the vocal-level fader to maintain an even performance, but this requires a lot of concentration and is generally only a partial solution. A better option is to use a compressor, which does essentially the same job as the engineer's hand on the fader but much faster and more accurately. If you have mix automation, this can be used to fix any peaks that the compressor fails to control fully.

In order to get the maximum level into the recorder, whether analogue or digital, it is sometimes desirable to compress the vocal signal prior to recording, but keeping in mind what I said earlier about inappropriate processing ruining an otherwise good take, I find it safer to apply rather less compression than I think I'll ultimately need and then add more when the song is mixed. A maximum gain reduction of around 6dB is usually plenty.

Different types of compressor produce a different sound – some act as almost transparent gain levellers while others add their own character to the sound, often described as warmth or thickness. Which one you choose depends on the compressors to which you have access and to your artistic taste, but a lot also depends on how the compressor is set up.

For the most transparent sound, try a soft-knee compressor, use a low ratio of around 2:1 and set the threshold so the gain reduction is around 6dB on the signal peaks. (This can be read directly off the gain-reduction meter.) Usually a fast attack time is combined with a release of between 100ms and 250ms, although if an auto attack/release function is available, this is likely to produce even more natural results, as it will adapt to the nature of the material being processed.

For a more obvious compression effect, use a compressor with a hard-knee characteristic and set a higher ratio of between 3:1 and 8:1. Set the threshold to produce up to 10dB (or even higher) gain-reduction on peaks and reduce the release time until you can actually hear the compressor changing the gain. This effect is known as *pumping*, and if used sparingly, it can make a rock vocal seem more exciting and powerful. However, if overdone, the sound becomes unsettling to listen to, so let your ears make the final decision.

A Happy Singer Is A Good Singer

Before you start to record a vocal, try to make sure the singer is comfortable, by which I mean the room temperature must be conducive to singing and the headphone mix must give the singer the balance they require. Some singers like a lot of reverb on their monitor mixes while others prefer them drier, so always ask them, and take the time to set up the monitor mix exactly as they like it. Some people perform better if the lighting is turned down, and a horde of onlookers can also stifle a performance, so ask the singer if they'd rather you sent the rest of the band to the pub for an hour. Always offer encouragement, and be diplomatic when criticising work, or a nervous singer might just get worse and worse. For example, if a take is really bad, play it back to the singer and ask if they feel it could be done even better. Don't tell them it was flat and sounded dreadful.

Give the singer chance to warm up by playing the tape through a few times, but always leave the track in Record, just in case you pick up a really good performance. (It's surprising how many singers deliver their best work when they think the red light is off.) This run-through will also give you a chance to optimise the recording levels.

Monitoring Without Phones

For those people who don't like singing with headphones on, there is a technique you can try using loudspeakers, shown in Figure 2.6. The principle relies on feeding a pair of identical loudspeakers from a mono source and then reversing the two wires feeding one of the speakers – it doesn't matter which one – so that the speakers are out of phase.

A microphone positioned midway between the speakers will pick up an equal amount of each, and because of the phase reversal, the sound will cancel out, resulting in very little remaining audio signal. However, the singer will hear plenty of level because the human hearing system uses two ears, not one, and although the out-of-phase nature of the sound might be a little odd, it's quite adequate for monitoring the backing track while overdubbing.

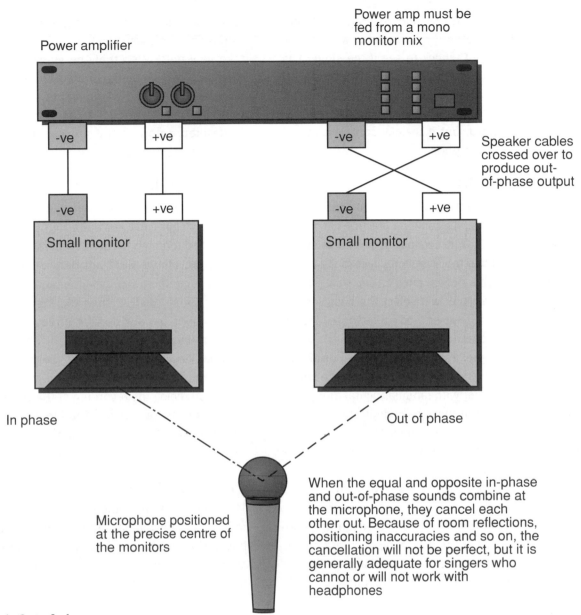

Power amplifier

Power amp must be fed from a mono monitor mix

-ve +ve   -ve +ve

Speaker cables crossed over to produce out-of-phase output

-ve +ve   -ve +ve

Small monitor   Small monitor

In phase   Out of phase

Microphone positioned at the precise centre of the monitors

When the equal and opposite in-phase and out-of-phase sounds combine at the microphone, they cancel each other out. Because of room reflections, positioning inaccuracies and so on, the cancellation will not be perfect, but it is generally adequate for singers who cannot or will not work with headphones

Figure 2.6: Out-of-phase vocal-monitor speakers

The benefit of using this system is that the singer can have a reasonably loud monitor mix over the speakers and can perform more naturally, yet a high degree of isolation is maintained. A little fine-tuning of the microphone position is required to get the best spot for cancellation, but although the degree of cancellation may not be perfect, due to the asymmetry of the speaker set-up and room surfaces, the degree of isolation that can be obtained is surprisingly good.

Performance Problems

Most performance problems are best dealt with by having the singer redo the offending part, and the simplest way is by dropping in a new word or phrase 'on the fly' by punching in and then out again, with the tape (or tapeless recorder) running. It's usually best if the singer starts from a line or two before the faulty section, and before going for a take you should get the singer to rehearse the part a couple of times so that you can check that the recording level is the same as it was for the original part. If not, check to see if the singer has changed position relative to the mic. The rehearsal will also give you chance to judge the best places to punch in and out. Sometimes you can capture just a single word, but it usually sounds better if you go for a whole phrase.

Vocal Compiling

In professional circles, whenever multiple spare tracks are available, it's common practice to compile a 'best' vocal track from sections of several complete takes. For example, the singer may record the whole performance half a dozen times on separate tracks, and then the producer will select the best version of each single phrase and compile these onto a single track for use during the mix.

With analogue recorders, this is done by bouncing the chosen phrases onto a spare track, but it's rather easier with modular digital multitrack machines as most of these have dedicated facilities for transferring precise sections of recording from one track to another. Alternatively, if you have access to a system with mix automation, it may be easier to use the automation to bring up the desired parts, then simply record the result onto a spare track. Automation has the advantage that any level changes at the punch-in/punch-out points can also be compensated for. Compiling in this way is easiest of all when using audio software, such as a sequencer.

Use A Lyric Sheet

When compiling, or even when patching up a single track by punching in and out, a copy of the lyric sheet and a highlighting pen are musts if you're to keep track of what you're doing. If you don't have a photocopier, you can run the original lyric sheet through a fax machine set to Copy. My procedure is to highlight all the sections that need redoing and then cross them out as they're completed successfully. A further tip is to handle all the punching in and out manually, if you can, and use any autolocation facilities you have to enable you

to get back to the start of the section as quickly as possible. This way you'll be able to redo a faulty take very quickly so that the singer doesn't lose the feel of what's being worked on. If you have to set auto punch-in/punch-out points and maybe even pre-roll times, spontaneity can easily be lost. Try to develop a flow to the process and everything will go much more smoothly.

Vocal Pitching

Occasionally, you'll come across a word or phrase that the singer can't get quite right, often because it's pitched too high for their vocal range. Obviously, the singer should warm up before recording, and maybe some throat spray will help, but if that note refuses to materialise, then the first and simplest trick to try is to slow down the recording by a few per cent by using the Varispeed function on the recorder. Now you can attempt the part at a lower pitch, and although the timbre will change slightly when you replay the recording at the correct speed, this is likely to be more acceptable than a flat note. Obviously, the less speed change you need to get the job done, the more natural the result will be.

Pitch Shifting

There are times when the singer is not available to redo a part and you have to make do with what you have. The technology is now available to fix up almost any tuning and timing problem, but anything more than minor surgery takes a lot of time and skill. The simplest high-tech technique for pitch correction is to use a digital pitch shifter that can be controlled via the MIDI pitch bend wheel on a synthesiser. If you have a time-code track or MTC output from your recorder, so much the better, because then you'll be able to run a sequencer in sync with your recording and record the MIDI data generated by the pitch-bend wheel.

The idea is to use the pitch-bend-controlled pitch-shifter to compensate for the tuning inaccuracy of the original performance, and if this occurs on a single word or phrase, you should be able to rehearse the necessary wheel movements reasonably well. When the wheel is left in its centre position, no pitch shift will take place, but as you move the wheel, the pitch of the processed sound will change accordingly. If you're recording to a sequencer, you then have the option of going into Edit mode and tweaking the data if you think the result can be improved further.

Because all but the most expensive pitch shifters tend to change the sound quality to some extent, it's probably best to record the phrase containing the corrected section onto a separate track and then arrange to use just the word (or words) that have been processed in the final mix. The rest of the vocal is taken from the original track. This may be achieved by compiling, track-bouncing or simply by using the mixer's Mute buttons during the mix. Again, automated mixing makes this easier.

Sophisticated Pitch Correction

We now have a whole generation of new and more powerful processing tools, many of which are provided either as standard or as plug-ins for hard-disk-based computer recording systems. Because 'audio plus MIDI' sequencing systems are now so powerful and so affordable, many of these techniques are accessible to the recording musician, as well as to the audio professional.

By way of pitch correction, some software packages include graphical pitch editors, where a pitch envelope may be drawn on screen to control the magnitude of pitch shift, and there are dedicated software packages that let you use a MIDI keyboard to play the note that you want the performance to be. The more advanced software processors have a number of adjustable parameters enabling some performance characteristics, such as vibrato, to be retained or removed as desired.

A few of the more up-market effects processors also provide this feature, either as standard or as a plug-in expansion card. In all cases, some skill and experience is required as no singer sings perfectly chromatically – natural singing includes lots of vibrato and glissando – but in most cases, it should be possible to fix flat or sharp notes quite satisfactorily. In this respect, software-based systems are generally more flexible than their hardware

counterparts as on them you can decide how much of the original feel to leave in. Automatic pitch correctors such as Auto-Tune work best when you enter the required scale and then set the correction rate to a moderate rather than fast setting.

Formant Correction

One of the main problems with simply pitch-shifting vocals is that the voice changes timbre – move the pitch up too far and the singer starts to sound like a cartoon character. That's because the human voice contains what are known as *formants* – frequencies due to such factors as chest resonance and vocal-tract dimensions, which remain fairly constant regardless of what note is being sung. If you pitch-shift something by simply speeding it up (and a basic pitch shifter effectively speeds up short sections of sound and then splices them back together), the pitch of the formants also increases, making the person sound physically smaller.

With the pitch-shifting technology available on some hard-disk audio recorders, it's quite feasible to copy a vocal line and then shift each note by the appropriate number of semitones to produce a musically correct harmony, but if the formants of the original are also shifted, the result can sound rather unnatural. Fortunately, it is now possible in many systems to shift pitch without shifting the formants of the sound being processed, and this is known as *formant-corrected pitch-shifting*. At the time of writing, formant correction is available in most MIDI-plus-audio sequencers, many hard-disk audio workstations and some high-end hardware processors, but the majority of multi-effects processors still use uncorrected pitch-shifting. This will no doubt change, but the point of formant correction is that it's now possible to shift the pitch of vocals (and some instruments) by a considerable amount without sacrificing their natural character. This is obviously useful when creating realistic-sounding harmonies.

Not only can we pitch shift without changing the natural formants of a sound, it's also possible to apply the process the other way around and change the vocal formants without changing the pitch. Used to its extreme, this allows male vocals to be made to sound female and vice versa, but if used more subtly it can be used to add extra depth to a male voice, for example, or to add variety to the sound of harmony vocals created from the same original voice.

Timing

There's very little that can be done to correct timing problems when you're working with simple analogue recorders and mixers, although it is possible to patch in a digital delay in order to pull back something that's been sung just a little too early. However, on a computer-based hard-disk recording system, it's generally possible to select individual segments and then move or copy them anywhere you want them. It's common practice for producers to select the best version of a chorus or backing vocal and then copy that to all the choruses in the song, but much smaller adjustments can be made to make the occasional phrase or word come in a faction of a second earlier or later to suit the feel of the song.

Audio Quantise

The better audio-plus-MIDI sequencers also enable audio to be quantised using intelligent time-stretch algorithms. You might think that these would work only on percussive sounds, but in practice, as long as the original sound doesn't need to be moved too far, the process can work surprisingly well on instrumental and vocal sounds, too. However, the more you compare original and quantised performances, the more you realise that it's the subtle timing differences injected by a good performer that create the musical feel of a piece. Indiscriminate quantising of audio or MIDI usually makes the performance sound stilted and unnatural.

Vocal Reverb

You've invested in a good reverb unit, and now you're determined to make it work for a living, but very often the processed vocal ends up sounding muddy or unclear. Try as you might, it doesn't sound properly 'produced', like the vocals on records. So what's wrong?

No pop record would be complete without additional reverberation, but many of the demos I hear have been spoiled simply through too much having been added. While reverb does make a voice more comfortable to listen to, it also has the effect of pushing it into the background, and a reverb with a long decay time can also use up all the valuable space in your mix. Excessive reverb can also reduce the intelligibility of your lyrics.

Separating the reverb from the vocal using a pre-delay of between 50ms and 100ms can help, as can selecting a shorter reverb-decay time. Listen to a selection of pop records with a view to studying the way in which the producer has used reverb. If the record has a very up-front vocal sound, the chances are that either the level of reverb is fairly low or the decay time is short. Longer reverbs can work, but only in songs where the arrangement has been designed to leave space for it. Even budget reverb units are extremely good these days, and in most instances it's mainly down to choosing the right type of reverb and then adding just the right amount of effect. Reverb units also vary considerably in sound quality, especially host-powered plug-ins, some of which lack the hardware density of DSP-powered effects.

Most of the obvious vocal-recording problems have been covered here, and the lesson should be: if in doubt, keep it simple. If you improvise a fairly dead area to record in and use a good mic with a pop shield, you should have little more to do other than add a suitable amount of compression and reverb. Indeed, with the right choice of mic, you probably won't even need to use EQ. While there is a lot of technical trickery available to help you polish an imperfect performance, getting the singer to redo the offending part is generally faster, more satisfying and more natural-sounding than spending hours sitting at a computer trying to make a silk purse out of a sow's ear.

Working With Drums

Unbelievable though it is, I've heard numerous stories concerning professional bands in top commercial studios where they've spent the best part of three days in getting just a decent bass-drum sound. If getting a decent drum sound is something you have problems with, here are some pointers – and a few cheats.

As emphasised in the previous chapter, a good drum sound starts with a good-sounding drum kit played by a good drummer. In particular, the heads need to be in good condition and properly tuned.

Drum Tuning

Visiting drummers should be able to tune their own kits, but when you're working in a project studio, this isn't always the case. If you need to intervene, here are a few tips you should find useful.

- A drum has a natural pitch. If you over-tighten the head, the tone will become hard and lose its depth, whereas if the head is too slack, the sound will lose its power and resonance.

  Ensure that the head is tensioned evenly all around. You can check this by tapping around the edges of the head with a stick while adjusting the tensioners until you have the same pitch all the way around. If you come across a flat spot, tighten the nearest tensioner slowly while tapping the drum.

- Tune each head by making small adjustments to first one tensioner and then the one opposite before moving around the drum. Single-headed toms are relatively easy to tune, while with double-headed toms the bottom head needs to be tuned to a similar pitch to the top head, and it may need a little damping to prevent it from ringing.

- The snare drum snare (bottom) head is traditionally tensioned slightly looser than the batter (top) head, although some drummers like the snare head slightly tighter. Because of their mechanical nature, the snare wires will vibrate in sympathy whenever another drum is hit, and although this may be reduced by careful tuning of the different drums, it is unrealistic to expect to be able to get rid of it altogether. However,

what sounds unacceptable in isolation may sound fine in a mix.

- If you're recording one drum at a time to produce samples, you can turn off the snares when they're not needed, or you can even work with just one drum in the room at a time if you want a really clean sound. Individual drums or other percussion instruments can sound good when miked in bathrooms or concrete stairwells.

If you have to record the whole kit in one go, you'll have to live with a few rattles and buzzes, and in my experience gating the individual drums doesn't help as much as you'd expect, because the rattles are also picked up on the overhead mics.

- If damping is needed, tape small pads of folded tissue or cloth to the edge of the top head of the drum. Internal drum dampers are seldom used by professionals. Meanwhile, some engineers simply prefer to use a loop of carpet tape. Whichever method you use, be careful not to overdamp. It's easy to become obsessed with eliminating rings and buzzes, but the sound soon dries up when you hear the drum sound in the context of the complete mix.

- Kick drums are invariably recorded via a hole in the front head. Don't remove the front head completely, however, as this risks distorting the drum shell. For damping, place a folded blanket inside the drum so that it contacts more of the rear head. Noise gates are useful when it comes to tightening up bass-drum sounds as a surprising amount of spill from the snare drum and toms finds its way into the bass-drum mic.

- The room has a significant effect on the sound of a drum kit and on how the player performs. If the room is too dead, place hardboard beneath the kit.

- Use an appropriate kick-drum beater for the style of music – wooden beaters work well for rock and pop while cork beaters are more suitable where a less attacking sound is required. Plastic patches are available to be stuck on the bass-drum head in order to produce a sharper attack.

- Oil pedals and stools using a silicone lubricating spray such as WD40. Even the smallest squeaks have a habit of being audible on the final recording! Rattling tensioner nut boxes may be silenced using lumps of plasticine or Blu-Tack.

Drum Miking

The main thrust of this book is on troubleshooting rather than basic recording techniques – I have other books covering those subjects – but there are a few basics of drum miking that I would like to include. There are many ways to mic a kit – for example, a stereo microphone pair (or even a single mic) placed between five and ten feet in front of the kit will do a reasonable job at capturing the way the kit really sounds in the environment in which it is being played. However, this approach probably lacks the power and punch demanded of a rock recording, so then you need to think about adding close mics – at the very least on the kick and snare drums.

Close-miking follows the same general method for all drums except the kick drum. You can use either capacitor mics or dynamics, cardioids or omnis, but most close-miking is still done using dynamic cardioids. It is, however, a mistake to use whatever happens to be left over for drum miking – you need good mics, and the same type and model of mic on each of the toms is recommended. If you have a slightly brighter mic than the others, use it on your snare drum, and for the kick drum use a mic with a good bass response. This should be positioned – using a boom stand – inside the drum, pointing towards the spot where the beater hits.

The usual mic position for the snare and toms is a couple of inches above the drum head, a couple of inches in from the edge and angled towards the centre of the head. Any damping should be positioned so as not to be between the mic and the drum.

Overheads

Using good overhead mics is essential for getting a good kit sound, as these have to pick up both the attack and the punch of the drums, plus the ring of the cymbals. You should use an identical pair of good back-electret or capacitor models, either cardioid or omni, and place them around three feet above the cymbals, spaced around four feet apart. Figure 2.7 shows a kit miked with both overheads and close kick and snare mics.

Percussion

Percussion instruments such as congas, bongos and so on are best miked from a couple of feet above, and the type of mic you should use depends on the type of percussion. Drum percussion works fine with dynamic mics whereas anything bright or metallic benefits from the extended high end of a capacitor or back-electret model.

Tracking Drums

To maintain maximum control when you come to mix, you need to spread your drums over as many tracks as is practical, but in any event, you should aim to keep the overhead mics on separate tracks to the close mics. If possible, keep the bass and kick drums separate, too. Ideally, the kit should be separated into kick, snare, stereo toms and stereo overheads, where the close tom mics are panned to the same positions as they appear on the overheads. It's perfectly possible to record all of the drums to two tracks, as a stereo mix, but this precludes any further balancing and the selective adding of effects, such as reverb.

TIP

For a traditional rock drum sound, balance the close mics and then add just enough overhead mic to the mix to give the sound life. For a more contemporary, 'natural' drum sound, use the overhead mics as the main sound source and then use small amounts of the close mic signals to balance the different drums in the kit. For example, if the kick drum is too quiet, bring up the close kick-drum mic slightly.

The overhead mics pick up most of the cymbal sounds and the ambient room sound of the drums. As a rule, bright rooms without excessive boominess work best. The mic positions should be adjusted to produce a good overall balance when only the overheads are used, and then the close mics can be added.

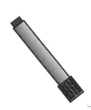

Overhead mics 3–6 feet (1–2m) above the kit

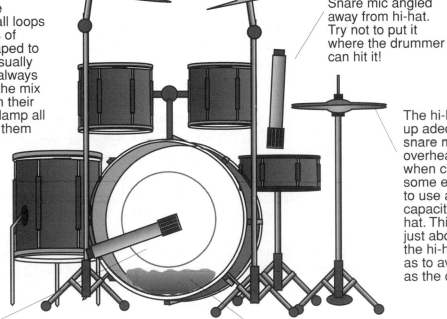

Go easy on the damping – small loops of tape or pads of folded tissue taped to the head are usually sufficient. Kits always sound drier in the mix than they do on their own, so don't damp all the tone out of them

Snare mic angled away from hi-hat. Try not to put it where the drummer can hit it!

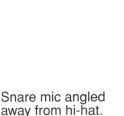

The hi-hat usually picks up adequately over the snare mics and overheads, though when close miking a kit some engineers prefer to use a separate capacitor mic for the hi-hat. This should be set just above or just below the hi-hat cymbals so as to avoid the air blast as the cymbals close

The kick-drum mic should be positioned on a boom stand inside the shell, pointing towards the centre of the rear head. Some people rest the mic on the blanket, but this leaves no scope for later adjustment

Note: The choice of kick-drum mic makes a significant difference to the sound. Dedicated kick-drum mics usually produce the best results, especially if you like a sound with a lot of depth

Blanket for damping

The front kick-drum head is fitted but has a large hole cut in it. If the head is removed altogether, the uneven tension can damage the shell. If the hole is too small, the remaining head material will ring

If the room is too dull, putting hardboard under the kit can help

Figure 2.71 Drum kit miked with both overheads and close kick and snare mics

Machines And Samples

While getting a good sound from an indifferent drum kit can sometimes be hard work, both drum machines and sequenced samplers provide a means of getting fully produced drum sounds with no buzzes, no rattles and no separation problems. When working with a sequencer, it is usually easiest to program drum parts in layers rather than trying to record the whole kit at once. Each pass can be recorded on a different track and then merged when all the parts are complete.

Having said that, many an otherwise good recording has been spoiled by an indifferent or wooden sequenced drum part. These machines need to be programmed by someone with a good feel for percussion, and it may be better to get a drummer to play the drum part in real time, either from a MIDI keyboard or from some form of MIDI drum-pad system. Inexpensive transducers are also available which may be attached to acoustic drums, allowing them to be used in place of pads.

TIP

If you want to use programmed parts, it often sounds best if you quantise the basic kick and snare parts but leave the hi-hats and drum fills as played. In order to preserve the feel of the unquantised parts, the quantised parts should be recorded onto one sequencer track and the unquantised parts onto another. If you put them all on the same track, the same quantisation will apply to everything. It can also sound far more natural if you mic real cymbals and hi-hats and then use these to replace the sequenced ones. The same is true of even the best electronic drum kits – real cymbals sound better!

Drum-Sound Replacement

Sometimes you record a great drum performance but the sounds just aren't good enough. In such cases, consider replacing the kick and/or snare using samples. To do this effectively, the drum or drums you want to replace will need to be on separate tracks, and in any event you'll probably need to gate the sounds in order to eliminate any spill. Gates with key filters are usually better able to reject spill from drums or cymbals of a different pitch to the one you're trying to separate.

The output from the gate may be fed into a pad-to-MIDI converter or into the trigger input of a suitable drum module. It is desirable that the trigger system allows the user to set a retrigger-inhibit time, which prevents a sample from being triggered twice in quick succession due to spill breakthrough or a careless stick bounce. Most trigger systems can be made responsive to the loudness of the triggering signal, but in the majority of pop work the bass and snare levels need to be kept even, so it may be advantageous to turn this facility off or to make sure that the input is always high enough to ensure that the sample is played at or near its maximum velocity. Figure 2.8 shows a typical arrangement.

If the original performance contains small stick bounces or grace notes that you want to keep and which the gate can't track adequately, try mixing the sampled snare sound with the original so that some of the original detail is still audible.

All MIDI instruments, including drum modules, introduce a small delay between receiving the trigger signal and the sound being produced. If the original track was produced on a hard-disk recorder or modular digital multitrack, it may be possible to dial in a small negative track delay to compensate for this. By monitoring the delayed drum sample against one of the undelayed drum tracks, it should be possible to adjust the timing for the best feel.

Hard-Disk Tricks

Recorders based on MIDI sequences with integral hard-disk audio often have numerous powerful signal-processing tricks at their disposal, which can be quite useful when you're sorting out an imperfect drum part. Perhaps the most obvious useful feature is cut and paste. If you have a regular drum part where some of the bars are performed better than others, it's a simple matter to copy the good bars and then use these instead of the suspect ones.

If you use the same bar of drumming through every verse, you'll end up with a slightly unreal, mechanical feel, but for some types of music this is

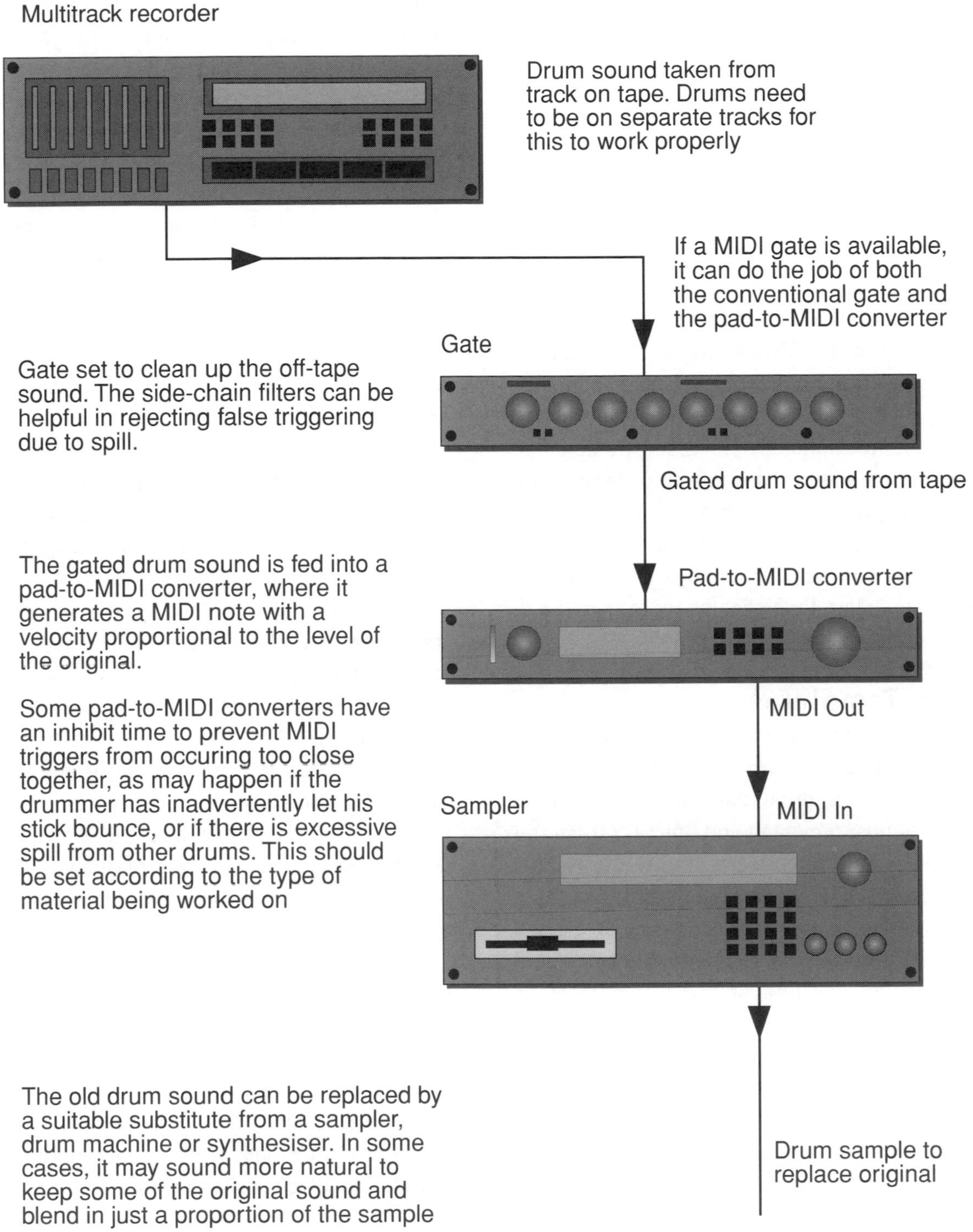

Multitrack recorder

Drum sound taken from
track on tape. Drums need
to be on separate tracks for
this to work properly

If a MIDI gate is available,
it can do the job of both
the conventional gate and
the pad-to-MIDI converter

Gate

Gate set to clean up the off-tape
sound. The side-chain filters can be
helpful in rejecting false triggering
due to spill.

Gated drum sound from tape

The gated drum sound is fed into a
pad-to-MIDI converter, where it
generates a MIDI note with a
velocity proportional to the level of
the original.

Pad-to-MIDI converter

Some pad-to-MIDI converters have
an inhibit time to prevent MIDI
triggers from occuring too close
together, as may happen if the
drummer has inadvertently let his
stick bounce, or if there is excessive
spill from other drums. This should
be set according to the type of
material being worked on

MIDI Out

Sampler

MIDI In

The old drum sound can be replaced by
a suitable substitute from a sampler,
drum machine or synthesiser. In some
cases, it may sound more natural to
keep some of the original sound and
blend in just a proportion of the sample

Drum sample to
replace original

**Figure 2.8: Drum-sound replacement setup, including
gate, converter and sampler/drum machine**

exactly what's needed. Even so, for most 'human-sounding' music, it's best just to patch up only the bits you really have to. You may also be able to import ready-made drum loops from sample CDs and use these either instead of your own percussion, or in combination with it.

Tempo Changing

Part of the problem with conventional samples and audio recordings is that you can't change their tempo without changing their pitch unless you process them in some way. For example, if you want to slow down a drum part without changing the pitch of the drums, you can use a time-stretch pitch-shifting facility to do it, but you'll only be able to change the tempo by a certain amount before the result starts to sound unnaturally processed. Some of the modern time-manipulation algorithms are surprisingly good, so as long as the change is no more than a few percent, you should have no problems. If you need to change the tempo of sample loops more than slightly, try to use REX or Groove Control sample material.

Groove Templates

A major feature provided in the better audio-plus-MIDI sequencers is the ability to quantise audio. This works best on drums but can be used on all kinds of sounds, providing you don't try to go too far. If you simply quantise a sloppy drum part, you'll probably find it sounds too stiff, but there are commercially available libraries of groove templates extracted from the performances of real players. If you use one of these templates to quantise your own drum recording, you may be able to tighten up the performance without losing the feel.

An alternative approach is to use the facility whereby a groove can be extracted from an existing audio or MIDI performance. Either take the bar from the drum recording that has the best feel and then use that to create a template for the other parts, or play in a drum-loop sample with the right feel, extract the groove and use that to modify your own audio or MIDI recordings.

Electric Guitar Sounds

Sound from synths, sampler, drum machines and other electronic instruments are straightforward to record – you just plug them into a mixer – but getting the right electric guitar sound onto tape can be more of a challenge. That's because the electric-guitar sound wasn't invented, it evolved, and it evolved in several different directions at once, which means there's no such thing as the definitive electric-guitar sound.

Of course, a good guitar sound starts at the guitar, so before any important session, ensure the guitars are properly set up and have new strings fitted. Sadly, may potentially good sessions are ruined by improperly set-up instruments, so before discussing the problems of recording, it's worth looking at what setting up a guitar entails.

Guitar Setup And Tuning

Although you occasionally come across a rogue instrument that simply refuses to co-operate, most tuning problems can be traced back to the way in which the instrument is set up, the way in which the strings are fitted and how the instrument is stored or transported. If you don't have the expertise to set up your own instrument (as described later in this chapter), it's probably best to hire the services of a really good guitar tech, and if you have an instrument that sees a lot of use, it's probably as well to get it checked over a couple of times a year. On the other hand, if you are reasonably practical and can lay your hands on a few simple tools, there's a lot you can do yourself.

Changing Strings

The next time you change strings, give the guitar a good clean, and that includes the fingerboard, where dirt tends to accumulate next to the frets. There's a lot of talk about silicon-free waxes and special polishes, but I usually use aerosol furniture polish and it's fine. Give the polish a few minutes to loosen the grime, then wipe clean with a piece of cloth.

Fitting the strings correctly is important for tuning stability, and unless you've already developed a preference for a different gauge, for most rock/pop work a set of 9–42s will work fine. These are thin enough to bend easily but still heavy enough to produce a decent tone. With most electric guitars, the strings thread through the bridge, so pull the strings through as far as you can and then feed them through the hole in the tuning machine peg. Some players like to wind the string over itself, but providing you leave enough slack so that the string goes around the peg just two or three times once it is tuned up, the tuning should remain stable. My own preference is to make a right-angled bend in the spare end of string where it leaves the peg to discourage it from slipping.

When all six strings are in place, snip off the excess using wirecutters so that you don't stab yourself in the eye, then use your tuner to check the intonation.

Intonation

Tuning up after fitting new strings can be a slow process if you have a tremolo unit fitted to the guitar because, as you tune up one string, the tremolo springs will stretch a little and all the other strings will go slightly flat. As a result, you might have to go around all the strings several times before they finally settle down. I find it helps to grasp each string in the middle of its length and give it a good tug before tuning up. This ensures that the strings are pulled fully through the holes in the bridge, and it also tightens the strings on the tuning machine pegs.

You'll notice that, when you check the pitch of a string with your tuner, the pitch will go slightly flat after the initial pick. This is quite normal, so wait a second or two until the note settles down before finally tuning it.

Once the open strings are in tune, play the octaves on the twelfth fret of each string and see if these read the same as for the open strings. If the octaves show up sharp on the tuner, adjust the bridge saddles so that they move slightly further away from the neck. Conversely, if the octaves are flat, move the saddles closer to the neck. Retune the open string every time you adjust the bridge saddle, then check again. Once the intonation is OK, it shouldn't need to be changed again, as long as you stick with the same gauge and brand of string.

Guitar Action

How low you would like the action of your instrument to be depends a lot on your playing style, but there comes a point where you can lower the action no further or the strings will buzz against the frets. My own preference is for a medium rather than very low action, because when the action is positioned very low, your fingers tend to slide over the strings whenever you try to bend a note. On a low action, you'll also hear the notes choking or buzzing when you perform bends on the higher frets. Before adjusting the action, you should check the straightness of the guitar neck to see if the truss rod needs any adjustment.

Fret Dressing

If the guitar has excessively worn frets, it may buzz no matter how carefully you set the action, in which case it is advisable to have the guitar serviced by a guitar technician. However, if you feel confident enough to do a little DIY work, small irregularities due to minor fret wear can be corrected using a carborundum stone. However, in the case of badly worn frets, the only solution is to have them replaced. If you have never dressed frets before, practise on an old guitar before you work on anything too valuable!

The technique is to hold the stone flat so that it is pressed up hard against several frets at the same time and then run it gently along the length of the neck so that any high spots are removed. As the fingerboard and frets generally have a curved profile, you'll need to work your way across the frets, taking care to remove only a small amount of material at a time. I find it helps to wet the stone with soapy water, and you can see where material has been removed by the fine marks left on the surfaces of the frets. When there are no low spots left, the tops of all the frets will show marks from the stone.

Finally, the stone should by held flat and then rubbed gently across the width of the neck to remove any abrasion marks. For more serious restoration, a fret file is necessary, but these really are for experts only!

Truss-Rod Adjustment

Contrary to some beliefs, a guitar neck shouldn't be absolutely straight but instead should be slightly concave – a vibrating string moves more in the centre than at the ends. As a consequence, the fingerboard needs to follow a shallow curve in order to allow the string to vibrate freely without buzzing. How curved the neck needs to be varies from guitar to guitar, but as a general guide, if you hold both ends of your bottom string down against the first and last frets, the gap between the middle of the string and the nearest fret should be around the thickness of a credit card or slightly less.

If the neck is more curved than this, you can tighten the truss rod to straighten it slightly, and if the neck is too straight, slacken the truss rod very slightly. This isn't a difficult job, but you do need to make very small adjustments, retune and then wait a few minutes to see how far the neck has moved. Patience is the main skill you'll need here. Most truss rods can be adjusted either using an Allen key or special spanner, and these should be supplied with the guitar. Access to the end of the truss rod is either from the tailstock end (sometimes under a small plastic cover) or from the end of the neck where it joins the body. Usually, it's enough to turn the truss rod a quarter of a turn at a time, but be sure to wait a few minutes and check the result before you do any more adjusting. If the truss rod isn't causing you any problems, however, don't mess with it!

A small adjustment to the truss rod can make a significant difference to the action, so you'll probably have to readjust the heights of your bridge saddles after you've got the neck curvature right. You'll also have to retune whenever you adjust the truss rod or the bridge saddles. It's important that the guitar is already tuned up when you adjust the truss rod, as the string tension needs to be correct.

Nut Problems

A lot of tuning problems can be traced back to poorly cut nut slots or nuts made from unsuitable materials. If the nut slots are cut too deep, the strings will rattle on the first fret, but if they are too shallow, the strings will have to be pushed down harder before they touch the frets, resulting in a sharpening of pitch because of the increased tension. Obviously, manufacturers don't want to deliver guitars that buzz, so they tend to leave the nut slots cut insufficiently deep. The result is a guitar on which the open strings are in tune but the fretted strings play sharp. The strings will also be harder to fret than they would be if the nut slots were cut properly.

You can deepen the slots with a fine mini-hacksaw blade, but check the results every few strokes, or you might find you've gone too far. To see how deep to cut, check the gap between the open string and the first fret and compare this with the gap you see at the second fret when you hold the string down at the first fret. The clearance between the open string and the first fret should only be marginally greater than that between the fretted string and the second fret. If you do cut the slot too deep, you can fill it with a drop of glue and a pinch of baking powder. This combination soon hardens sufficiently so that you can recut the slot.

The other major nut-related problem is strings sticking in the nut slots rather than sliding freely through them. To find out if you have sticky nut problems, try this test with your tuner. Tune the open string so it is precisely in tune, then do a few string-bending exercises. Has the string gone flat? If so, get hold of the string at the other side of the nut and pull it to one side, then check the tuning again. If the pitch has come back up, you're suffering from the strings sticking in the nut slots. Replacing your nuts with some made from graphite compounds can help cure this problem, but a quick and dirty cure is to use a strip of plumber's PTFE or Teflon tape over the nut before you fit your strings. This is very thin and the strings will pull it down into the slots without affecting the action, but the co-efficient of friction of this material is so low that it will act as an effective lubricant and prevent sticking.

Some people suggest rubbing graphite from a pencil into the bridge slots, but this falls out very quickly, leaving you back where you started. For a more permanent cure, fit a graphite-impregnated nut, and if you're having string-breakage problems, buy a set of bridge saddles made of the same material. Graph Tech parts are particularly good.

To make the strings last, clean them after playing using a string-cleaning spray and a clean cloth. If you don't clean them, your acidic perspiration will weaken the strings and deaden the tone.

Tremolo Setup

The most popular guitar in world must be the Fender Strat, and then there are the thousands of competing designs based on it. On a standard Strat or Fender Squier Strat, the tremolo is either pivoted on two posts fixed into the body or on a row of screws running along the front edge of the tremolo assembly. The tension of the strings is balanced by means of a set of springs inside the guitar body and provision is generally made to fit up to five springs. However, the usual number of springs to use is just three, and these can be adjusted in tension by means of the large woodscrews passing through the metal plate which holds the ends of the strings furthest from the tremolo unit.

With the correct gauge of strings fitted and tuned to pitch, the tremolo plate should float just above and roughly parallel to the guitar body – the type fixed with screws should have a space of maybe 3mm or 4mm under the end of the tremolo plate furthest from the neck. If the tremolo is pulled down hard against the body by the springs, or if it is floating too high, adjust the springs to bring it about halfway back to where you want it to be, retune all the strings and measure again. Repeat this procedure until the tremolo is sitting in the correct position with the strings tuned to concert pitch.

Guitars And Noise

If there is too much interference noise from the guitar or hiss from the amp, a gate can be used at the mixing stage to maintain silence during pauses or between phrases. As a rule, set the gate attack to its fastest setting and make the release time long enough so as not to chop off the end of sustained notes. Also, ensure that the gate's threshold is set as low as is possible without the noise breaking through, as this will mean that the gate is less likely

to chop out wanted parts of the sound, such as quiet notes.

As a rule, use the gate when mixing, not when recording, as a good take can be ruined by unsuitable gate settings. If you make a mistake while mixing, all you have to do is reset the gate and try again. If you must use a gate when recording, use a dedicated guitar gate and place it in the signal chain before any delay effects, as shown in Figure 2.9. This will prevent the gate from cutting off any reverb or delay decays.

Use the same tuner for all members of the band (or at least make sure that the various tuners agree) and check the tuning before each take. Find a position in the room where other equipment interferes least with the guitar signal and turn off any computer monitors that are close to the guitar. Guitars with single-coil pickups (for example, Fender Stratocasters), are particularly susceptible to picking up hum and buzz from transformers, striplights, VDUs, TV monitors and so on. Sitting on a revolving chair is a good way to find the quietest position – you simply rotate until you find the position of least hum. Replacing VDUs with flat-screen monitors helps significantly.

Guitar-Sound Evolution

The guitar sounds we hear at concerts and on record today evolved from sounds created by the inadequacies of amplification and speaker technology at the time when the electric guitar first became popular. Nobody designed the distorted guitar sound; it just happened. The quest to build amplifiers that distorted intentionally came later. Solid-state amplifier designers have been trying for years to unravel the mystery of the tube-amplifier sound, and to compound the problem American-built guitar amplifiers tend to have different tonal characteristics from European models.

All guitar amplifiers are voiced – or, to put it another way, the frequency response isn't flat but is modified to sound good, usually by adding mid- or high-frequency boost. Different models use different voicings, which all adds to the variety of sounds available. To complicate the issue further,

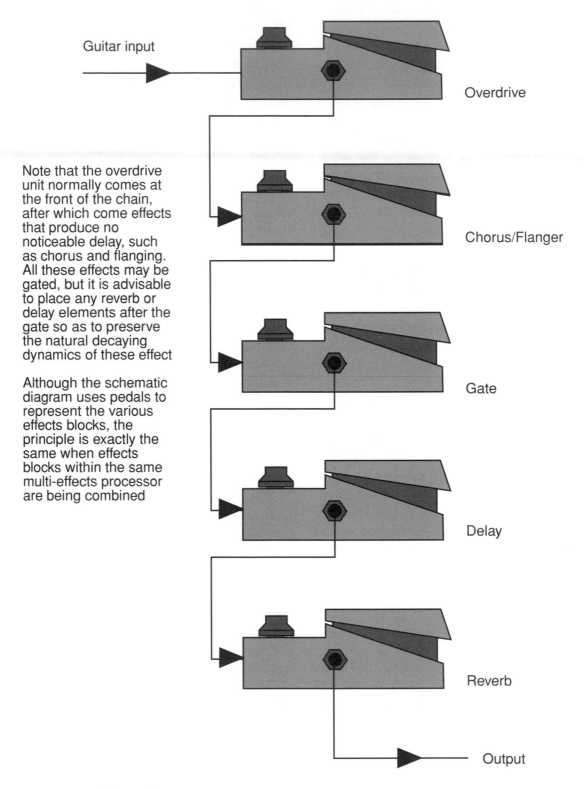

Guitar input

Overdrive

Note that the overdrive unit normally comes at the front of the chain, after which come effects that produce no noticeable delay, such as chorus and flanging. All these effects may be gated, but it is advisable to place any reverb or delay elements after the gate so as to preserve the natural decaying dynamics of these effect

Chorus/Flanger

Gate

Although the schematic diagram uses pedals to represent the various effects blocks, the principle is exactly the same when effects blocks within the same multi-effects processor are being combined

Delay

Reverb

Output

Figure 2.9: Guitar effects with a gate (after overdrive, before delay and reverb)

the sound of an overdriven guitar amplifier depends on the voicings used both before and after the overdrive circuitry.

Elements Of Guitar Tone

Before looking at the common problems associated with recording a good electric-guitar sound, it's important to realise that the result depends on a combination of the guitar itself, the amplification, the loudspeaker system used, the room acoustics, the type and position of the recording microphone and, most importantly, the way in which the instrument is played. The amplifier and speaker together make a profound contribution to the sound, which is why so many people still prefer to mic up guitar amps rather than rely on speaker simulators, guitar multi-effects units or recording guitar pre-amps.

Having made that point, I've used both approaches, and the better pre-amps and speaker simulators come very close to the sound of a miked-up guitar amp, and in situations where the acoustics are less than ideal, or where the choice of mics is limited, pre-amps and simulators often sound better.

So why does a guitar amp sound so special? Guitar amps nearly always use 10- or 12-inch speakers, either singly or in multiples, mounted in cabinets that are fully sealed (as in stack cabinets) or open-backed (as with most combos). The distinctive overdrive sound is caused by having a pre-amp with sufficient gain to overload one or more of its gain stages, and possibly the power amp stage too, resulting in significant levels of harmonic distortion. These artificially generated harmonics are then low-pass-filtered by the limited frequency response of the speaker and its enclosure.

The Speaker As A Filter

The low-pass response of a typical guitar speaker removes most of the upper harmonics (rolling off above 2kHz or so) introduced by the overdrive circuitry, and without this filtering effect the result is invariably thin-sounding and buzzy. This is a very common problem: if a guitar overdrive pedal or combo pre-amp-out signal is DI'd into a mixing console, the benign low-pass-filtering effects of the speaker are missed, which is why the sound seems so raspy and unnatural. Ironically, although most traditional engineers would go to any lengths to avoid this type of sound, some contemporary bands are using it as an alternative to traditional rock-guitar sounds. Of course, this is purely an artistic decision, but if you're after an authentic rock-amp sound and you're ending up with something that sounds more like a bee in a bottle, this is most likely what's happening. The solution to getting an authentic DI'd sound is either to use a guitar pre-amp with a built-in speaker simulator or to use a stand-alone speaker simulator after your pre-amp or pedal.

Speaker Simulation

Throughout the rest of this book, I've resisted the temptation to mention specific pieces of equipment by name, as gear dates very quickly, but I'm going to make an exception for speaker simulators. The best one I've used to date is the Palmer Junction Box, a simple and relatively inexpensive passive device that can take either a pre-amp-level or speaker-level signal at the input and deliver a mic-level, balanced signal at the other, with extremely authentic speaker cab coloration.

If the unit is being used with a power amplifier, it must be connected between the amplifier and its speaker or between the amplifier and a suitable dummy load. Because the box is passive, it requires no power and adds no noise. I've even found it improves the sound of several other pre-amps that have their own speaker simulators built in. I simply turn off the internal speaker simulator and pass the signal through the Palmer Junction Box instead. Of course, there are other speaker simulators on the market, and they all sound slightly different. As guitar sounds are so personal, you may find that you prefer the sound of a different model.

Of course, the most convenient method is to use a digital-modelling guitar pre-amp that combines amp and speaker-modelling with effects. These are DI'd, usually in stereo, and the sound you hear over your studio monitors as you play is the sound you get on your recording.

Clean Guitar Sounds

Most of what we perceive as being clean electric-guitar sounds are actually still very distorted by hi-fi standards. What we interpret as clarity and ring is probably due to a generous helping of second-harmonic distortion and power-supply compression! However, there are occasions on which a very clean electric guitar sounds perfect, but even if you accept that you can do without distortion or a speaker simulator, you can't just plug an electric guitar into a mixing console mic or line input, because an electric guitar only works properly into a high input impedance. Sure, you'll get a sound out of the thing by plugging directly into the mixer, but the chances are it will be dull and lifeless.

A simple active DI box makes a world of difference, and you'll be surprised at how beautiful the electric guitar can sound without effects or EQ of any kind. Of course you can add effects, as with any other recorded sound, and a little compression will improve the sustain even further. If you're after a more natural, clean sound, use a clean setting on your recording pre-amp or mic a clean amp.

Miking Amps

Miking guitar amps isn't difficult, but it's surprising how many people don't end up with the sound they're after. There are two main reasons for this. One is that the amp is being set up to sound right to the player standing in front of it, whereas you should always listen to the miked signal coming over the studio monitors and then adjust the amp controls until that sounds the way you want it. The other is that guitarists seem to expect the recorded sound to have the same bass-end kick and punch that their stack does. This simply can't happen. A domestic 10W hi-fi playing through a couple of six-inch speakers can never recreate the low-end energy of a 100W guitar stack powering a pair of 4x12 cabs, so what you should be comparing your recorded sound with is the guitar sounds on other records, not with what's coming out of the amp.

Amplifier Size

Unless you have a huge room in which to record, a small combo is often easier to coax a good sound out of than a stack, partly because a small combo will produce a more natural overdrive when run hard than a large master-volume amp just ticking over. I use a little Fender tube combo in my own studio and it sounds exactly right, either when miked or when played through the speaker simulator. In fact, it's surprising how close the miked and DI'd simulator sounds are.

Guitar Mics

All microphones sound different, so your choice of mic will affect your final sound, as will the location of the mic. Dynamic microphones are the most common choice, and even a budget cardioid will usually give quite adequate results as there's very little high-frequency energy to worry about, and there's certainly no shortage of level. Even so, a capacitor mic will produce a brighter, slightly thinner sound than a dynamic model, and part of the reason why American records sound different from UK ones is that US engineers seem to prefer to use capacitor microphones to dynamic models for this application. It's also true that American-designed amplifiers sound slightly different to British amplifiers, and talking in very broad strokes, rock-guitar sounds can be categorised as Fender-type (US) or Marshall-type (UK).

Mic Position

The position of the mic relative to the guitar speaker probably makes just as big a difference as the choice of microphone, and the brightest, most direct sound comes from placing the mic very close to the centre of the speaker. If the sound is too bright, move or angle the mic to one side slightly to see how much difference it makes before resorting to EQ. Figure 2.10 shows some close-miking options.

Even with a sealed cabinet, a surprising amount of sound comes from the back and sides of the box, so to find the best spot, get someone to move the mic around while you listen over the control-room monitors. With an open-backed cabinet, as much

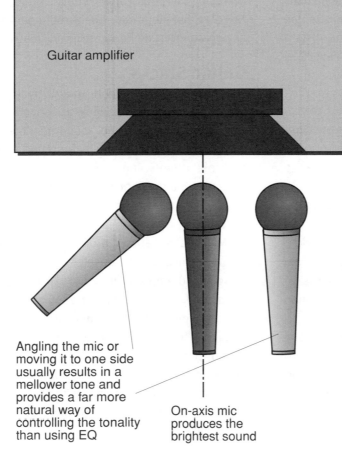

If the cabinet has two or more drivers, listen for the best one and mic that. There's often quite a difference in sound between supposedly identical speakers in the same cabinet

Guitar amplifier

Every amplifier, mic and room setup sounds different, so try miking the back of the cabinet or adding a back mic to the front mic, both with and without phase reversal

Compare what you hear over the monitors with records, not with what you're used to hearing on stage, and listen with effects added, even if it's just a little reverb to create the illusion of space. If you listen to the raw off-mic signal, it will probably sound unnaturally dry because close miking excludes virtually all room ambience

Angling the mic or moving it to one side usually results in a mellower tone and provides a far more natural way of controlling the tonality than using EQ

On-axis mic produces the brightest sound

Adding an ambient mic further back in the room can sound great in a good room, but unless you're recording somewhere special, you're probably better off faking it with a good reverb unit

Figure 2.10: Miking the electrical guitar amp, showing different mic angles

sound comes from the back as from the front, and just occasionally you can get a better sound by miking the back.

TIP

If you're working on your own, put on a pair of sealed headphones monitoring the mixing console, then try the mic in different positions while monitoring the result in the headphones. Even though the headphones won't give you perfect isolation from the amp, they should give you a good idea of which mic position produces the best sound.

Using Two Mics

You've probably read that some engineers use a combination of both a close mic and a more distant ambient mic, but when you try it, the results aren't great. Here are a few tips to help you improve things.

TIP

When any two mics are picking up the same sound source from different distances, some phase cancellation takes place, which will modify the frequency response of what you hear. Sometimes the results are great, sometimes not, so if you feel the sound isn't as good as it could be, get somebody to change the distance of the furthest mic as you listen. Also, try inverting the phase of the distant mic, as this will also make a difference, especially if the two mics are mixed at similar levels.

TIP

Try changing the height of the amp from the floor by placing it on a stand or a chair. Some sound is bound to reflect from the floor and find its way to the more distant mic, and because the path length of the reflected sound is greater, phase-cancellation will occur here, too. Changing the amp height will change the path length and hence the sound picked up by the more distant mic. Even the sound from the close mic can be affected if the amplifier is on the floor. Figure 2.11 shows the sound paths when two mics are used.

Occasionally, a good sound may be had by miking both the front and rear of an open-backed cabinet. Strictly speaking, the phase of the rear mic should be inverted (using the Phase button on the mixing console) so that its output is in phase with that of the front mic, but try both options and decide which sounds best. If you don't have a phase-inverting button, you can make up a phase-inverting lead by

swapping the wires going to pins 2 and 3 inside the XLR plug that plugs into the microphone. Ensure that any phase-reversing leads are clearly marked as such!

Guitar Stacks

To get a big-stack concert sound, try miking from ten feet or more and playing at concert level. This way, you capture the direct sound from the speakers, including any phase-cancellation effects caused by multiple drivers, and you also get the sound reflected from the floor, which, because of the longer path length, creates further comb-filtering or phase-cancellation effects.

Miking at a distance produces a warm, powerful sound quality, but it doesn't sound as bright as a close-miked amp and may not cut through a busy mix as well. For this reason, the signal is often mixed with the sound of a close mic aimed at one of the speakers in the cabinet. Speakers can differ in sound, so try all four in each cab until you find the best-sounding one. As in the combo-miking example, if the sound of the close mic is too bright, it can be mellowed by moving the mic towards the edge of the speaker.

A distant mic 'hears' the performance more as an audience would hear a real backline, but few

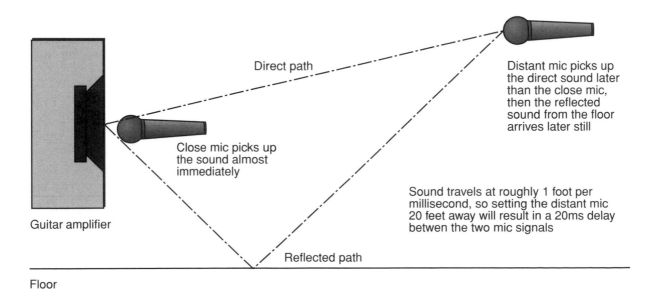

Direct path

Distant mic picks up the direct sound later than the close mic, then the reflected sound from the floor arrives later still

Close mic picks up the sound almost immediately

Sound travels at roughly 1 foot per millisecond, so setting the distant mic 20 feet away will result in a 20ms delay betwen the two mic signals

Guitar amplifier

Reflected path

Floor

Figure 2.11: Showing direct and floor reflections and the effect of miking a guitar amp at a distance (ambient mic)

home studios have the space to work this way, especially when several members of the band are playing together. Furthermore, in a session where several players are working together, separation becomes a major problem unless the microphones are placed as close to the guitar amps as possible. For this reason, only studio with very large recording spaces tend to record in this way.

Guitar Treatment

Once you've recorded your guitar sound and you're satisfied with the performance aspect, you can make further modifications using EQ, compression and effects.

Some additional EQ may be needed to achieve the desired tone, but it's worth trying to get the best sound you can by moving the mics around rather than trying to compensate using EQ. Of course, if you're DI'ing from a pre-amp, then you'll have to use the EQ controls on either the pre-amp, the console or both to shape the sound. A common problem with inexperienced bands is that they record guitar parts using far too much distortion. It's often better to use rather less distortion and then to use compression to restore the sustain and power.

Guitar Effects

In the case of the guitar, any effects such as pedals are modified by the character of the amplification system itself, so it might be wise to record these live rather than try to duplicate them while mixing. Also, the player responds to the sound being created, and effects are an integral part of the sound. This is particularly true of wah-wah, overdrive or echo. Don't compromise the performance by insisting that you add all the effects during the mix.

Close-miked or DI'd guitars always need a little reverb to provide a sense of space, but you'd be surprised how little you need to do the trick. Short ambience settings can create an intimate feel without cluttering the mix, so add heavy amounts of reverb only if you have an artistic reason for doing so. Also, consider mixing echo with reverb if you want a strong effect. Lastly, don't discount the spring reverbs found in guitar amps. These have a unique

tonality that works supremely well with some guitar styles. If the sound is good, don't dismiss it as being too low-tech.

Separation

Keeping two or more guitar parts sounding separate and distinct can be a major problem when mixing, and much of the blame usually rests on the song arrangement. Ideally, choose as different a sound as possible or rearrange the song so you haven't got two or more guitars playing overdrive chords all the way through everything!

Of course, if you're faced with a tape to mix and the guitar tracks are both busy and similar-sounding, you can use EQ to remove excess bass end and to peak up the presence part of the sound in different parts of the spectrum for the different guitars – for example, one guitar could be boosted at 2kHz while the other might be peaked up at 3.5kHz. Once you've done all you can to make the sounds a little different, you can pan them to different sides of the mix to separate them that way. However, don't rely on this method as your only means of separation, as some people may be listening in mono.

The DI Fallback Option

Although guitar players need to be able to respond to the way their amp sounds, there are times when it would be nice to be able to take that same performance and hear it through a different amplifier. Some engineers manage to do exactly this by using an active DI box to split the signal feeding the guitar amp such that a clean DI feed can be recorded onto a separate track of the recorder. Figure 2.12 shows how this is done. The guitar amp is miked or DI'd and recorded as normal, but the guitar signal going via the DI box is completely untreated, which means that the clean track can be played back through any amplifier or DI pre-amp at the mixing stage and either be used to replace the original guitar amp recording or be added to it. This is a useful technique for when the guitarist refuses to play with less overdrive.

If facilities permit, it is even possible to play the

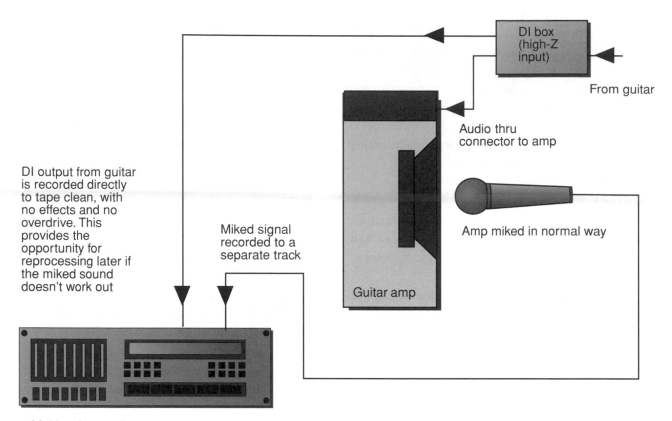

DI box (high-Z input)

From guitar

Audio thru connector to amp

DI output from guitar is recorded directly to tape clean, with no effects and no overdrive. This provides the opportunity for reprocessing later if the miked sound doesn't work out

Miked signal recorded to a separate track

Amp miked in normal way

Guitar amp

Multitrack recorder

Figure 2.12: Recording a DI guitar onto a spare track

track back through an amp set up in an unusual acoustic environment, such as a concrete stairwell, a bathroom or even a different building altogether. For example, by exploiting the flexibility of modular digital multitrack, you could take the recording to any location and then, with the aid of a simple mic pre-amp, a few leads and a different guitar amp, re-record the track in the new environment. Figure 2.13 shows a workable arrangement.

This same technique may be used to modify guitar tracks recorded conventionally, but there will be less flexibility as the original sound is already defined, and it is impossible to remove any overdrive that has already been added. Even so, you can liven up a sterile-sounding DI'd track by playing it through a real guitar amp and then remiking it, and an unpleasant solid-state overdrive sound can sometimes sound better after a real tube amplifier and speaker has a had a chance to smoothe the rough edges off it.

TIP

If a guitar track has been recorded using an amplifier that clips unpleasantly rather than distorting smoothly, play the tape track back via a good speaker simulator. This will help smoothe out the sound, although you may need to use a little EQ to put the bite back. This technique is more fully described in the section on mixing.

Bass Guitar

You'd think that recording the bass guitar was easy – after all, you can mic the amp, you can use a DI box, you can record via a dedicated bass pre-amp or you can plug an active bass straight into the mixing desk. Even so, it's all too easy to end up with a sound that seems fine on its own but doesn't really cut it when the rest of the mix is in place.

While the way in which you record does make a big difference to the sound, most serious tonal problems can usually be traced back to poorly set-

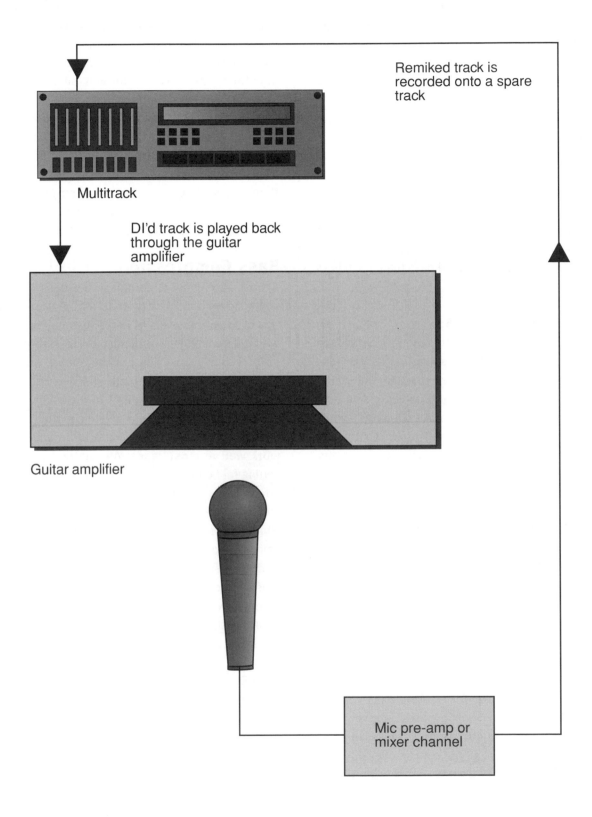

Multitrack

Remiked track is recorded onto a spare track

DI'd track is played back through the guitar amplifier

Guitar amplifier

Mic pre-amp or mixer channel

Figure 2.13: Remiking a DI'd guitar track

up instruments or poor playing technique. If you want a bright bass sound, then don't expect to get it from very old strings, and if you want a powerful, punchy sound, the instrument has to be played positively. Any rattles or buzzes should be sorted out by either adjusting the action or taking the guitar to a qualified technician before bringing it into the studio.

As with conventional guitar, the way that the string is 'attacked' by the player determines the harmonic content of the sound, and unless the instrument is played with confidence, it will never sound big and powerful. I'm a firm believer in using real instruments wherever possible, but I'd rather hear a good-sounding sampled bass than a real bass played poorly!

Direct-Injected Bass

First off, just like electric guitars, non-active basses don't interface well with mixer-line inputs, because the mixer impedance is too low to match that of the pickups. The result is a dull and unresponsive tone that will never sound good. To DI such a bass, you'll need either a high-impedance DI box (most active DI boxes will do the job), although you may prefer to use a bass pre-amp with on-board effects, such as EQ and compression. Active basses and guitars can be plugged directly into a desk because the active circuitry effectively functions as a DI box.

Bass Equalisation

Like a regular guitar amp, a bass-guitar amplifier doesn't have a flat frequency response but is instead 'voiced' to suit the instrument. To emulate this when you use a straight DI box, you'll need to add some form of EQ, either from the console or from an external equaliser. Graphic or parametric equalisers offer the most flexibility for creating bass sounds. There's little point in boosting much above 5kHz, however, as this will only bring up hiss and fret noise, but you need plenty of control over the bass and mid-range. If you DI the bass flat, it will probably sound very nice on its own, with a deep, round bass end and a nice wiry top. The problem is that, in a mix, the deep bass end becomes an indistinct

rumble and the top end starts to sound very thin and probably accentuates finger noise. To give the instrument definition, you'll probably need to add some lower mid, and the best way to do this is to monitor the bass sound on very small speakers, then EQ it until it sounds as big as possible within the whole mix. To increase the attack, you may need to boost at between 1.5kHz and 4kHz. Because the final EQ treatment depends on the rest of the mix, it's generally best to record the bass dead flat and then apply EQ during the mix. Using a speaker simulator when DI'ing may also help clean up the top end of the sound while giving it more body.

Bass Compression

Almost all engineers compress the bass guitar to some extent as a matter of course. Not only does this even up the levels of notes that may be played with different styles – pulling, picking, slapping and so on – but it also fills out the sound, making it project through the mix more effectively.

Initial compressor settings of a 5ms attack time combined with a 0.2–0.5s release time usually sounds about right, and a ratio of around 4:1 will work well in most cases. Alternatively, the Auto setting found on some compressors often gives very good results on bass. Higher ratios may be used to create a more tightly limited sound, while soft-knee compressors provide a more natural, less obviously compressed sound. Adjust the threshold control so that the gain-reduction meter is reading between 6dB and 10dB on signal peaks, then fine-tune the settings by ear. As with vocals, you may prefer to apply a little compression during recording and then add more as you mix.

Bass Pre-amps

The number of guitar and bass recording pre-amps on the market seems to increase weekly – some are relatively simple and emulate the pre-amp in a typical amplifier, while others combine the traditional pre-amp functions with compression and a full-blown effects section. Most conventional bass sounds require only EQ and compression, but a degree of overdrive helps add power and penetration to rock tracks. A gentle chorus works well on fretless basses but may also be used to good effect on conventional fretted basses, especially for slower songs. Reverb should be used very sparingly with bass for fear of muddying the sound, but a short ambience setting helps give the instrument a sense of place. As with chorus, the slower the song, the more effect you can generally use.

Wait Until The Mix

Because the bass may appear to sound rather different in the context of a mix, it is as well to leave as many options open as possible, so if you have a bass pre-amp complete with all the bells and whistles, consider recording the bass flat and then running the track back through the pre-amp when you mix. If you don't, you may add too much of something at the recording stage which you can't

take off again. Another valid reason for adding effects last is that you only need to feed in a mono track to get a stereo effect out. To record a stereo effect in the first place, you'd need to use up two tracks.

TIP

If you have to record the bass with effects, either because of track restrictions or because the player needs to hear the effects while recording, consider recording a dummy bass track early on with what you believe to be the right sound, then replace it later once the rest of the mix has been recorded. That way, you'll be able to choose a more appropriate sound.

TIP

If you have to work on a tape where the bass sound has insufficient punch, try feeding the track back

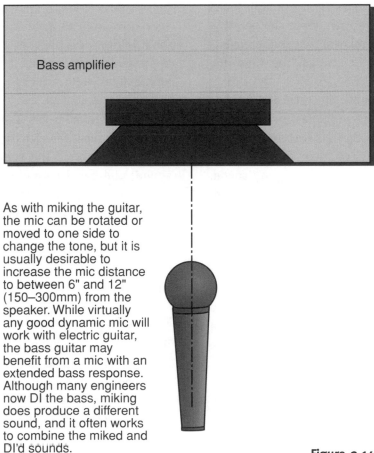

Bass amplifier

As with miking the guitar, the mic can be rotated or moved to one side to change the tone, but it is usually desirable to increase the mic distance to between 6" and 12" (150–300mm) from the speaker. While virtually any good dynamic mic will work with electric guitar, the bass guitar may benefit from a mic with an extended bass response. Although many engineers now DI the bass, miking does produce a different sound, and it often works to combine the miked and DI'd sounds.

Figure 2.14: Miking a bass guitar

through a bass amp or even a small guitar combo and then miking it up. The technique for miking bass amps is similar to that for conventional guitar amps, except the mic is usually positioned between 6 and 12 inches from the speaker grille rather than pushed right up against it. (Figure 2.14 shows a typical bass-miking arrangement.) Even so, experiment with mic distances and see which sound you prefer – every combination of bass, player, amplifier and microphone is unique.

As an alternative to miking the amp, DI the pre-amp output (or the speaker output, if your simulator will handle it) via a speaker simulator. Remember that, with any speaker simulator, unless it includes a dummy load or power soak, you'll need to leave the amplifier's own speaker connected. Figure 2.15 demonstrates this arrangement for both guitar and bass.

Acoustic Guitars

Try as you might, your acoustic guitar doesn't sound like what you hear on records. What can be going wrong? Assuming the instrument is in good condition and is fitted with good strings, the following techniques may help.

Acoustic guitars may be recorded in the traditional way, using microphones, or if they are fitted with a transducer pickups system, they may be DI'd. Good results are possible either way, but common problems include a hard or boxy sound, lack of brilliance, unwanted hiss, excessive finger squeaking or too much bottom end. However, by following a few basic rules, you should be able to get professional results, even when using fairly basic equipment.

As with any recording, quality starts with the instrument itself, and even though you can get good results from a modest instrument, it must be properly set up and fitted with good strings. If the strings are old and dull, no amount of EQ will inject life back into the tone, and if the strings are too light, the sound will lack body whatever you do. Light strings may also buzz excessively while unduly heavy strings produce a tight, rather tubby tone and are uncomfortable to play. The ideal gauge depends

on the player and the instrument. There's also no way to disguise fret buzz, and while a certain amount of fret and finger noise is part of the organic sound of the instrument, too, too much can spoil an otherwise good performance.

Acoustic DI

If your instrument is fitted with a piezo-electric pickup system (usually built into the bridge), and if that system has it's own on-board pre-amp, you can plug the guitar straight into the line input of a mixing console and get a decent result with very little effort. Having said that, I've never yet found a pickup system that sounds as natural as miking the guitar, especially at the top end, so some engineers like to combine the DI'd sound with conventional miking. A piezo pickup won't work well if plugged directly into a mixing console because the impedances won't match – if your guitar doesn't have an on-board pre-amp (if there's no battery, there's no pre-amp), then you'll need to use a specialised acoustic guitar pre-amp, with a very high input impedance, between the guitar pickup and the mixer. Many a dull, hissy acoustic-guitar sound has resulted from a piezo pickup being plugged directly into a console mic or line input.

If the instrument has on-board EQ, adjust this carefully as small changes to the settings can make a big difference to the sound. For a good solo sound, pull back the mid-range slightly so as to emphasise both the high and low end of the instrument. However, if the guitar part is just one layer in a mix, try rolling off some bottom end to thin the sound out a little. If you have no EQ on the instrument's own pre-amp, use whatever EQ you have on your mixer.

The Playing Environment

To help prevent tuning problems, the guitar should be placed in the studio for as long as possible before recording, and the studio temperature should also be reasonably constant. Tuning should be checked, using an electronic tuner, before very take.

The environment also affects the perceived sound of the miked instrument, because microphones pick

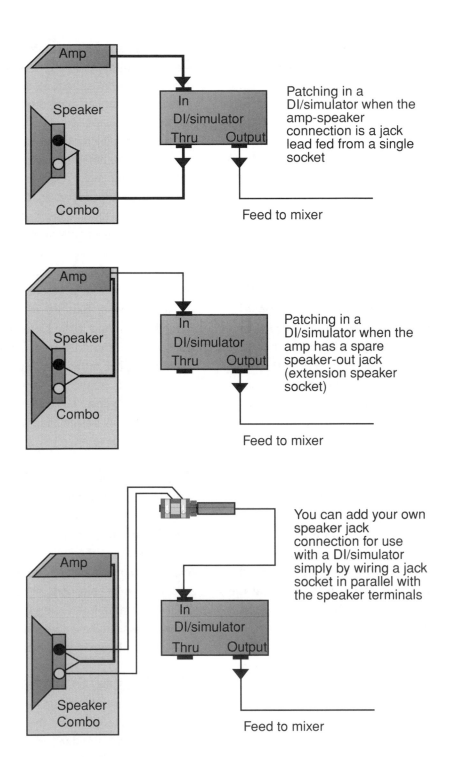

Patching in a
DI/simulator when the
amp-speaker
connection is a jack
lead fed from a single
socket

Patching in a
DI/simulator when the
amp has a spare
speaker-out jack
(extension speaker
socket)

You can add your own
speaker jack
connection for use
with a DI/simulator
simply by wiring a jack
socket in parallel with
the speaker terminals

The connections illustrated assume you have a speaker-simulator
unit that does not include a dummy load. Never disconnect the
speaker when using these devices as some amplifiers can sustain
damage if run with no load. If you have a model with a built-in load,
you can use it in place of the existing speaker, which enables you to
work quietly

Figure 2.15: Recording/reprocessing via a speaker simulator

up both the direct sound from the instrument and reflected sound from the walls and ceiling. One of the most common mistakes is for people to attempt to record the acoustic guitar in a dead, acoustically unsympathetic room. If you have to work in a carpeted room, try placing a sheet of hardboard or similar hard material on the floor beneath the performer. If you have a great-sounding bathroom or hallway, it's worth the effort to run some long leads out there in order to capture a good acoustic sound.

The second most popular mistake is to place the mic too close to the soundhole of the guitar in an attempt to capture as much level as possible. If the guitar is small or has a rather thin sound, you might get away with this, but as a rule, miking close to the soundhole results in a boomy or boxy sound that is difficult to cure using EQ. If you have to deal with a track recorded this way, try cutting the lower mid and rolling off some bass, but don't expect to get a perfectly natural result.

A better approach is to select a mic position that picks up sound directly from the strings, from the front of the guitar body, and includes some room reflections. In general, this usually means keeping the mic 12–18 inches from the guitar and pointing towards either the bridge side or the neck side of the soundhole. If the mic is too far away, you'll end up with plenty of live ambience but little of the original sound of the instrument. Furthermore, the more distant the sound, the quieter it is and the more noise problems you're likely to encounter, especially with cheaper microphones.

For stereo use, a coincident pair pointing either side of the soundhole usually sounds good. Here's a tip, though: the acoustic guitar sound can vary a lot depending on mic position, so I like to set up a pair of good-quality enclosed headphones to monitor what the mic is picking up, then I move the mic while the player plays and listen to the result via the phones as I make adjustments. That way, I soon find the best sounding spot.

Acoustic-Guitar Mics

So far I've covered the room acoustics and the mic position, but problem number three usually stems from using an inappropriate model of microphone. Acoustic guitars produce harmonics right up to the top of the audio spectrum, so to capture these you need a mic that has a good high-end response. Back-electrets and capacitor mics are significantly better than dynamic microphones in this respect, although you can sometimes get acceptable results from a good dynamic mic.

In most instances, cardioid (unidirectional) microphones tend to be used to reduce the spill from other instruments or external sources of noise, but omni mics invariably produce a more open, natural tone. Whichever you choose depends on the mics you have available and on your artistic taste.

In all cases, I try to record with little or no equalisation, and if the tone is very wrong for any reason, this should be corrected (if possible) by moving the mic rather than by reaching for the tone controls. This applies to all aspects of recording – if you get a good sound at source, the end result will always be better than you'd get by trying to equalise an unsatisfactory sound.

Mono Or Stereo Guitar?

Different engineers will argue the merits of stereo or mono miking, and if you're going to add artificial reverberation, even a mono miked recording will have a stereo image in the final mix. From my experience, mono miking produces the best-focused sound, even for solo work, although stereo can sound wider and more interesting if you get it right. In my view, unless you have a real need or desire to record in stereo, mono will give more predictable results.

The Singer/Guitarist

If a singer/guitarist is recording songs in one take (as opposed to recording the guitar part separately), spill between the guitar and vocal mics is an obvious problem. If you have access to only cardioid-pattern mics, get the guitar mic as close as you can without compromising the guitar tone and put the vocal mic no more than 12 inches from the mouth, with a pop shield between the mic and the mouth. Inevitably, some guitar sound will pick up on the vocal mic and vice versa, but this may not be too serious a problem and can even be used to create the illusion of stereo if the guitar mic is panned a little to one side and the vocal mic to the other.

If, however, you need better separation, the figure-of-eight microphone can be a useful ally because of its total insensitivity to sounds coming 90 degrees off axis. By using one figure-of-eight mic on the vocal and another on the guitar and by angling the mics carefully, as shown in Figure 2.16, it is possible to create quite a high degree of separation between the guitar and vocal. Of course, a figure-of-eight-pattern microphone picks up sound just as well from the rear as it does from the front, so the contribution of the room ambience will be greater. If room reflections are proving to be too obtrusive, a piece of foam rubber or a duvet can be used to shadow the back end of each of the figure-of-eight microphones. It may also help to hang a blanket in front of the performer and to rely on the floor and rear wall to provide the necessary ambience.

Sitting In The Mix

Although it's safest to record with little or no EQ, the sound may benefit from a little subsequent equalisation to make it sit properly in the mix. For example, an acoustic guitar used in a rock mix often sounds better with the low end filtered out, so as to prevent conflicts with vocals, electric guitars, pad keyboards or other mid-range sounds. If the sound is too boxy for any reason, a low-mid cut often helps, and if more brilliance is required, a little boost at around 6kHz usually does the trick.

The recorded sound almost always benefits from additional reverberation, but don't use too much. A common problem with inexperienced musicians is that they add a lot of reverb to make something sound impressive on its own, but when it's added to other instruments, many of which also have reverb added, the mix can get very cluttered. In most cases, a short, bright setting will add sparkle and create a suitably convincing stereo effect, even if the original recording is in mono.

Where adequate live room ambience has been recorded along with the guitar, an early-reflections or ambience setting may still be used to add stereo width to a mono recording without making the sound significantly more reverberant.

Acoustic-Guitar Compression

Compression is often used to make an acoustic-guitar track sound more even, but as long as the playing is proficient, the amount of compression required may be quite small. Unless you're experienced at using compressors, use a soft-knee model with an auto-release function if at all possible. If not, use a conventional compressor set to a 3:1 ratio with a 10ms attack time and a 200ms release time. Adjust the threshold until the sound is right, at which point you'll probably be registering around 6dB of gain reduction on signal peaks.

The main aim is to get a well-balanced tone, a good performance and a little ambience or reverb to provide a sense of space. As touched upon earlier, it's also possible to combine the output of a guitar pickup with a mic, one possibility being to pan the pickup sound to one side and the miked sound to the other to create a pseudo-stereo image.

Acoustic-Guitar Fixes

If a recorded acoustic-guitar sound is boomy or boxy, try cutting the mid range at between 150Hz and 250Hz. If the sound is dull, boost at between 5kHz and 8kHz or use an enhancer/exciter (sparingly) to restore the edge. A bright reverb patch with pronounced early reflections will also give the guitar sound more life. If the sound is hard or aggressive, cut at between 1kHz and 2kHz. If you want to add edge to dull strings, use an exciter.

If the sound is uneven, use compression to smoothe it out – this will also add sustain. For a rhythm guitar part that isn't perfectly in tune, try pitch-shifting the sound slightly (just by a few cents) and add this to the original for a subtle chorus effect. Where the original part is flat, shift it sharp, and vice versa. Hopefully, the chorused final sound will centre around the desired pitch.

At various points in this book I'll remind you not to try to cover flaws by using effects – though I'll probably go on to suggest ways in which you might do it anyway!

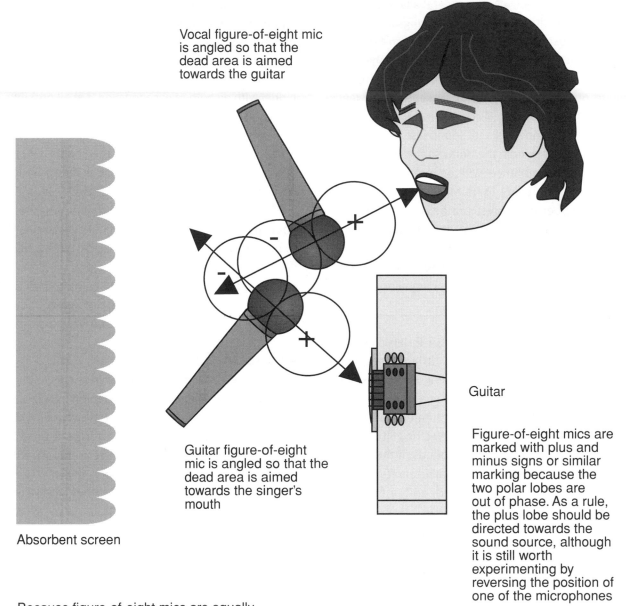

Vocal figure-of-eight mic is angled so that the dead area is aimed towards the guitar

Guitar figure-of-eight mic is angled so that the dead area is aimed towards the singer's mouth

Absorbent screen

Guitar

Figure-of-eight mics are marked with plus and minus signs or similar marking because the two polar lobes are out of phase. As a rule, the plus lobe should be directed towards the sound source, although it is still worth experimenting by reversing the position of one of the microphones

Because figure-of-eight mics are equally sensitive front and rear, some form of absorbent screen may be required to reduce the effect of room reflections

Figure 2.16: Recording guitar and vocals using figure-of-eight mics

Other Instruments

Occasionally you'll come across and instrument you haven't recorded before, and if you don't know where to put the mic, there are a couple of strategies you can adopt. One is to assume that the player always hears a reasonable sound from the instrument, so if you put up a mic pointing over the player's shoulder from behind, the mic should collect pretty much what the player hears. When recording French-horn players, choose the shoulder without the horn!

Another tactic is to estimate the length of that part of the instrument that produces the sound and then to put the mic the same distance away. For example, a wind instrument with holes in the body produces sound all along its length as well as from the open end, so if the instrument is 18 inches long, try putting the mic 18 inches away. Pianos and drum kits are much larger, so you'll need a longer mic distance if you're going to record them with a single mic (or with a coincident stereo pair). On the other hand, the human voice comes mainly from the mouth, so you can afford to close-mic in that case.

The reason why this method works is because it gives the mic a chance to capture the different components of the sound coming from different parts of the instrument. If you get too close, you focus in on just one part of the sound, whereas if you get too far away, the room influences the sound too much and you may lose too much level.

Earlier in the chapter, I mentioned the trick of wearing enclosed headphones to enable you to monitor the sound as you adjust the mic position. By picking one of the two techniques mentioned and then performing the final mic adjustments while monitoring over phones, you should end up with a useable sound no matter how odd the instrument.

3 MIX TECHNIQUES AND PROBLEMS

Getting a good mix is no easy task, and a lot of people have problems in this area. We've all done it – spent hours working on a mix only to feel like tearing it all down and starting again. The more work you put in, the worse it seems to get. What's more, it seems that, the more sophisticated the equipment at your disposal, the more difficult it is to get a satisfactory mix. How is it that four- and eight-track demos done with virtually no outboard equipment can sound so good but once you get more tracks, add a MIDI sequencer and then patch in a few effects units and processors the job seems so much harder?

If your equipment is simple, you're forced to work simply – you record as few parts as you need to make the song work. You may have reverb as your only effect, and your mixing facilities may well only have treble and bass EQ. The outcome is that you record the individual sounds more or less as they are – you balance the result, and that's about it. In my case, my first reverb was a spring unit that was so twangy that I had to use as little of it in the mix as possible. Any guitar effects were added during recording and were usually confined to chorus or echo, and because there were no DI solutions to guitar recording around at that time, I miked up my amplifier.

In these technologically advanced times, many problems stem from the recording process being too open-ended, and there's an almost overwhelming urge to tinker with everything, whether it needs it or not. MIDI also has a lot to answer for – in pre-MIDI days, you might record one keyboard part and overdub a second, but now it's quite common to find a 16-track recorder stuffed with live takes locked up to a sequencer with 16 or more tracks of electronic stuff going on. No wonder the mixes sound confused and cluttered! There's also the temptation to use wooden-sounding, quantised drum parts rather than a real drummer, and if the rhythm section of a song doesn't have a groove, it's never going to work.

Keep It Simple

So what does this reveal? If you record the various elements of a good performance and then adjust the balance without adding any effects or EQ, the result will be at least acceptable and at best excellent. It's largely down to sensible musical arrangement followed by the clean recording of a competent performance. It's true that some things can be improved by using EQ and other forms of processing, but a good rule is to record everything at least with no EQ. That way, if the mix isn't working out, you can easily get back to a clean slate by resetting the channel EQs to their flat positions.

Some engineers insist on adding EQ when recording, and if that works for you, fair enough, but I don't feel entirely comfortable with this way of working, because you don't really know what EQ a sound finally needs until you hear it in context with the rest of the mix. As most mixes are built up in layers by overdubbing, how can you possibly know what EQ you'll eventually need? What's worse is that, if you do make a mistake, it's virtually impossible to change an already EQ'd sound so that it sounds as it did originally. The only possible exception is the electric guitar (and electric bass), which have no natural sound and so may need some EQ to get the sound into the right ballpark. Even so, I'd still avoid over-equalising, as you may still need to make further adjustments during the mix. It's always easier to cut frequencies using EQ than to add them, so at the very least you should ensure that you have enough top end in your recordings.

Keep It Clean

A typical problem with mixing is that unwanted noises that you never noticed before start to appear on the master, such as rustling papers or creaking chairs on the vocal track, the sound of an electric guitar being put down at the end of a song, unerased material on sections of track that should be quiet and so on. It makes life a lot easier if, before settling down to the mix, you listen to each track in isolation and erase all those unwanted glitches, pops, squeaks and ill-timed comments from the drummer. While this is hard work in a tape-based environment, it's easy using audio software.

The Arrangement

A good mix starts with a good performance of a suitable musical arrangement, and unless everything is in tune and in time, there's virtually nothing you can do to fix it short of sampling the few bits that work and building a new arrangement out of the rubble. However, one very common problem you can do something about is arrangements that get too busy, resulting in all the sense of space and separation being lost. As mentioned earlier, the options offered by MIDI make it very easy to over-orchestrate a song. A good arrangement will also take account of what instruments are playing at the same time so that you don't end up with three things playing at once, all occupying the same space in the musical spectrum. Again, MIDI instruments can be a problem in this, because many patches are designed to sound as big and impressive as possible.

Ensemble instruments such as brass and strings blend nicely so you can afford to layer patches from different instruments in order to get a rich ensemble voice, but the end result will still be treated as a single sound that has to find its place in the mix.

On the other hand, if you have a middly bass guitar, a low, thick synth pad and a woolly sounding rhythm guitar, then the chances are that the mix is going to sound confused. Some engineers tackle this problem by trying to make similar sounds appear different by using heavy EQ, and this works to a limited extent, but the only really satisfactory approach is to choose the right sounds at the outset. EQ should be regarded as a tool for fine polishing, not as a large hammer and chisel. Invariably, there are exceptions to this rule when you start getting creative, but when it comes to making instruments and voices sound good, I've always found that the less EQ you can get away with, the more natural the results.

If the mix includes sequenced instruments, MIDI gives you the choice of changing sounds right up to the last moment, but even this is a double-edged sword as much time can be lost trying out different patches. In choosing the best sounds for any particular job, you need to be careful – many modern synths sound so rich and impressive that they can take up all the space in your mix, especially factory presets that are designed to sound impressive when played on their own in the shop. Creating thinned-down versions of some of the factory presets can be a good idea, and if you're inclined to create your own patches, you'll probably find this more satisfying than using sounds that appear on everybody else's songs.

Choice Of Sounds

Continuing on the subject of sounds, you may find that, with instruments like electric guitars and basses, you have far less control over the sound than you thought you would once the recording has been made. For example, it's virtually impossible using a conventional desk EQ to thin out a humbucking guitar sound to produce a single-coil sound or vice versa. On the other hand, hearing sounds in isolation is of little help, because they appear so different when everything else is up and running – only experience will enable you to judge what sounds are going to work together.

If you're recording a band with two guitar players,

you should really get them to play together in the studio so you can see how the sounds work together. This is even more important if you are planning to record the guitars independently. A common mistake made by bands with little studio experience is that they use far too much guitar overdrive. While this may be fine live and for studio solos, two guitars playing wall-to-wall fuzz power chords all the way through a song is a sure recipe for a migraine at mix time. This problem isn't confined to rock bands, either – a lot of indie guitar bands use heavy distortion to fill out their sound when performing live, but if this is carried over into the studio, the sound can end up as an uncontrollable mess.

TIP

If you have enough tracks, use a DI box to split the output from the guitar so that you record one track by miking up the amp (or using a suitable recording pre-amp) and the other is the clean feed straight from the DI box. If the miked-up sound doesn't work out, you still have the option of running the DI'd track through a guitar amp or recording pre-amp while you mix, which gives you the opportunity to use any overdrive and amp EQ setting you like. This new sound may then be used in place of the original track or mixed in with it.

Listen In Context

What goes for the guitar goes for the bass too, and you often find that a bass that sounds rich and punchy on its own sounds dumpy or soggy when everything else is happening. What's not often appreciated is how important the lower-mid frequencies are in making a bass sound full, and if you don't believe this, listen to a good record on a small radio or mini hi-fi. You'll get little real bass from such a system, but what's going on in the 80Hz–150Hz region still provides the illusion of depth. If you can get the bass player to play along with the guitarists or whatever else is in the mix while you listen to the result from the control room (or from a test recording), you'll get a better idea of how things are going to sound. If you're DI'ing the bass via a DI box, adding compression can improve the sound

significantly, but there are occasions when miking the amp is the only way to get a good sound. If you have enough channels of compression at your disposal, compress the bass only slightly when recording it, then compress more as you mix.

Playing Technique

One very important point is that the sound of an instrument changes very significantly depending on how it is played. Put two drummers on the same kit and they'll sound quite different. If you hit drums hard, then it sounds as though you're hitting them hard, but you can't make a quiet drummer sound loud simply by turning him up in the mix. If this sounds like it's going to be a problem, don't be afraid to talk it over with the musicians. Bass guitars also suffer dreadfully if they aren't played with confidence and power. No amount of EQ, compression or anything else will help, so again, have a word with the player before recording.

The Importance Of Balance

Once you've got the required tracks on tape, you have to set a balance, and the more tracks you have to play with, the more there is to go wrong. If the vocal keeps drifting in level, you should consider compressing it, and in a typical pop mix I like to hear a good balance between the bass, drums and vocals before I start to add the other instruments. It's here the musicians' egos can become a problem, however, because you'll sometimes find that there are parts that can best be used very low down in the mix, but if the player in question is feeling insecure, he may be wondering why he isn't as loud as the other guys in the band. That's one advantage of working with a sequencer – computers don't have attitude problems.

Don't rely entirely on the pan controls to keep your sounds separate – get the mix working in mono first. Only then should you pan out the various elements. This will also help you to ensure that your mix is mono-compatible, although you must check this again after adding any effects. Once you've got a rough balance in mono using no EQ, you can start to fine-tune things a little.

Contrast And Perspective

Another common problem is that, in trying to get all the sounds in your mix to stand out, the end result gets cluttered. That's because naturally performed music doesn't normally exist along an imaginary line drawn from left to right – some of the performers are nearer the front than others. However, when panning a sound between two loudspeakers, all you're doing is moving it from left to right, not from front to back.

The early reverberant reflections produced when a sound occurs in an enclosed space have a significant effect on how near or far the sound appears to be from the listener. Intuitively, it seems reasonable that a more distant sound will contain a greater proportion of reverberant sound than a near one, but the spacing and rate of build-up of these reflections also appears to be important.

TIP

If you have a reverb device that allows you to change the characteristics of the early-reflections patterns, or the rate at which they build up, it's worthwhile experimenting to locate the settings that produce a definite sense of closeness or distance. Small-room, ambient or closely spaced reflection patterns that build up rapidly seem to create a sense of closeness or intimacy while a slower reverb build-up suggests distance. If you have the option to turn down the level of the reverb tail independently of the early reflections, this can help to prevent the sound from becoming too 'wet'.

TIP

Make up-front sounds slightly brighter and sounds in the background slightly less bright. Exciters can be useful for bringing sounds forward in a mix, but to maintain the contrast between main and supporting sounds, don't process everything or all your sounds will be competing for first place again!

Once your mix is set up, check for mono compatibility, as the changes in phase produced by some stereo-miking techniques or stereo effects can radically change the way that the mix sounds in mono.

Panning Checklist

- Pan bass instruments and bass drums to the centre of the mix. Snare drums tend also to work best when panned near the centre, but the toms and overhead mics may be spread (not too widely) from left to right.

- Keep the lead vocals close to the centre of the mix, as they are the focus of the performance, but experiment with positioning backing vocals to the sides.

- When you pan an instrument away from the centre of the mix, don't always feel you have to go hard left or right. Try to paint a picture, with your sounds spreading across the stereo stage. Your key sounds should be nearest the centre, supporting the sounds panned to either side, and artificial reverberation should be panned the widest.

- Don't pan stereo pianos, drum kits or synths hard left and right or they'll sound unrealistically wide.

- Unless you're specifically trying to create a special effect, pan the outputs from your stereo reverb unit hard left and right and ensure that they are the same level in the mix.

- Use your discretion when panning the outputs from stereo effects units such as delays and chorus units. Consider panning them over just half of the stereo soundstage – between dead centre and hard left, for example.

- Always check your mix in mono, just in case the way you've used stereo effects changes the balance by an unacceptable amount.

EQ Influences Perspective

The other reason for not getting too hung up on EQing sounds until everything is playing is that, in order to create a sense of perspective, some sounds must take a backseat role, which may mean they sound slightly uninspiring when heard on their own.

Of course, that doesn't matter because they're not going to be heard on their own, but there's still a temptation to solo every sound, then try to make it as strong and up-front as possible. Obviously, the vocals will need to be somewhere near the front of the mix, and the rhythm section will need to be right behind it if you're working on an upbeat song or dance track, but rhythm guitars and keyboards play a supporting role. Thinner guitar sounds – such as those you get from a single-coil-pickup instrument – leave plenty of space in a mix and cut through effectively, even when they're quite low in volume. The thicker sound of humbucking pickups can be overpowering while still having a tendency to merge in with other sounds, although cutting some lower-mid EQ can help lighten the sound.

Mixing And Effects

Before you switch on an effect, ask yourself, 'Why am I doing this?'. Once you've paid out for a good multi-effects unit, there's a temptation to use it wherever possible, but you must resist. Effects are there to create illusions, and before you can start, you have to decide what illusion you wish to create and why it would benefit the mix. Most Western music is designed to be heard indoors, so the first illusion to construct is that of an indoor environment, and for this you need only a little reverb.

The Importance Of Reverb

Other than concert halls and bad venues, few listening rooms have huge amounts of reverb – you just need enough to create the effect of your music existing in three-dimensional space. Add too much reverb and your sound will recede into the distance.

Another consequence of adding reverb to instruments indiscriminately is that the space in your mix starts to disappear, and as has often been quoted, the spaces in music are as important as the notes. If you don't have a reason to use it, turn it off, and if you do need to use it, use it sparingly. Similarly, if the lower-mid section of your mix seems awash with confusion, switch off the reverb returns for a moment and listen to how much your use of reverb is contributing to the problem. The same is

true of echo effects, and while chorus is less likely to steal your space, it can have the effect of putting the treated instrument 'out of focus'.

Note that some reverb units clutter the sound more than others, and the ability to maintain clarity within a busy mix is one of the more important factors that separates budget reverbs from top-end pro units. Even so, a budget unit applied with care can produce seriously good results. One tip is to use a short, bright reverb with plenty of early reflections if you want to create ambience and space without flooding the mix with reverberation. It may also be useful to patch an equaliser before the reverb so as to take some of the low end out of the signal being processed. This will help to keep the low frequencies under control, resulting in a cleaner mix. Where the early-reflection balance can be adjusted separately, it's worth experimenting with higher levels.

Chorus Effects

Chorus creates the illusion of movement and a wide, dynamic stereo image, but it also has the effect of pushing sounds further back in the mix. The repetitious modulation can get annoying if the chorus effect is too strong, but if used with care chorus can be used to help build the front-to-back perspective of a mix. It works well for rounding out pad sounds and also suits some guitar parts, but it doesn't usually work well on vocals. Once again, before adding it, think about the kind of effect you want to achieve – don't chorus the rhythm guitar simply because you always chorus the rhythm guitar.

Here are a few tips to get you out of trouble when adding effects to a mix.

- If you find that a reverb patch is making the vocal appear sibilant, edit the patch so that it has more high-frequency damping, You may need to bring it right down to 3kHz or even less to clean up the sound. Alternatively, patch a de-esser into the reverb-send signal path.

- Sometimes you may need to add reverb to a complete track that's already been mixed, in which case the bass instruments will probably get over-treated and become muddy-sounding. You can get around this by putting an equaliser before the reverb input to cut off anything below 150Hz or thereabouts. Use a short-ambience setting to avoid cluttering the mix and add the reverb sparingly. If your unit has an early-reflections-only or dedicated ambience algorithm, try that instead of conventional reverb.

- To add interest to an otherwise static-sounding reverb, try feeding the effect send though a chorus or flange effect before feeding it into the reverb input. The modulation of the chorus/flange effect will add movement and interest to the reverb patch but will leave the original sound untouched, so you won't end up with a gimmicky result. This effect works for all kinds of music.

- For more radical musical styles, try effecting the sound heavily before it's fed into the reverb. You could use a pitch-shifter, for example, to push the reverb feed up or down by an octave or even a fifth. You could use a distortion box before the reverb or even set up a multitap delay with loads of feedback so that all the individual delays get transformed into their own little cloud of reverb. Distorting the reverb send can sometimes be useful in creating vintage R&B guitar sounds and may reduce the amount of overdrive you need to add to the dry sound.

- If you feel a sound needs more reverb, but adding more makes the mix sound messy, consider increasing the reverb level but shortening the reverb decay time. This makes the sound seem more like it's being produced in a real space without flooding everything in a wash of reverb. You can also roll off some bottom end from the reverb return by coming back in via two mixer channels panned hard left and right, or you could increase the low-frequency damping, as long as this doesn't make the reverb sound too cold.

- Lastly, you might have an old effects unit that you feel sounds unnatural by today's standards. Don't bin it, however, because some of those trashy old sounds are great in a creative context. Don't judge everything by how natural it sounds – look how much vintage gear appears on modern records.

Mix Compression

Once the mix is set up and you've compared it with a commercial CD of a similar musical style, you might find that your mix still lacks energy. In addition to the routine compressing of vocals, bass guitars and so on, some engineers like to compress the whole mix, and this is one way of increasing the average energy contained within. This is quite valid, but you have to be a little choosy about the model of compressor you use, as some tend to dull the sound or cause it to pump unacceptably.

As a rule, a good-quality soft-knee compressor will work well, and you'll need to increase the attack time until high-frequency transient sounds come through without being 'squashed' every time there's a kick-drum beat. Compressors, with auto-release settings are usually the best at dealing with the complex dynamics of a mix, but if you have a manual compressor, set a release time of around 0.3 seconds and then increase this slightly if you can hear too much gain-pumping. An attack time of around 10ms should be adequate. Ratios in excess of 5:1 can also cause pumping problems, as can unnecessarily low threshold settings. Ideally, you should only need to compress enough to see gain reductions of around 5dB registering on the signal peaks.

Important: When doing an A/B test by switching the compressor in and out, make sure that the subjective level of the compressed signal is adjusted to be the same as the bypassed level. If you don't do this, whichever sound is loudest will almost certainly appear to sound best!

Mixing With MDM

DAT has established itself as a standard stereo-mastering medium in both the semi-professional and professional markets, but rather than mix directly to DAT, MDM (Modular Digital Multitrack) owners have another, more flexible option. If you mix directly onto two spare tracks of your MDM, rather than to DAT, the master stereo recording and the original tracks are always in the same physical place, so it's easy to keep track of your material. Furthermore, if you have two or more MDM machines, when you clone your master tapes for safety purposes, you also clone your masters.

Modern MDMs handle drop-ins or punch-ins by creating a very rapid crossfade, which results in a seamless edit. In the context of mastering, this means that, if you've done a mix and it hasn't all gone according to plan, you don't have to go back to the top and do it all again; you can simply set up your mixer to correct the offending part and then punch in and out at the appropriate places. Most of the time, a manual punch-in and -out will be fine, but if you have the capacity for automated punching, you can be as surgical as you like.

Working in this way, you can achieve the sort of results normally associated with automated mixing – any song can be mixed in as many different sections as you like. An example of this might be a song where you require a different mixer set-up for the choruses and yet another for an instrumental solo. A sensible approach might be to mix the whole song in one pass with the mix set up for the verses and then go through again, dropping in all the choruses with the chorus mixer setting. Finally, the solo can be replaced with the correct mix.

With a sequencer, you can automate the entire mix and then record it back to a couple of free tracks, ideally keeping it at 24-bit resolution. This way, you retain the maximum quality through to the mastering stage.

Cleaning Up

Two serious shortcomings of DAT when it comes to mastering are that you can't easily top and tail songs (ie erase unwanted material at the start and end) and you also can't change the order of the songs or introduce precise spaces between tracks. With digital multitrack, the automatic (or even manual, if you're confident) punch-in and -out can be used to record silence right up to the start of the song and again at the end, and if you have two or more multitracks you can digitally transfer your mixed masters from one machine to the other in any order and with appropriate gaps between tracks. (ADAT/BRC users are particularly well catered for when it comes to working this way.) Once the mix is completed, it may then be transferred to DAT either via a suitable digital interface or via analogue connections. If an analogue transfer is required, this would be a good time to do any other analogue post-production work, such as using EQ, tube processors or compression. Note: Don't clean up the song start if there's a chance you'll be using digital de-noising later, as you'll need to take a noise 'fingerprint'.

Monitoring

If you find that your mixes always sound great in the studio but awful on everybody else's music system, there may be something wrong with your monitoring. However, before jumping to that conclusion, have you made a point of playing other CDs through your monitors to get an idea of what you should be aiming for? It's a great temptation to monitor everything loudly in the studio, and when you combine this with the excitement of mixing (and possibly with a temporary hearing shift caused by listening to loud music all day), you may produce a bad mix, even if the monitors are OK. If possible, don't mix on the same day as your recording session, or at least take a break beforehand.

If things seem to be going badly wrong, first check your speakers are wired in phase and that they aren't mounted too close to corners. If the room is fairly small, you should also be using small to medium-sized monitors – anything bigger may just emphasise the room problems. The next step is to play a few CDs over the system to check that they sound OK. If they do, your monitoring system is probably useable, but if they don't, look again at your choice of speakers and/or room acoustics. If you have a graphic EQ connected between your mixer and power amplifier, try switching it out of circuit – in my experience, they generally make things worse rather than better.

Next time you set up what you think is a good mix, take the time to play a similar-style CD and compare the CD with your own work. Listen particularly to the sounds at the bass end – many mixes go wrong because of the temptation to add excessive bass in order to compensate for using small monitors. Also, the nearer you can work to your monitors, the less the room character will interfere with what you hear. For more details on monitoring, refer to Chapter 5, 'Monitoring And Room Problems'.

Mix Philosophy

Ultimately, a mix is just a balance of instruments and voices that provides a pleasing result, and the more you process and manipulate the various elements without reason, the less natural the result is likely to sound. It's rather like photography – put a good subject in front of a camera, make sure the lighting is OK and you have a respectable picture. If you then start to touch up that picture using something like a computer-graphics program, you may be able to change the colour balance, move trees out of the background and give the donkey on the left two heads, but unless you're a real expert, it's never going to look as natural as the original.

When it comes to the arrangement, if an instrument or voice can't justify being there, why have it? It's rather like cooking – if you throw in the entire contents of your spice rack every time you cook, you'll never get any variety and the flavours will be confused. Having said all that, mixing is an art, and in art you can break all the rules you want to, providing you get a result. Keep things simple to start with, but as you gain more experience and confidence, you'll develop a method of mixing that works for you.

More About Panning

You have a mixer full of inputs and a couple of stereo effects units, but when it comes to the mix, do you know where to pan everything, or do you just hope for the best?

Mixing music is an art, and as such any rules are made to be broken, but before you can break them with confidence, you really need to know what they are! Because we were born with two ears, we live in a stereophonic environment, so when it comes to music, a mono recording can sound rather one-dimensional. That's because it lacks the spatial cues that allow our brains to estimate the distance and direction of natural sound sources.

By analysing the slightly different sounds that arrive at each ear, the human brain can deduce a surprising amount of information about the source of the sound and about the physical environment. No recording/replay system yet invented offers more than an approximation of the way in which we hear sound naturally, although a stereophonic loudspeaker system used in conjunction with stereo-miking techniques or thoughtful use of panning can still be impressive.

Pan Pots

Pan, in the context of terms such as 'pan pot', is short for *panorama*, and by changing the balance of a mono signal between the left and right speakers, it's possible to reproduce some of the cues that give us our aural sense of direction. Pan pots may able used to position mono sound sources at various positions between the loudspeakers to imitate a natural, stereo soundfield, but this is still an extremely crude approximation of real life, as this means that only some of nature's audio cues are mimicked. The result is really panned mono, not true stereo – although in all fairness most 'stereo' pop records rely extensively on panning rather than on stereo-miking techniques.

Rules Of Panning

When using pan controls, it's wise to place bass-heavy sounds and lead vocals in the centre of the mix so that their load will be shared equally by the two speakers. Apart from maximising the available power from the end user's stereo system, placing key sounds in the centre creates an anchor point for the rest of the mix.

Panning is often used to approximate the way in which performers might be arranged on a stage. The main vocals will be in the centre, along with the bass guitar, bass drum and very often the snare drum, too. Panning may be used to widen the rest of the drums in the kit, but don't be tempted to pan the toms hard left and right or the drum kit will sound unnaturally wide. The same is true of pianos and stereo keyboards – pan them, by all means, but pan then half left and half right or full to one side and centre rather than spreading them right across the whole mix.

The same is also true of any stereo effects, such as chorus, that are applied to individual instruments, although how you apply these depends on how many mixer channels are sharing the same effect and where in the mix the original sounds are panned. We've grown accustomed to hearing very wide stereo effects on record for some years now, and although the results are rather larger than life, there's no reason not to use them if they work on an artistic level. However, if you are using more than one stereo effect, it might be more effective to pan one between hard left and centre with the other panned between hard right and centre.

Guitars, keyboards, brass and so on can be panned to either side, as can backing vocals. Outputs from stereo reverb units are normally left panned to the left and right extremes.

TIP

Don't get too concerned that you're not making full use of stereo simply because so many of your sounds are located at or near the centre of a mix. You need to move only a couple of sounds out to the sides to create a sense of space, and the addition of stereo reverb will greatly add to the sense of width.

TIP

If you have a multitrack system with only a few tracks, you'll probably have to do a lot of track-bouncing to make everything fit. This usually means that you end up with mono mixes on each track rather than having everything completely separate. To create a sense of space, add effects in mono as you bounce tracks, but when you come to mix, add a very short stereo reverb to each track that you

feel needs it. This shouldn't increase the overall impression of reverb very much, but the stereo nature of the effect should make the mono effects in the mix sound more spacious.

Digital And The Illusion Of Space

Stereo digital-reverberation units are both sophisticated and affordable, and it is largely thanks to these devices that the gap between the results that can be achieved from home and professional recording studios is now so small. Digital reverberation is still only an approximation of what happens to sound in a real room, but it can create a believable illusion of space and width.

Digital reverberation is usually created from a mono input with digital processing used to synthesise a stereo output where the two channels carry slightly different signals. Even FX units with stereo inputs tend to use a mono mix of the left and right inputs to create the reverb, with only the original sound being passed through in stereo. The outcome of this is that, no matter where in the mix the original signal is panned, its reverb will come equally from both sides. This is exactly what happens in real life – a performer in a concert hall will generate positional cues based on the direct sound, but any reverberant sound bouncing from the walls will seem to come from all sides equally.

Natural Space

Because the reverb level is equal in the left and right channels, it tends to 'dilute' the effect of panning the original sound, but as I've said, this is quite natural. However, if you demand a more tightly localised sound, there's nothing to stop you using a mono reverb and panning this to the same position in the mix as the sound being treated. The result won't be natural, and it won't have stereo width, but it can still be effective in a pop mix.

The pragmatic way of looking at it is that, when you add stereo reverb (with the stereo reverb outputs panned hard left and right), you trade off a degree of stereo localisation for a sense of stereo space. Adding a short plate or ambience reverb to a panned mono sound is generally the most effective way of giving it a sense of space without making it seem unduly effected.

Fixing Mix Problems

So far, I've tried to pinpoint problem areas to help you keep out of trouble, but at some time or another you're going to need to rescue an unsatisfactory session at the mixing stage. Furthermore, you may be called upon to pick up work on a poorly recorded job that was started elsewhere. That's where your skills are really put to the test. There's only a limited amount you can do to fix a bad recording, but as long as things aren't disastrously bad, it's usually possible to make some improvement.

Replace Or Repair?

If a track sounds wrong, either musically or technically, then the most satisfactory solution is to re-record it. While this option may not be open to professional producers working with busy international artistes, it's not usually too difficult if you're working in your own studio with your own material. Even when it's possible to patch something up – say, by copying and pasting within a hard-disk multitrack recording system – it's still usually quicker and better just to play the offending part again. Of course, re-recording is not always possible, but many seemingly insurmountable problems can be fixed with a little ingenuity.

The most obvious technical problems relate to noise, distortion, EQ, poor overall sound, spill, etc, while the more artistic considerations include the wrong choice of sounds, poor timing, bad singing, out-of-tune notes or just plain wrong ones. As you might expect, the more serious the problem, the more difficult it is to do anything about it, but by using samplers and hard-disk recorders, even out-of-time and out-of-tune playing can be improved, if you have the patience.

Tackling Noise

Probably the most common technical problem is noise, which includes tape hiss, instrument-amplifier hiss, amplifier hum and general digital background noise from budget synths and effects units. You can

attack noise on several different levels, and if the contamination is serious, you may need to use two or more of the following processes in combination.

Gating

A noise gate is a very effective tool for removing noise during the pauses between sounds, and you'd be surprised at how much you can clean up a mix by gating any channels containing parts that aren't playing all the way through the mix. For example, if the lead guitar solo pops up only in the middle of the song, you don't want any background noise on that track contributing to the mix the rest of the time, so use a gate on it. It's also often worth gating vocals, because there are usually pauses between words or phrases where nothing useful is happening. However, don't feel you have to gate out all traces of breath noise, or the vocal track may well end up sounding unnatural. If you have the drums on separate tracks, you'll get a cleaner sound by gating the kick and snare drums, and if the kick drum or toms ring too long, a gate with a fast decay time can help to tame them.

With any slowly decaying sounds, make sure you set an appropriately long gate-release time. Even if some gated sounds appear to be slightly unnatural, there's a good chance that they'll sound OK when you add reverb, especially when the rest of the mix is playing. Never gate a sound once reverb has been added, however, unless there's no other choice, and even then, consider adding a little more reverb to the gated result in order to prevent the decay from sounding unnaturally abrupt.

Less obvious is the trick of gating effect sends. Very often, effects add more than their share of noise to a mix because the aux send includes mix-buss noise from all the mixer channels.

MIDI Muting

Closely related to gating is MIDI muting, and if you have a mixing desk with this facility, it can really be of help in cleaning up your work. Although it isn't usually practical to use MIDI muting to clean up tiny pauses between individual words or phrases, it's very useful nonetheless for shutting down tracks when they're not needed. Again, the obvious uses are muting the guitar solo until it's needed and vocal tracks during instrumental sections. Mutes can also be used to ensure that each track is completely silent until needed – even in a busy mix, there are usually some tracks that don't start playing right away, so why allow them to add noise to your mix?

A word of warning, however. Some MIDI mute systems operate so quickly that they can cause clicks if a channel is switched on or off while a signal is passing through it. In this case, either arrange to switch the mute when no signal is present or switch on a snare-drum beat to hide any click that might occur. If you're fortunate enough to have a mixer with fader automation, this may also be used to silence tracks when they're not needed, as well as to allow you to automate balance changes while the track is running.

Single-Ended Noise Reduction

A more subtle alternative to gating and muting is the single-ended noise-reduction unit. Gates and mutes can remove noise only when they're shut down – they can't do anything about noise that's audible over the top of the wanted signal – but single-ended noise-reduction units (SNRs) employ variable-frequency low-pass filters that open and close according to the level and frequency content of the music being treated. Although by no means the perfect solution to noisy signals, a well-designed SNR can significantly reduce audible noise, both during pauses and when material is playing, without inflicting too much damage on the wanted signal.

The trade-off is that, if you ask it to rescue an excessively noisy recording, side-effects will show up. These side effects can include audible dulling of the signal (if you try setting the threshold too high) and the over-processing of reverb tails. For this reason, it's best to route signals through an SNR prior to adding reverb if at all possible, and if you have several channels that you think would benefit from the treatment, route them all to a stereo subgroup and put the SNR in the group insert points. Although it's possible to use an SNR on a complete stereo mix, you normally have to be satisfied with

a modest amount of noise reduction in order to avoid audible side-effects.

Corrective EQ

An often-forgotten ally in the war against noise is the equaliser, but the EQ in a typical mixing desk might not be flexible enough to do the job properly. A graphic equaliser is more versatile, but for the ultimate in control you need a good parametric EQ. Changing the EQ of a signal is obviously going to have some effect on the overall sound of that signal, but quite often you'll find that your mix includes sounds that occupy only a limited part of the audio spectrum. For example, overdriven electric guitar contains no really deep bass and the top end rolls off very quickly above 4kHz or so because of the limited response of guitar speakers. This being the case, you can apply a sharp top cut above 4kHz and a low cut below 100Hz without changing the sound too significantly. You'll have to experiment to find the exact frequencies, but you'll find this technique very useful, not only with guitars (and bass guitars) but also with warm synth pads from cheap or vintage instruments. Careful use of EQ may also help to reduce the effect of finger noise on stringed instruments.

TIP

When treating noisy overdrive guitar sounds, try sending the off-tape signal through a speaker simulator. This may change the sound of the track slightly, but you'll probably lose less bite than if you try to use the EQ on your desk to roll off the top end. You may also find that adding a little upper-mid boost on the console restores the tonal balance without allowing the noise back in. Not only does the speaker simulator reduce noise, it can also take the rough edge off a poorly recorded guitar sound and even disguise minor clicks or crackles.

Gate Filters

If you don't have a parametric equaliser, you can use the side-chain filters of a gate as equalisers simply by leaving the gate in Key Listen mode. Most gates with side-chain filters utilise a steep filter response, allowing the shelving filters to be used to 'bracket' the wanted sound without changing it too much. The Low filter will keep out bass rumble and hum while the High filter will reduce hiss or digital noise. Some equalisers also include variable-frequency shelving filters, and these may be used in exactly the same way.

It's vitally important to keep in mind that noise is cumulative and that, although individual tracks may sounds reasonably clean, when you bring all the faders up, the background noise can end up being quite significant, especially if you have 16 or more tracks (including virtual MIDI tracks) feeding into the mix. Anything you do to reduce the noise contribution will greatly improve the clarity of your mix.

Software De-Noising

Many of the more serious hard-disk recording systems now offer digital de-noising, which tends to be far more effective than the simple analogue processes discussed so far. Such systems divide the audio spectrum into a large number of frequency bands and treat each independently, enabling the effect of background noise to be reduced greatly without significantly compromising the original signal integrity. SImpler systems may allow you to reduce the overall level of noise by as much as 5dB or 6dB without audible side effects, while the more sophisticated systems can probably double that figure.

Once the signal has been split into a number of frequency bands, a software algorithm is used to decide how much noise is present in each band. A corresponding amount of energy is then subtracted from each band, almost like having separate intelligent noise gates working in each of several hundred very narrow frequency bands. The process threshold on the simpler systems relies on a short sample of noise being analysed by the system, although more advanced de-noisers continually re-evaluate the noise characteristics as the material is played.

If excessively noisy material is being treated, audible side-effects may be evident as narrow bands of noise become audible through the narrow filters,

causing a tinkling sound almost like distant wind chimes. Again, the more advanced systems are less likely to suffer from this problem, but if you hear it, at least you'll know what it is.

Such digital solutions can be applied to individual tape tracks (or sections of tracks) by copying them from tape onto hard disk, along with their time code references. Here, using time code is a good idea – if you don't use it, you may find it difficult to copy the processed audio back onto the multitrack in the right place after you've cleaned it. Ideally you should put the processed audio onto a spare tape track, but if you don't have any, you might have to risk recording it back over the original. If synchronising the cleaned-up audio is a problem, you might be able to load the cleaned-up sound into a sampler and then fly the offending parts back into the mix that way.

Noise-Reduction Essentials

- All noise-reduction techniques work better when applied to individual tracks rather than to entire mIxes, although digital noise-reduction systems and SNRs can be used on complete mixes, providing the amount of processing is carefully controlled.

- To clean up a reverb, try putting a gate or SNR on the reverb input. Most allegedly noisy reverb units are actually victims of noise coming from the effects buss. Any attempt to treat the reverb output is likely to result in the reverb decay being modified in an unnatural way.

- Even if you think your recording is reasonably quiet, you'll probably still hear an improvement if you gate or otherwise mute mixer channels when the track isn't playing anything.

- Always switch your noise treatment in and out to hear what difference it's making to the wanted part of the sound. Listen in particular for 'noise breathing' (the effect of the noise-floor level changing as the noise gate or mute opens) and, in the case of EQ and SNRs, listen for high-frequency timbral changes, especially at the ends of decaying sounds.

Non-Random Noise

Mains hum or buzz from striplights can be a serious problem because, as well as the fundamental frequency of 50Hz (or 60Hz, depending on which country you live in), it also contains a whole string of related harmonics that run right across the audio spectrum. High-pass filtering may well take away the hum component, but you'll still be left with an irritating buzz. Some software and hardware based digital SNRs employs a series of digital filters that creates narrow notches in the frequency spectrum corresponding to both the odd and even harmonics of the fundamental hum frequency. Depending on the system, these filters may track the offending hum frequency automatically, or you may have to tune it in manually. However, attempting to attenuate the hum by too great a degree can cause 'phasey' side-effects as the notch filters start to affect the wanted audio signal.

Parametric EQ

A simpler approach to hum removal is to use a multiband parametric equaliser with the lowest band tuned to the fundamental hum frequency and the following filters tuned to double, three times and four times that frequency. The filters should be set for highest Q and the cut applied gradually until the hum problem is reduced. This method will be only partially successful, because there won't be enough filter bands to tackle all the harmonics, but you should be able to make a noticeable improvement. In most situations, the fundamental plus the first few harmonics will be the loudest, with the higher harmonics being much quieter. Each filter will have to be tuned in by ear, and it may be useful to bypass all the filters apart from the one you're tuning so that you can hear exactly what effect each filter is giving you. Once you've optimised the individual filter settings you can switch all the other filters back on. Once the signal is as clean as you can get it, gating can bring about a big improvement.

Distortion

Distortion is a particularly difficult problem to deal with, and I don't know of any technique that's entirely successful for rescuing a distorted lead vocal or acoustic instrument sound, although there are several that can reduce the perceived degree of distortion. In theory, there are elaborate digital processes that could be used to reconstruct distorted waveforms, and some low-cost click-removal software also helps to hide distortion, but if these facilities aren't available, there's the choice of replacing the distorted section with material from elsewhere in the song (or an outtake) or using an equaliser to smoothe out the sound.

Before reaching for the equaliser, though, look for other solutions that avoid using the distorted material altogether. For example, can you re-record the section or do without it altogether? If the distortion occurs in only one or two places, you could look for identical passages or bars elsewhere in the music. If these exist, you can sample them and then replace the original sections with the samples. Of course, this is easiest if you have a sequencer synced to your recorder.

TIP

When you're replacing a section containing repeating riffs or drum patterns, don't let your sampler do the looping or you may find that your sample drifts out of time with the original recording. It's always better to use short samples of one or two bars in length and then trigger these from the sequencer so that each starts exactly at the beginning of the bar.

Even if your original song didn't start with a MIDI sequence, as long as you have some means of syncing a sequencer to your multitrack recorder, it can still be used to trigger samples. However, unless you have the facility to tap in a new tempo map, you'll have to turn off the Quantise function and record the sample-trigger points manually. In other words, the sequencer is simply being used as a recorder of MIDI data with no reference to the sequence tempo, bar lines or quantise grid. This makes correcting timing errors more difficult, as trigger notes have to be moved by ear rather than by simple quantising, but anyone with a reasonable sense of timing should be able to manage.

It's advisable to work on a spare track using a copy of the original part if at all possible, because it's very easy to make something sound even worse if the punch-in doesn't go as planned. If you have access to a hard-disk system, this is where you'll come to appreciate the joys of cut-and-paste editing, although modular digital multitrack tape machines can do the same sort of thing (only rather slower), as long as you have at least two of them.

Understanding Distortion

If you have to use the distorted section of the recording, you'll have to resort to processing, but to tackle distortion successfully, you need to understand a little about what it is. Distortion is caused when a circuit is driven into clipping or when an analogue tape is driven into saturation, and the usual outcome is that a whole series of harmonics are generated during the period of clipping, some of which can sound very unpleasant. In extreme circumstances, a clipped transient can sound like a click. Because the harmonics are higher than the basic pitch of the sound being distorted, it's sometimes possible to reduce their effect by applying high-cut filtering, but in most instances this will also affect the wanted sound. Even so, a slightly dull acoustic guitar might sound better than a distorted one, and I've used the High filters of a gate with side-chain filtering on more than one occasion to 'skim off' some of the distorted top end from a signal.

In practice, any variable-frequency, low-pass shelving filter with a slope of 12dB per octave or greater will do the job, and if you want to create a sharper filter you can patch the two filter sections of a dual-channel gate in series. In theory, this will double the filter roll-off, providing greater attenuation of frequencies immediately above the cut-off point. A parametric equaliser that includes a shelving low-pass filter will also work nicely. Using a speaker simulator may also smooth out a badly distorted sound, although if this is used on an acoustic guitar, some top-end loss is inevitable. Digital de-noising systems designed to remove vinyl crackle and clicks may also be effective in improving the sound of distorted material.

De-Essers Against Distortion

Another ploy is to use a de-esser to attenuate distorted peaks. Because distortion causes an increase in high-frequency harmonics, it may be possible to set up a de-esser to trigger from the distorted sound and pull the gain down briefly in that part of the audio spectrum. A split-band compressor may be used in a similar way, but the success or otherwise of this approach depends largely on whether the harmonic content of the distorted section is high enough in level to trigger the de-esser reliably. It's also a fact that most de-essers can be heard working, so if the sound being treated is very exposed at this point in the mix, it may be impossible to hide the processing.

Remiking

Tape tracks containing instruments like electric guitars or basses may also be played back through guitar combos and remiked – the speakers will act as filters while the amp EQ will also give you chance to polish up the basic tone. The same technique can be used with distorted synth sounds, but please realise that this is a last resort and that distorted parts should always be re-recorded if at all possible. Just occasionally, you'll find you can hide distortion by applying even more distortion to the whole track, but this is more likely to work on an artistic level when used on guitars and synths than it is on, say, vocals or piano. Having said that, distorted drums and even vocals can be useful in certain styles of dance music, although you're very unlikely to get away with it if you're mixing a ballad.

Don't Try To Hide It!

It's rarely possible to hide a serious error by recording something over the top to distract people – nine times out of ten, it won't work. If it's a drumstick click, you might be able to overdub more percussion, such as a tambourine, but it has to be artistically appropriate, and even then it will work only if the flaws being covered are very minor. In the '70s, engineers used to joke that, if they had a lousy mix, they could at least flange the whole thing – but they weren't entirely serious.

Dull Sounds

It can be very frustrating when the sounds you hear on professionally produced albums literally sparkle but, when you try to recreate the same quality, the instruments sound dull and lifeless. This shouldn't happen if you're using the right recording techniques and good equipment, but in a budget situation you often have to compromise on mics, instruments and signal processors, in which case you may need a little help. Exciters are useful allies in restoring missing top end to a sound, because they can actually synthesise new harmonics rather than simply attempt to boost what was never there using EQ. Over-use can cause the sound to become harsh, but if used with care an exciter can bring back that 'new string' zing to acoustic guitars, add edge to cymbals recorded using budget mics or add a breath of intimacy to vocals.

Uneven Sounds

With pop music, we're used to hearing very controlled sound levels, but in reality, people tend to inject a lot of dynamics into their performance, and if they're not well trained, the dynamics they inject may not be entirely predictable. Vocals almost always require the use of some compression to keep them under control, but it's also common to compress bass guitars, rhythm guitars and drums. (See the chapters on individual instruments for more details.)

Musical Problems

Sometimes the material has been recorded well enough but somehow still doesn't seem to want to work. In these cases, the problems can usually be broken down into three main areas: the musical arrangement, the choice of sounds and, most importantly, the performance itself.

Starting with the arrangement, there's no hard-and-fast rule as to what makes a good arrangement – getting it right is an art, and you'll find that some people can do it brilliantly while others can't do it at all. Most of us fall somewhere in between. In pop music, arrangement can usually be subdivided into the literal arrangement of the song components – verse, chorus, intro, solo, bridge and so on – and the instrumentation used for each part. A good arrangement for a traditionally structured pop song will be properly paced to create a sense of anticipation before a catchy chorus, and the best way to test an arrangement is to listen to a demo in front of critical friends. They won't need to say anything – you'll feel yourself squirming at any over-long links and solos or over-repetitive sections! Fixing this is usually a case of being ruthless and making every section of the song justify its existence – if it isn't needed, shorten it or get rid of it altogether.

Hard-Disk Editing

If you're dealing with ready-recorded material, you might think that changing the arrangement isn't an option, but now that basic hard-disk editing is starting to appear as standard on so many sequencers it's quite feasible to chop up a song into sections and then reassemble them in a different order without the joins showing. As long as you choose your edit points carefully – usually to coincide with a drumbeat – it should be possible to make the end result sound as natural as the unedited version. In many cases, it's best to mix the entire song as arranged and then edit the resulting stereo mix, although if you have a hard-disk multitrack system you might be able to transfer the whole song into it from the multitrack master tape, which will give you a lot more scope when it comes to moving parts around or replacing substandard parts with sections copied from elsewhere in the song.

Instrumentation

Looking at the instrumentation, you can't completely reorganise this if you're remixing existing material (unless you've been given a clear brief to re-record parts), but you do have the option to use EQ in order to reduce the level of parts. You can also mute parts and, in the case of drums, there's sometimes the possibility of replacing sounds. If you have a copy of the sequencer file that accompanied the original recording, you may also be able to replace any MIDI instrument parts with different sounds.

As touched upon earlier in the chapter, EQ is a useful tool because it can be used to thin out sounds that are taking up too much space in a mix. For example, an acoustic rhythm guitar used in a busy pop mix might benefit from radical bass cut so that you end up with a thin sound, almost like a musical hi-hat in terms of its role in the music. Similarly, if a bass guitar is too boomy, you could try a combination of mid-range boost and low bass cut to harden up the sound. Gating can also help tighten up the sound by creating gaps, and hence contrast, between the notes.

As I explained earlier, the sense of aural clutter comes from two or more instruments playing at the same time and occupying the same parts of the musical spectrum, and as before you can use variable-frequency high- and low-pass filters (such as gate side-chain filters) to 'bracket' the sound to make sure that it doesn't spill too far outside its allocated section of the audio spectrum.

A less well-known application of EQ, however, is simply to take a little top off a sound while only the conflicting part is also playing. Again, this is best illustrated by example. If you have a distorted rhythm guitar, you might find that it obscures the lead-guitar riff, and the instinctive reaction is to pull down the level of the rhythm sound while the lead is playing. The problem with changing levels is that it might cause a noticeable drop in energy, so as an alternative, try simply backing off just the high-frequency EQ on the rhythm-guitar sound when the lead is playing. This should provide more space for the lead guitar to cut through without losing any low-end energy.

There are few other rules governing the use of EQ, apart from judging whether or not it sounds OK, but in general you should use cut rather than boost

where possible and avoid over-equalising natural sounds such as lead vocals unless you want to create a specific effect. It's also worth noting that a good-quality equaliser sounds significantly better than a cheap one, and you're likely to be able to modify the signal far more radically without the result sounding unnatural.

Performance Problems

Performance errors include poor timing, poor tuning, wrong notes or even wrong lyrics! As explained earlier, there's only a limited amount you can do about any these, unless you have a hard-disk multitrack system and you're prepared to spend a lot of time experimenting, but now that most sequencer packages come with multitrack audio capability, such techniques are open to a greater number of people. If you can get your tracks onto a hard-disk system, you have the option of copying and pasting the best-played riffs, the best-sung choruses and so on. Samplers are also useful in this application, which has a lot in common with remixing.

However, even without resorting to hard-disk editing, there are a few tricks you can do involving samplers and rack effects that can help fix minor problems.

Tightening Up The Timing

In a mix where some parts are played just slightly out of time, you might be able to tighten up the bass guitar and drums by using the kick drum to key a gate through which the bass track is being fed. You'll need to set the gate-release time by ear, but at the very least this patch will ensure that the bass guitar only comes in with the bass drum and never comes in before it. Figure 3.1 shows how this works.

Those with hard-disk audio-plus-MIDI sequencer systems that include a 'quantise audio' facility may be able to reconstruct the offending parts to conform either to the sequencer quantise grid or to a 'groove template' grid taken from another piece of audio that was played correctly. However, unless you're just fixing the occasional part, this could take a long time. If possible, it's a lot quicker to find a similar part elsewhere in the song that is played properly,

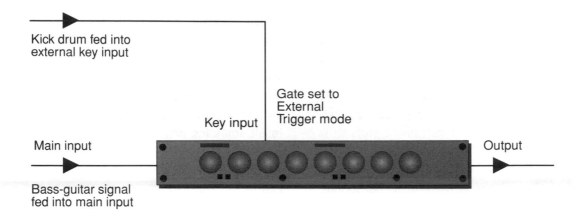

Kick drum fed into
external key input

Gate set to
External
Trigger mode

Key input

Main input

Output

Bass-guitar signal
fed into main input

The bass guitar at the output is gated so that it attacks when the bass drum is hit and then decays at a rate set by the gate's rate control. If either a drum hit or a bass note occur on their own, there will be no output – in this respect, the gate provides a logical AND function, which requires both inputs to be present in order for there to be an output

- If the bass plays slightly early, the drum will gate it on time, creating an artificial attack

- If the bass plays slightly late, the gate will have little effect, but hopefully the drum attack will help to disguise the fact!

- If the bass player puts in additional notes between the drum beats, these will be gated out altogether

Figure 3.1: Bass drum keying a bass guitar

copy it and then paste it in place of the faulty section. Similarly, if you have a dodgy phrase in a guitar solo, see if you can edit it out to shorten the solo without ruining the musical feel. If you can't shorten the solo, repeating a phrase from elsewhere in the solo may work.

Bass-guitar timing errors can be fixed in a sequencer or other multitrack audio program by splitting the part into short sections (one bar or less) and then visually aligning these with the kick-drum track.

Drum Timing

If you're working with a modular digital multitrack system and you've got a drum track that seems to be dragging, you could use the track-delay facility to delay all tracks except the drum track by a few milliseconds. Quite often, a small adjustment is all that's needed to improve the feel of a piece significantly. If, however, the drummer's timing is at

fault in an inconsistent way and the drum kit is recorded on several tracks, you may be able to gate the bass-drum and snare-drum parts and then use these 'cleaned up' sounds to trigger a drum-sound module with a trigger-to-MIDI facility, as described in the previous chapter. This is the patch often used to replace drum sounds with nicer-sounding samples – and this is something you might want to do anyway – but if you first record the MIDI data into a sequencer locked to tape, you have the opportunity of moving offending beats around to tighten up the timing. If the sound was originally played to a sequencer click track, you'll be able to use the sequencer's own quantise grid, but even if it was played free, all is not lost – you can still sync up a sequencer, tap in the tempo manually as the song plays and then use the re-bar facility (found in most modern sequencers) to create a new tempo map to match your manual 'tap' track automatically. You have to be a pretty accurate tapper to get this dead right, but once you've done it, you can quantise any MIDI data in the knowledge that it will be in time with your song on tape. Figure 3.2 shows a taped drum track being recorded into a sequencer via a gate and a trigger-to-MIDI interface.

Replacement Drum Samples

Once you've got the relevant drum parts into the sequencer, you can decide whether to trigger samples taken from the original drum recording or pick a new sampled sound altogether. Whatever you decide, keep in mind that the trigger-to-MIDI process takes a small amount of time and that triggering a sample or drum machine also takes a finite time, so you could end up with your triggered beat coming back a few milliseconds later than it should. The subjective delay will probably be very small, but it may be enough to upset the rhythmic feel, in which case entering a negative track-delay facility in your sequencer should enable you to get the timing back to where it should be.

Tuning

If a track is slightly sharp or flat compared to the rest of the band, you can shift it back to pitch in a number of ways. The simplest is probably to use a pitch-shifter – even the cheapest models are virtually glitch-free when performing small shifts, although you might find some general tonal degradation from budget models. Hard-disk recording systems offer slightly more scope with their on-board time- and stretch-shifting algorithms. As a rule, the hard-disk-based, off-line shifters produce much more natural results than rack-mounted, real-time units.

Some of the latest audio-plus-MIDI sequencers have very advanced facilities for pitch manipulation, and there are also third-party plug-ins designed specifically for fixing out-of-tune recordings. The more sophisticated of these track the pitch of the original monophonic signal and then automatically pitch-shift it to the nearest semitone.

If the part is only slightly sharp or flat, you may be able to 'fake it' by adding a pitch-shifted version of the original to create a chorus effect. For example, if the track is 10 cents sharp, you could add a −20

cents pitch shift, which would create a doubling part 10 cents flat. When played together, you'd hear a chorus effect centred around the correct pitch. Whether you can use this or not depends on the part at fault – strings or pads are usually OK but other instruments or voices may simply sound wrong with added chorus. The further you have to shift the sound, the stronger the chorus effect will be.

If just the odd note is out of tune, you can use a stand-alone pitch shifter with real-time MIDI control and use a synth pitch-bend wheel to control the amount of shift. Once again, if you can record the control data into a sequencer , you can tweak it until the tuning is spot on. Because the tone may suffer when the signal is passed through a pitch shifter, you may want to replace just the offending notes or phrases by recording the shifted part on a spare track and then bouncing this to the original track in the same way as you'd do a punch-in.

Basic Stereo-Mix Sweetening

If you're asked to try to sweeten an existing stereo master, the main tools are EQ and compression. Compressing a complete mix will reduce the dynamic range and increase the average energy of a mix, but because this increases the average signal level you might find that you've squeezed all the space out of the mix, which is rarely a good thing. Mix compression was covered earlier in this chapter, but it's worth adding that numerous engineers like to use tube processors at the end of a digital recording chain simply to inject a little warmth into the proceedings. Recording the digital master onto an analogue stereo recorder can also warm up the sound nicely, after which it may be re-recorded back to DAT or some other digital medium. The amount of analogue warmth is dictated by the level at which the signal is recorded, and with analogue machines it's quite common to have signal peaks drive the VU meters several decibels into the red.

Global Warming

Even if your mix is correct in the first place, the judicious use of a good equaliser may be able to improve it further. Music can be made to sound

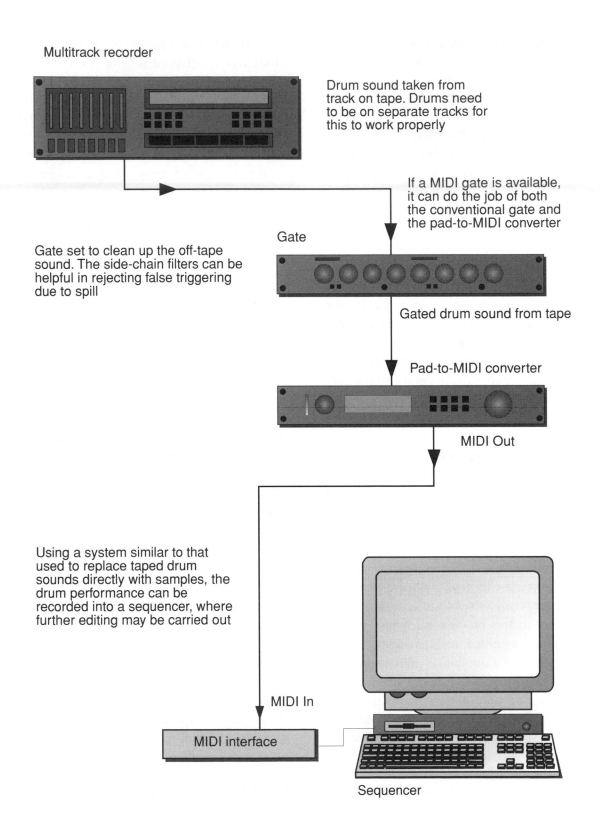

Multitrack recorder

Drum sound taken from
track on tape. Drums need
to be on separate tracks for
this to work properly

If a MIDI gate is available,
it can do the job of both
the conventional gate and
the pad-to-MIDI converter

Gate

Gate set to clean up the off-tape
sound. The side-chain filters can be
helpful in rejecting false triggering
due to spill

Gated drum sound from tape

Pad-to-MIDI converter

MIDI Out

Using a system similar to that
used to replace taped drum
sounds directly with samples, the
drum performance can be
recorded into a sequencer, where
further editing may be carried out

MIDI In

MIDI interface

Sequencer

**Figure 3.2: Drum track being recorded into a
sequencer via a gate and trigger-to-MIDI interface**

'louder' by gently cutting the mid range to simulate the human ear's response at higher sound levels, and it's quite common to treat a whole mix with an exciter or a dynamic equaliser to add sparkle and detail. Having said that, my own opinion is that mixes need contrast, which can be better delivered by using an exciter on selected subgroups within a mix.

When processing a finished mix, make sure you audition the result on several different stereo systems, including the car cassette player, just to check that your new mix will travel. I also favour checking mixes on headphones, as these are much better at revealing low-level distortion and noise than speakers. They're also good for identifying artefacts from signal processing such as single-ended noise reduction.

The Realities Of Mixing

Every mix is different, so there are no hard-and-fast rules, only suggestions and hints. What I've documented are tricks that I use myself and by other engineers I know, but any attempt to salvage a substandard mix is likely to come second best to re-recording the offending part, unless you have a multitrack editing system that will allow you to take only the good parts and rebuild the song from those. Here are a few tips on how to proceed if you come across that difficult mix.

- Without using EQ or effects, set up a mono balance and get the mix sounding as good as you can. Once the mono balance is close to being right, you can use the pan controls to create a stereo image. Build up your mix from the rhythm section and make sure that bass and drums are working together before you add more layers. If the kick drum sounds limp, try triggering a sample and use this to augment or replace the existing kick-drum sound. Gating the kick and snare drums usually helps create a tighter, cleaner sound.

- If the result is obviously cluttered, see if you can drop one or more parts completely without losing anything musically important, or at least see if you can drop the level. For example, a pad keyboard part might work at an almost subliminal level, whereas at a higher level it would just swallow up all the space. You can also use the trick of turning off the top end of a track just while the part it's clashing with is playing.

- Another cause of cluttering is microphone spill between tracks. If this is a problem, see if you can patch a gate into any tracks that are suffering excessive spill so as to keep them quiet when they're not actually contributing to the mix. It's surprising how much rubbish is picked up by the kick-drum mic, so gating this track is a good first step. If you have MIDI muting, use it to keep all tracks silent when nothing is playing.

- Use EQ to reduce the overlap between parts that conflict, but don't over-EQ vocals or critical acoustic instruments. EQ cut invariably sounds more natural than boost. A good parametric EQ is an essential tool for sweetening; console EQs are rarely flexible enough and budget graphics invariably sound plain nasty in this role!

- If the guitar parts sound unconvincing, fizzy or just plain gutless, try playing the track back through a guitar combo and then mic the result. You can either record this to a spare track or use it live in the mix. The same applies to limp bass parts.

- When it comes to adding effects, don't apply too much delay or reverb because this is yet another way of losing all your space. As a rule, the more effects a sound has on it, the further back in the mix it sounds. If a sound needs reverb, try a shorter decay setting to keep the sound up front.

- An exciter-type device shouldn't normally be used as a salvage tool – they're designed to make good things sound better, not to rescue poor work – but such enhancement can create a sense of space and separation in difficult situations, as well as adding top end to sounds that have been recorded without enough in the first place. Applying too much processing usually gives the mix a harsh edge (and brings up noise), which can be fatiguing. Combining gentle excitement with mid-range cut from a parametric EQ sometimes produces more acceptable results than an exciter used on its own.

- If the mix sounds well balanced but is still lacking punch, try overall compression. You can also use a good parametric to bring up the bottom end, but be careful not to make the mid range muddy. Sometimes, combining low-bass boost with low-mid cut can help add both power and clarity.

- Use compression to keep sounds at an even level, especially vocals and bass guitar.

- Finally, if you still have problems, take a rest before you start again – your ears will work better for it! Also, compare your mixes with known good CDs as you progress.

Mix Automation

Go to any trade show where automated mixers are on show and you'll see whole rows of faders rippling up and down, but in reality mixes seldom work like this. In most mixes, the rhythm section needs to keep to a fairly constant level, or the mix will sound as though somebody is just turning the level up and down. My usual method of working is to get a basic mix that works reasonably well without level changes and then to use the automation to control the levels of solo instruments as required and adjust the vocal level to make it sound more even. If the chorus has a radically different mix to the verses, run the song all the way through with the level set for the verses, then reset the faders for the correct chorus balance, run the song again and punch in the automation on the required mixer channels just for the choruses. This is quicker and more accurate than trying to move the faders to their new positions every time a chorus comes around.

As long as the backbone of the song is solid, you can gently push the levels of other instruments by a decibel or two to make room for other instruments or vocals, but don't feel that, just because you have 24 or more automated channels, they all have to be working all the time. Also, don't expect automation to make mixing quicker – clients invariably want to make more changes, so the job actually takes a lot longer!

Once the mix is running the way you want it, use the automatic mutes to kill any track that isn't playing. This can really help to clean up a mix, but try not to operate a mute in the middle of a sound, or you may end up with an audible click or glitch. If you must mute or unmute during a sound, make the mute action coincide with a drumbeat so as to mask any undesirable side-effects.

Save your automation data in case you need to do a remix, and if your EQ isn't automated, make a note of the settings. The same applies to any external effects patches and aux settings, if these aren't remembered.

Cassette Multitrack Workarounds

While handling a mix done on an eight- or 16-track multitrack recorder can be tough, sorting out a mix done on a cassette multitracker can be an even greater challenge, especially if the machine has very basic facilities. While such machines provide a great introduction to multitrack recording, the onboard mixers are usually quite limited, especially on the cheaper four-track models. If you've made a particularly good recording, you may be able to get a better result by mixing via a separate mixer, but sometimes the recorder's facilities conspire to make this very difficult.

Separate Track Outputs

If you're working with a machine that provides separate tape outputs for all four tracks, this is no problem, but what if you have a machine where you have to go via the internal mixer and you only have a stereo output? With a little lateral thinking, you may be able to find more outputs than you originally thought you had.

Left output carries mainly the signal from channel 1, though there will be a small contribution from channel 4 due to the need to leave the fader partly open

Right output carries mainly the signal from channel 2, though there will be a small contribution from channel 4 due to the need to leave the fader partly open

Pre-fade send carries only the signal from channel 3

Post-fade send carries only the signal from channel 4

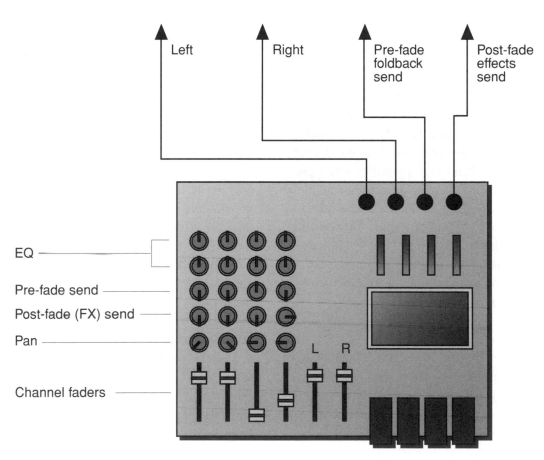

Left

Right

Pre-fade foldback send

Post-fade effects send

EQ

Pre-fade send

Post-fade (FX) send

Pan

Channel faders

L   R

Although not a perfect solution, this technique makes it possible to separate the tracks from a basic cassette multitracker in such a way that three of the tracks are completely separated while one of the remaining tracks includes a degree of crosstalk from one of the separated tracks

Channel 4's fader must be left partly open to allow an adequate level of signal to be routed to the output of the post-fade FX send, so some of the signal will also be mixed in with the main outputs carrying channels 1 and 2. The Pan control determines whether this unavoidable crosstalk is added to either channel 1 or 2

Figure 3.3: Outputs being taken from the left, right, pre-fade and post-fade sends of a multitracker

The solution you ultimately arrive at may well be a compromise, but you'll probably still have more flexibility than you originally thought. The main stereo outputs cab be used to output two of the tracks, so let's assume that tracks 1 and 2 are panned right and left and fed to the stereo output as normal. The faders are set at their unity gain position – usually about three-quarters of the way up – and any aux-send controls are fully down on both channels. This leaves us looking for a way out for tracks 3 and 4.

Aux Sends As A Way Out

A useful avenue for further exploration is the aux sends. Only the most basic of notepad machines will have no aux sends, in which case your best bet is to borrow a more sophisticated multitracker (making sure it has the same type of noise-reduction system). However, if you have a machine with a pre-fade or foldback send control on each channel, this may be used to send one of the remaining tracks – say, track 3 – to the foldback output. This may be a separate output jack or it may be the headphone socket. If it's the latter, simply use a stereo-to-dual mono adaptor plugged into the headphone socket and take the appropriate side to your mixer's line input. You may have to adjust the phones level a little, but it should work fine.

To use the pre-fade send, channel 3's main fader or level knob must be fully down, the pre-fade send knob needs to be around three-quarters of the way up and the master pre-fade send level (if fitted) also needs to be around three-quarters of the way up. This leaves us with only channel 4 to worry about.

If you have a post-fade effects send, there is another dodge you can try, and although it seems to be quite a compromise, I've actually used it quite successfully. To separate track 3 on a machine that has only a post-fade effects send, the track is panned either left or right but the fader or level knob is set only around a quarter of the way up. The aux-send control is set fully up and the output is taken from the aux-send socket.

The reason why the channel fader is partly up is that the effects send takes its feed from after the level control, so if you turn off the channel level

completely, there's no post-fade output at all. The way I've described will give you plenty of post-fade level, but the compromise is that, by leaving the fader partway up, a small amount of track 3's signal will be mixed in with either track 1 or track 2, depending on which side you've panned it. Even so, as long as you don't actually need to be able to mute track 3 in the mix, the degree of separation achieved should be adequate to allow you to EQ and effect each track relatively independently.

If you need further isolation and are prepared to try something a little more complicated, you may be able to take a split feed from the post-fade aux send, invert its phase and use it to cancel out the unwanted track 3 component in the relevant multitracker output. However, in most situations, this degree of complexity won't be necessary.

If you have a machine with both pre- and post-fade sends, a combination of the main outputs, the pre- and the post-fade outputs should allow you to separate all four tracks – accepting of course the compromise that a little of the output from the post-fade send will also be mixed in with one of the main outputs. Figure 3.3 shows outputs being taken from the left/right pre-fade and post-fade sends.

Sync Output

If, however, you don't have both pre- and post-fade sends, you can always look at the sync output (if fitted) as another way out for track 4. This is normally used to allow the user to record time code onto track 4 and then play it back while bypassing the EQ and noise-reduction circuitry. Because the noise reduction is probably disabled when the machine is switched to Sync mode, try settings the Sync switch to Off while monitoring the sync output via your external mixer and see if that produces the right result. If your machine doesn't allow you to get a normal-sounding signal out of the Sync socket when replaying a recording that was made with noise reduction, you may have to re-record track 4 with the noise reduction switched off and put up with the extra tape hiss. This can be compensated for to some extent by using a single-ended noise-reduction system or a simple noise gate.

Improvising Stereo Returns

There are several models of basic cassette multitrackers that have only single, mono effects returns, which are of little use if you wish to use a stereo effects unit. However, if you have the patience to solder together a few sockets and resistors, you can get around this limitation surprisingly simply, and without modifying your machine.

Figure 3.4 shows a simple passive, stereo mixer that may be used to combine the output of a typical multitracker with another stereo line signal, such as the output from an effects unit. The effects unit is fed from the post-fade effects send in the usual way (you can use a direct tape out as an effects send if you need to add effects to just one track) and the amount of effect added is set using the output level

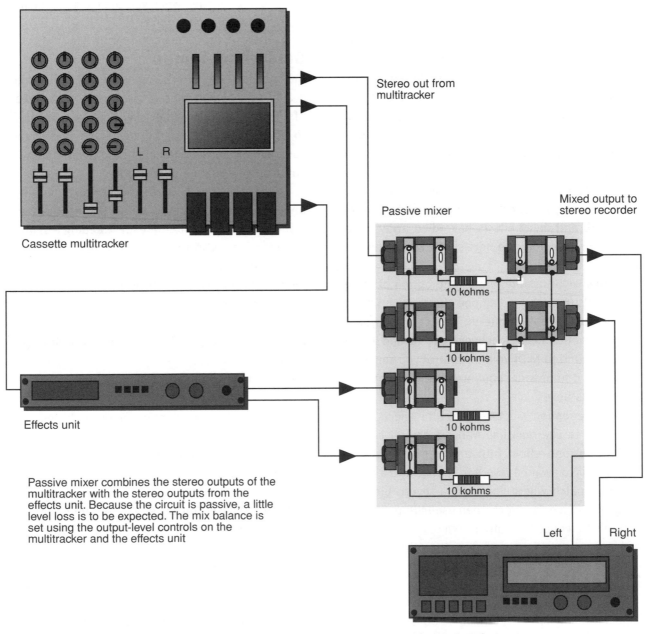

Stereo out from multitracker

Mixed output to stereo recorder

Passive mixer

10 kohms

10 kohms

10 kohms

10 kohms

Cassette multitracker

Effects unit

Passive mixer combines the stereo outputs of the multitracker with the stereo outputs from the effects unit. Because the circuit is passive, a little level loss is to be expected. The mix balance is set using the output-level controls on the multitracker and the effects unit

Left   Right

Master recorder

Figure 3.4: DIY passive stereo effects return mixer

control on the effects unit itself. The dry/effect mix must be set to effect only, as usual.

The only real compromise of working in this way is that any fade-outs must be handled using the input gain controls of the master stereo recorder; if the master fader on the Portastudio is used, the mix will fade but the effect won't! You'll probably also find that you experience a slight drop in level when the mixer is inserted, so you may have to increase the record level on the master recorder slightly.

Effects And Timing

Most digital effects units allow you to create and store patches, which may be changed manually or via MIDI program-change messages. However, if you need to change an effect setting in the middle of a mix, you need to be aware that the vast majority of effects units mute their output for up to a second when changing patches so as to allow old data to be purged from their delay memories. The outcome is that you don't get a smooth changeover, so you need to plan your effects changes to come in after all reverb and delay effects have died away but a second or so before the next signal to be effected is due to start.

If this isn't possible, there's the option of using two effects units and fading one effect's return down as you fade the other one in. This can give you a lovely smooth transition between effects, and if your units respond to MIDI volume control you can even automate it from your sequencer, but it does tie up two effects boxes.

A further option is not to change the effects patch at all but to use real-time MIDI parameter control to 'morph' one effect into another instead. For example, if you want a reverb to change into a delay, set up a patch where you have a reverb block in parallel with a delay block, then use MIDI parameter controls to reduce the output from one effects block as you increase the output from the other.

Zipper Noise

Although even budget effects now tend to offer real-time MIDI parameter control, some do it better than others. The problem is that digital algorithms can't

change smoothly like analogue circuits do; instead they change in a series of small steps, and sometimes these steps are coarse enough to be audible, especially on things like filter settings. If you have the time and the inclination, hook up your effects unit so you can change parameters from a synth mod wheel or similar source, then listen carefully to find out which parameters change smoothly and which ones don't. A poorly designed unit may produce a sound like ripping cloth or a zipper being fastened when you change a parameter, hence the term *zipper noise*.

Delay And Tempo

Delay effects often work best when the delay time is a multiple of the tempo of the song, and a number of effects units allow the delay time to be synced to MIDI clock. This has the advantage that, if the song includes a tempo change, the delay time will automatically change to match it.

Where you need to set the tempo manually, divide the desired tempo by 60 to find out how many beats per second there are. Keeping a simple calculator handy in the studio is a real help here. The easiest way to set up the delay is to use the formula shown below, which gives the required delay time in milliseconds:

Delay Time = (30,000/bpm)ms for two delays per beat

Delay Time = (60,000/bpm)ms for one delay per beat

Delay Time = (120,000/bpm)ms for one delay per two beats

Delay Time = (240,000/bpm)ms for one delay per four beats

Triplet time based on 12 repeats per four-beat bar can be calculated from the following equation:

Delay Time = (20,000/bpm)ms for three delays per beat

For example, if you have a four-to-the-bar song where you need two echoes per bar, that means you need one echo every two beats. If the tempo is 135 bpm, the delay time you need is therefore 120,000/135ms, which works out at 888ms.

Be aware that delays that are physically locked to the song tempo may sound strange immediately following any abrupt tempo change. This is because a rapid change in delay time produces a brief period of pitch change.

4 POST-PRODUCTION CONSIDERATIONS

Once your master tape is mixed, further processing may be required before your album is ready to be duplicated as a CD or tape, and the tracks will also need to be placed in the correct order with gaps of the correct length between them. There are many potential problems that can occur at the mastering stage, so the aim of this chapter is to look at key stages in the mastering process and to point out the most common problems and ways in which they may be avoided or corrected.

Digital Recording Levels

A common concern amongst those new to digital recording is how best to set the recording levels, especially when several songs are to be recorded on the same tape and the relative levels need to match. Unlike analogue machines, it isn't permissible to go into the red on a digital recorder, yet there is a potential problem due to the fact that our ears perceive sound based on average level while a DAT machine's meters read peak levels to warn of clipping. Because of this, it isn't practical to set a notional point on the meter that will work for every type of song, as every song has a different peak-to-average ratio. It is possible to balance the subjective levels of successive mixes on a DAT tape by making aural judgements of apparent loudness, but for this to really work the song with the highest peak-to-average energy ratio needs to go on first and then the other mixes referenced to that.

An alternative is to compress the songs that have wide peak-to-average ratios, but only if the compression doesn't compromise the way in which the song sounds. After all, the DAT machine is there

to record your work the way you want it – you shouldn't have to make artistic concessions just for the sake of getting more level on tape. When recording different mixes to DAT with a view to compiling an album, a good limiter can really help because it will allow you to push the subjectively quieter songs up in level without any fear of the peaks clipping. A limiter will produce a more transparent sound than blanket compression, providing you don't ask it to trim more than a few decibels off the peak signal levels.

Because most DAT masters destined for album release are recompiled on some form of editing system, it's generally safer to leave level-matching until that stage. Aim to set your programme peaks at two or three decibels below clipping. A number of hard-disk-editing packages include very good limiters for mastering purposes, so it's probably best to accept that your DAT recordings won't always match up in level and instead record each song at the highest level possible without processing of any kind and without allowing the peaks to clip. Not only does this produce the lowest background noise level, it also ensures the lowest possible distortion and the best signal resolution during quiet passages or fades. A professional mastering system may well have more bits of resolution to play with than the 16 bits used by the CD format so that, when level changes are made on the final master, techniques such as noise-shaped dithering can be used to ensure that low-level signals sound cleaner and more transparent than if you'd mixed them to DAT at that level in the first place.

Rather than fade out your songs at the mixing

stage, keep your initial mixes at maximum level, allowing the song to run on for at least 30 seconds to allow you to implement a smooth fade-out later on. Fades produced on a digital editor will be smoother and quieter than fades performed at the mixing stage.

Max Headroom

When recording a live performance, it's particularly important to leave sufficient headroom to cope with unexpected rises in level. In effect, headroom is the safety margin between the level you think you'll need and the point at which the signal level hits the end stops. Because you can't always predict the level of the highest peak, you have to decide how much headroom to leave, but this may vary depending on the type of music you're recording. For example, a dance track may have a very limited dynamic range, so you could get away with something like 12dB of headroom above the average signal level, but there's no way to guarantee this, as the peaks will be higher than the average level and in extreme cases may exceed the safety margin you've left. A safer alternative may be to ignore the average level and just concentrate on the peaks, then leave 6–10dB of safety margin to accommodate unexpected excesses. It's the peaks that matter, as far as the DAT machine is concerned, so keep a close eye on them.

More dynamic forms of music may need to be recorded with even greater headroom, but even if you've done a trial run, the chances are that the levels will change significantly during the actual performance. In this case, you might want to set your nominal recording level around 20dB below clipping and your peaks 12dB or so below, just to be on the safe side. Theoretically, this will compromise the signal quality to some extent, but because of the wide dynamic range of DAT, this is unlikely to be serious and, in any event, is far better than audible clipping. To make doubly sure, consider using a good stereo limiter when recording, just to provide a safety net, with the limiter threshold set 1dB or so below clipping. Although limiting isn't favoured by purists, it sounds a lot better than accidental clipping.

Sweetening

It's tempting to think that once you have a mixed stereo master, that's it – you can go ahead and put it on a record or CD. However, that's not the end of the story. If you're compiling an album, the tracks have to be arranged in the right order, with the right gaps and at the right respective levels. If you're working from DAT, hard-disk editing is the most practical way to do the job. If, on the other hand, you're working with an open-reel mastering machine, you may prefer to splice the tracks together physically, inserting a couple of seconds of blank tape or leader tape between the tracks. If you have access to a computer editing system that uses plug-ins, refer to Chapter 9, 'Computers And Audio', for advice on how to approach mastering.

Monitoring Problems

One of the problems with mixes originating from small private studios is that most have less than optimum monitoring environments, and this leads to mixes with tonal balances that need further work. To improve on this, you ideally need a really good parametric equaliser and a monitoring system that you know to be accurate and that you're used to working with. There's no reason at all not to use an analogue equaliser for the job, and some of the more esoteric tube models can inject a little of their own personality into a mix, but the digital equalisers included with the better hard-disk editing systems can be very good. What's really important is not which equaliser to use but what you do with it.

In the case of mixes done in rooms with poor monitoring systems or acoustic problems, the most serious errors tend to occur at the bass end of the spectrum, so you're likely to end up with a master that has either too much or too little bass. In a typical pop record, the bass drum sits in the 80Hz part of the spectrum, so you can do quite a lot to balance the subjective bass-drum level using a parametric or even a sweep filter tuned into this region. However, there's quite often stuff going on below 80Hz, and if there's too much down there, you can end up with a very ill-defined, rumbly bass end that's best treated using a shelving filter to attenuate everything below 50Hz or so.

Deep Bass

With some musical styles, the mixes may actually rely on deep bass sounds, but when you try to bring them up using a simple shelving control, the lower mid starts to get a bit boxy. A parametric EQ tuned to between 40Hz and 70Hz may produce the desired result, but if you have to use your desk equaliser, try adding around 8dB of shelving bass boost and combine this with around −8dB of lower-mid sweep tuned to between 150Hz and 250Hz. The lower-mid cut counteracts the bass EQ's tendency to spill over into the mid range, which enables you to add more deep bass without swamping the lower-mid range.

Sonic Detail

At the high-frequency end, lack of brightness or detail can be a problem, especially if the recording was made using analogue multitrack and several bounces were involved. It's tempting simply to turn up the treble control, but this will also bring up the noise and may not produce the tonal result you need. What can work better is to identify the high-frequency sounds that need help and then use a parametric EQ or sweep mid to lift these slightly. Sounds like cymbals and the pluck of an acoustic guitar can be enhanced by boosting between 4kHz and 8kHz, and because you're only boosting a relatively narrow band of frequencies, you bring up less background noise. Be careful when adding top, though, as it's too easy to make a mix sound harsh or aggressive, especially with budget equalisers. As a rule, the higher the boost frequency, the more 'air' you get around the sound. Boosting lower down – at 3–4kHz, say – can bring out the bite in electric guitars and similar sounds, but it also tends to make the top end sound harsh.

Exciters

The other popular way to bring out high-end detail is to use an exciter or enhancer of some kind. Most models work well if used sparingly, but the better models include an effective bass-enhancement system as well as a means of lifting the high frequencies. I can't emphasise too strongly that enhancement needs to be used with restraint, so keep switching your enhancer in and out as you're setting up to make sure you haven't gone too far. Comparison with records and CDs is recommended at this stage, too, as your ears easily get used to treble, and you could end up with a lethally bright mix without noticing that anything's wrong.

Compression

Some producers like to compress their finished mixes, while others claim that this always makes things worse. The truth is that it all depends on the type of material you're working with and how you go about applying the compression. Why might it help? Well, a regular comment from recording musicians is that their mixes don't sound as 'loud' as the ones on the radio, even though the meters say the level is the same. It isn't simply a matter of increasing the level on tape, however; it's more to do with dynamic range and average signal levels. In other words, the peaks may be as loud as everyone else's peaks, but the average level of the material may still be well below the average level you'd expect from a commercial album of similar material. You might imagine that, as everyone has a compressor in their studios, dynamic range would be no problem, but in the real world a great many recordings are compressed on an individual track basis, with more compression being added to the overall mix.

Compression Decisions

If you know that you're going to compress the overall mix, it makes sense to patch in a compressor at the outset so that you can hear the effects of the compressor as you mix. The reasoning behind this is that compression can change the subjective balance of a mix, so if you finish your mix before thinking about compression, you could end up with problems. However, if you ever need to do any post-production sweetening, you'll almost certainly be presented with a finished stereo tape, usually a DAT.

There are specialist compressors and limiters made specifically for mastering, some of which are excellent, but they tend to be very expensive. However, with a little ingenuity you can achieve good results by using two of the compressors in your everyday effects rack.

Dual-Stage Compression

A good soft-knee compressor is a good starting point because it's likely to be less obtrusive in operation than a fixed-ratio type. Try a fast attack and a relatively slow release time, combined with a low ratio (around 2:1), and set the threshold so as to produce around 6dB of gain reduction on the signal peaks. (This isn't a great deal of reduction, but you don't want the signal to sound squashed.) Soft-knee compressors may be unobtrusive, but what they offer in subtlety they sacrifice in assertiveness, and occasionally a peak comes by that they don't hold down firmly enough. To solve this problem, you can use a second compressor as a safety limiter, although this still won't be as fast as a dedicated limiter.

Set your second compressor – which should ideally be a hard-knee model, preferably with a peak-sensing facility – to a ratio of around 10:1 and use the Auto-Attack and -Release mode, if there is one. If you have only a manual model, set a fast attack and around 250ms release time. The threshold should be adjusted to produce about 4dB of additional gain reduction on the signal peaks so that the limiter isn't working too hard.

If one of your two compressors has a built-in limiter section, this can be used at the end of the processing chain as a final line of defence. By deliberately driving the limiter so that the Limit LED is permanently on and then gradually adjusting the threshold, you can set the recording level on the target DAT machine to fractionally under digital full scale. One this is set, reset the compressor output gain so that the Limit LED flashes briefly only on the very loudest signal peaks, then back it off just a hint more. In theory, the limiter is just there as a safety net, so the Limit LED should come on rarely, if at all. However, be aware that, while the combination of two compressors can work fairly transparently, the same can't usually be said of limiters.

You can now copy the original DAT to a new tape. If you've set the compressors carefully, you should notice the subjective sound is louder but without the dulling of transients that can occur when a single compressor is used to heavily compress a mix. There should also be no audible gain pumping, although, if you have a good parametric EQ, you might want to try to fine-tune the sound, as compression sometimes changes the apparent spectral balance. With any luck, your tape will be ready to send to the CD-pressing plant without further delay.

I've used this 'cascaded compressors' treatment on a number of occasions and put its success down to the use of two separate stages of compression backed up by a 'watchdog' limiter. The first compressor provides the bulk of the gain reduction and therefore has to be unobtrusive, which is why a soft-knee model is specified. The second model comes in to deal with only those peaks that the first compressor fails to bring under control, so you can afford to be a bit more heavy-handed. Either a soft- or hard-knee compressor can be employed, depending on what you have, although the type with a variable ratio is best, and hard-knee types tend to sound most positive.

Normalising

If you're working with a hard-disk recording system, you may be tempted to normalise the data to ensure that the highest signal peak comes right up to the digital maximum. If you do intend to normalise, there are a couple of points you should keep in mind. Firstly, always normalise after you've done everything else, or you may perform a subsequent process that increases the gain further, which means your signal will be forced into clipping. Even an EQ setting that produces only cut can increase the signal level slightly, simply because you may end up reducing the level of some frequency components that were previously helping to cancel out peaks at other frequencies. Apparently, this is also true of sample-rate conversion, because of the filtering involved.

Secondly, if you have the option, try to normalise to a decibel or so below the maximum peak level. For reasons similar to the previous example, clipping may occur when a normalised signal is passed through subsequent digital systems, such as oversampling DACs. In practice, this source of clipping rarely causes audible problems, but if you have the option, why not be a perfectionist?

Digital Resolution

Every time you manipulate the level of a signal in the digital domain, some resolution is lost. For example, if you add EQ, the signal level is likely to be increased, so it has to be scaled down again to fit into the original 16 or 24 bits. The practical outcome is that, if you have several stages of digital processing to go through, low-level detail may suffer, resulting in reverb tails becoming less smooth or the stereo imaging becoming blurred. This problem may be countered by adding dither to the signal, which will improve low-level resolution but will also cause the signal-to-noise ratio to suffer slightly. A more sophisticated way to do this is to use so-called *noise-shaped dithering*, which is mathematically designed so that the added noise components appear at the high end of the audio spectrum, where the human ear is relatively insensitive. Many hard-disk packages now include noise-shaped dithering options, and these really do make a difference to low-level signal resolution. Where possible, record with a higher bit depth than you need for the master. For CD (16-bit), record at 24-bit and then reduce to 16-bit during mastering.

Noise

Good recordings shouldn't be noisy in the first place, but budget effects, noisy synths and ground-loop hums in home studios invariably mean that project-studio recordings will have some audible noise on them during pauses or quiet passages. A great improvement can be made by making sure that your track is completely silent until the music starts, and if you're splicing analogue two-track tape, this simply means taking care to make your splice half an inch or so before the song starts.

Rocking the tape over the heads manually is the best way to identify this point, and you can mark the back of the tape with a wax pencil to show you where to cut.

DAT tape is virtually impossible to cue up accurately, but if you're using a hard-disk editor, things are rather easier because you can actually see the waveform of the first sound in the song, so it's simply a matter of selecting the appropriate area and then using the Silence command to replace it with digital silence. At the end of the song, you can also perform a digital fade-out at the tail end of the natural decay of the last sound so that the song fades into true silence rather than hiss.

Noise occurring during the track is less easy to deal with, and in order to tackle serious noise effectively you really need a specialised digital noise-removal system. Again, quite serious packages are becoming available for computer-based audio systems at relatively low cost.

TIP

If you're not sure whether your material needs de-noising or not, listen to it back over headphones. Headphones show up noise more than speakers, so if the sounds played back over the phones are noticeably noisy, some kind of treatment may be advisable. If the headphone playback is acceptable, noise isn't going to be a problem.

Less severe noise contamination can be dealt with in the analogue domain using a single-ended noise-reduction processor. These units work by monitoring the input signal's level and frequency content. When a low-level signal with little or no high-frequency content is detected, a variable-frequency low-pass filter moves down the audio band to filter out the noise. Obviously, the filter has some effect on the wanted signal, so it's best to set up the unit so that it's only coming into action on very low-level signals. By switching the Bypass switch in and out, you can hear if the sound quality is suffering and adjust the threshold level accordingly. However, as a rule, if noise is to be reduced at the mastering stage, it is likely that a digital system will be more effective.

Artistic Considerations

When compiling an album, there are artistic as well as technical decisions to be made. For instance, the relative levels of the tracks need to be balanced so that they sound right – if you simply normalise all the tracks individually, any quiet ballad will sound unnaturally loud next to a heavy rock track. The only way you can get this right is to use your judgement, but a good guide is to make sure the vocal levels are subjectively similar from track to track. Listening from outside the room as one track plays into another will help you recognise any level problems.

A related problem arises if you're using tracks made at different sessions or even in different studios. Do you want them to sound different or do you want to EQ them to make them all sound similar in tonal character? Again it's down to you, but you'd be amazed at how different recordings of the same band can sound.

Finally, judging the length of the gaps between songs is an art in itself. The usual gap is between two and four seconds, but a lot depends on whether the previous track has an abrupt stop or a fade-out, and on how different the mood of the two songs is. Fortunately, the correct gap is usually pretty evident, and I've found that, even when several people are involved in a session, the chances are that they'll agree on the optimum gap length to within half a second.

Safety Copies

Don't forget to make a backup copy of the tape or CD-R before you send it away for duplication, and if you're making a cassette master then it helps if the two sides are as equal as possible, with side 1 being the longer. Leave a gap of at least two minutes between the two sides of the cassette, and if you're mastering to DAT then don't just wind the DAT on to create a gap; instead, record silence, or you might end up confusing the DAT machine at the duplicating plant. By recording silence, you're still recording a subcode, whereas if you simply wind on the DAT tape, you'll leave a section of unformatted tape.

If you're mastering for CD, you don't need to leave a gap between sides, although you should always leave a minute or so of recorded silence at the beginning of any DAT tape just to make sure you don't get any dropouts or errors. Also, try to make the master DAT at 44.1kHz sampling rate. If your machine works at 48kHz only, mark the tape clearly as such and you should have no problems – the duplication company will convert the sample rate for you. However, if you send away a tape for CD mastering containing mixed 44.1kHz and 48kHz sample rates, you only have yourself to blame if some of the tracks on your CD album play back ten per cent slow!

Pre-Emphasis

Another potential pitfall presents itself when you get a DAT tape to edit that was made on one of the older machines that use *pre-emphasis*, a simple kind of noise reduction whereby the digital data on tape actually has a significant top boost added during recording and which is filtered out again on replay. If you transfer tapes made on these machines into some digital editing systems, the emphasis flag is stripped out but the material isn't de-emphasised, so you end up with an unpleasantly bright master tape. Until now, the only solution to pre-emphasis was to go into the editing system via the analogue inputs so that the source DAT machine did the de-emphasising, but now some software-based digital equalisers include a de-emphasis filter that allows you to restore the original tonal balance of the recording.

CD-R

Many CD-manufacturing plants now accept CD-Rs as masters for duplication, but be aware that the master CD-R should include full PQ coding so that the CD player can locate individual tracks, read the number of tracks on the disc and display either elapsed or remaining time. Several software packages offer these facilities, but simpler systems may provide you with a playable disk that isn't in the correct format for professional duplication. If in doubt, consult your CD manufacturer before producing the master disc. If you only need a small number of CDs – for distribution to A&R departments and so on – then CD-R is financially viable for small runs.

It's important that CD masters are recorded in Disc At Once mode so that all the data is written in a single pass. This avoids introducing errors caused by discontinuities where the writing laster is being switched on and off.

5 MONITORING AND ROOM PROBLEMS

The importance of accurate monitoring has been touched upon in other parts of this book, but this section concentrates on the main points of choosing and setting up a monitoring system, paying particular attention to common problems and their solutions. If you don't have an accurate monitoring system, you can't know exactly what's going onto your master tape, so you shouldn't be surprised if your mixes sound completely different when played back elsewhere.

The technology underlying loudspeaker systems appears to have changed little since the '60s, other than the unsurprising fact that you can now buy better monitor speakers for less money than ever before. It can be argued that the lack of radical new ideas in loudspeaker design is an affirmation of the fact that a great deal of the pioneering work was right first time around, but, as in all other areas, there have been improvements.

Monitoring Criteria

The simple aim of a studio monitoring system is to provide an accurate reference by which we can judge out work with confidence, but how often have you mixed on an unfamiliar pair of speakers only to find that the mix sounded dreadful as soon as you got it home? Sadly, there's no such thing as a standard monitor loudspeaker, and even if there was, it would still sound different depending on its acoustic environment and position. Furthermore, the mixing engineer has no idea what the end user's speaker will sound like, so he has somehow to come up with a mix that will sound acceptable on the majority of consumer systems.

What's A Monitor?

Exactly what is the difference between a monitor loudspeaker and a hi-fi loudspeaker? Well, a monitor speaker must be as tonally accurate as possible, whereas a hi-fi speaker could be designed to flatter. Also, a studio monitor usually has to put up with more abuse from people wanting to monitor at high levels.

A perfectly accurate speaker would be capable of reproducing the entire audio spectrum with the minimum of distortion or coloration, although for smaller systems it's accepted that the low-frequency end isn't going to extent down as far as a big full-range system. However, I'm going to stick my neck out here and say that speakers with a limited bass response are easier to mix on, and for two reasons: firstly, the bass doesn't overpower the mid range, which is where all the important information is concentrated; and secondly, because few consumers have the budget or space for a full-range system.

Off-Axis Performance

While some speakers are reasonably accurate when you're standing directly in front of them, their off-axis behaviour is just as important. Why? Well, sound bounces off hard surfaces, and what we hear when we listen to a pair of loudspeakers in a typical room is a combination of the direct (ie on-axis) sound plus some off-axis sound that has reflected from the walls. If the off-axis sound is inaccurate in any way, that proportion of what we hear that's due to reflected sound will also be inaccurate. Indeed, it's largely because of the differences in off-axis performance that two similarly specified loudspeakers can sound so different in the same room. With a pair of good monitors, you should be able to move from one side of the room to the other and hear a nominally constant tonal balance. The high-frequency end will drop away once you move a long way off axis, but it should do so smoothly and unobtrusively.

The Room's Influence

Virtually all large-scale professional monitoring systems are designed to take into account the acoustic environment in which they are likely to be used. Indeed, if a studio is being built from scratch, the chances are that the monitoring system and the room will be designed symbiotically. Full-range monitors are generally built into wall soffits, although most near-field and mid-sized monitors are deigned to be used on stands positioned a little way behind the mixing console.

A professional studio designer will probably design a room to have a reverb time that is reasonably short and nominally equal at all audio frequencies. Domestic rooms can vary a lot in terms of acoustics, but one with fitted carpets, soft furnishings and curtains is usually damped well enough for mixing on smaller monitors. You can't expect to generate very deep bass in a small room, however, because the dimensions are incapable of supporting the very long wavelengths involved. A practical option for smaller rooms is to use a pair of speakers that have a flat response down to, say, 50Hz or 60Hz and that roll off gradually below this. A good two-way system with a soft domed tweeter usually works best in this role, and now that active versions of some small monitors are becoming more affordable, these are well worth considering, as they rule out all the guesswork in buying a power amplifier.

Monitor Position

The placement of monitor loudspeakers within a room can affect their performance to a significant degree because of the way in which low frequencies behave. At mid and high frequencies, the sound radiates from the loudspeaker in the form of a cone, but as the frequency gets lower, the radiation pattern widens

until, at very low frequencies, the speakers are almost omnidirectional, with almost as much energy being directed backwards as forwards. This low-frequency energy reflects from solid walls, passing through less substantial structures, and any walls adjacent to and behind the speakers will bounce energy back into the room, making the perceived bass level within the room louder. Sadly, this 'free' bass boost will occur at different frequencies, depending on the exact distances between the speakers, the floor, the walls and the ceiling, and if the speakers are too close to the boundaries of the room, the bass performance can become very erratic.

To ensure the smoothest and most accurate bass response, the distances between the speaker and the nearer surfaces should be different and as random as possible. This will prevent all of the reflections combining at the same frequency. For example, it would be bad to place a speaker in a corner, exactly midway between floor and ceiling, as this would produce a bass response that was interspersed with large peaks and troughs, resulting in some bass notes sounding much louder than others. If the distances from the speaker to the nearest two walls, the floor and the ceiling can all be made different, the reflections will combine in a more random – and, hence, more benign – manner.

Consult the manufacturer's recommendations that came with your monitors, but as a rule you should try to mount them at least a foot from the wall behind your mixing console and at least 18" from the side walls. Figure 5.1 shows a typical monitoring arrangement. In rectangular rooms, it's usually best to set up the speakers along the longest wall, but don't worry too much if this isn't possible.

I know that a lot of people place speakers on the meter bridge of the mixing console, and some are actually designed to work in this position, but most will sound more accurate if they're positioned on stands a little way behind the console. This is to reduce the amount of sound that's reflected from the hard surface of the console reaching the listener. When combined with the direct sound, this reflected sound causes comb filtering and can compromise the accuracy of what you hear.

Speaker distances from the side wall A and rear wall B should not be equal or direct multiples of each other. The speaker-to-floor and speaker-to-ceiling distances should also be unrelated to A and B. This precaution is necessary to randomise any peaks in the bass response caused by proximity to a reflective boundary. In the worst case, where the distances to the wall, floor and ceiling are equal, the response peaks will all occur at the same frequency, giving rise to a highly inaccurate bass performance

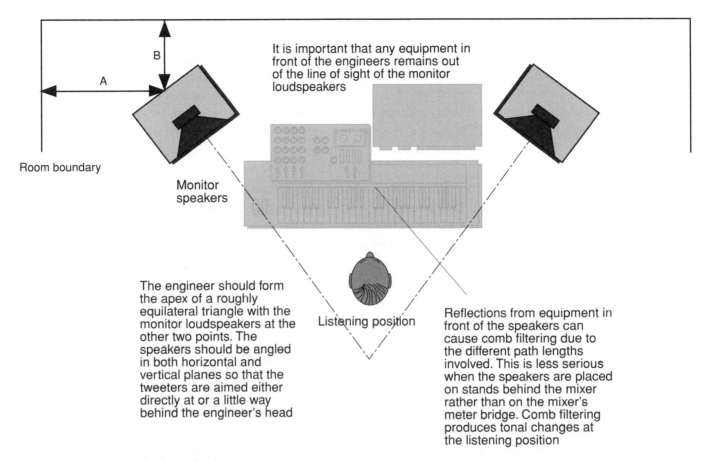

B

A

Room boundary

It is important that any equipment in front of the engineers remains out of the line of sight of the monitor loudspeakers

Monitor speakers

The engineer should form the apex of a roughly equilateral triangle with the monitor loudspeakers at the other two points. The speakers should be angled in both horizontal and vertical planes so that the tweeters are aimed either directly at or a little way behind the engineer's head

Listening position

Reflections from equipment in front of the speakers can cause comb filtering due to the different path lengths involved. This is less serious when the speakers are placed on stands behind the mixer rather than on the mixer's meter bridge. Comb filtering produces tonal changes at the listening position

Figure 5.1: A typical monitoring arrangement

The majority of monitors are intended to be mounted with the tweeter above the bass unit, not set on their side, as this provides the widest accurate listening area. Where the speakers have the bass units and tweeters close together, this isn't quite so important, but if possible you should use the speakers in the position and orientation that they were designed to be used.

It's important that the tweeters are pointed towards the head of the listener in order to ensure that the listener is on axis with the monitor, although to widen the 'sweet spot' a little, it may be better to have the tweeters intersect just behind the engineer's head. If arranging this geometry causes a problem, it's OK to stand speakers upside-down, with the tweeter at head height, or to angle the speakers using wedges.

In systems that use separate sub-bass speakers, the optimum placement can be found by first putting the sub where you normally sit and then moving around the room until you find a spot where the bass notes sound most even. You can then move the sub to this position.

Stands should be solid, with no tendency to vibrate, and the monitor may be mounted on soft rubber pads, or even on four small lumps of Blu-Tack to stop them from slipping and to decouple cabinet vibrations before they reach the floor.

Amplifier Power

Conventional wisdom used to suggest that buying a small power amplifier was the best way of protecting your speakers from overload, but in recent years the converse has been proven to be true. Most speakers will stand short periods of overload, providing the input signal isn't unduly distorted or clipped. However, an under-powered amplifier can easily be driven into clipping, resulting in a harmonically rich, clipped waveform being fed into the tweeters. Aside from sounding disgusting, this can easily overheat the tweeter's voice coil, causing it to burn out.

It's actually safest to buy the largest amplifier recommended for your speakers, ideally one with clip indicators to warn you if clipping is taking place. The ideal amplifier power depends on the efficiency of the speaker and on the level at which you like to work, but a reasonable estimate might be between 50W and 250W per channel. Amplifiers lower in power than 50W can very easily be driven into clipping, especially when used with less efficient speakers.

Speaker Wiring

A good speaker cable needs to have a very low resistance, so the main factor is weight of cable, although some proponents believe that using high-purity copper cable results in an improvement in sound. Using flimsy wire will compromise the sound of your speakers, but there is really very little to choose between one good-quality heavy-duty cable and another compared to the differences that other components in the system can make. Speaker-cable capacitance can affect the sound slightly, so speaker cable isn't all black magic and marketing, but don't get talked into buying anything too expensive. Keep speaker cables as short as possible and ensure that both speaker leads are the same length. Check that your speakers are wired in phase (red terminal on the amplifier to red terminal on the speaker), and check that the cable ends are firmly clamped at both the speaker and amplifier end. Active speakers bypass the problems associated with speaker cable and usually deliver a better-controlled bass, so if you're thinking of replacing your monitors, active models are worth seriously considering.

Balance

Getting a good balance can be difficult, especially if you've spent all day listening to the same song being recorded. Most professionals advise you not to mix on the same day as you record, but in a commercial environment there is pressure to get the mix done straight away. In the private recording environment, impatience usually wins out over logic. However, it always helps to play a couple of commercial recordings through your monitoring system in order to help you restore a sense of perspective.

Another very positive tactic is to listen to the mix from outside the room with the door left open. In this situation, level-balance problems become much more obvious. Once you've made any necessary corrections, the mix should sound right from both inside the room and outside.

Headphones For Monitoring?

Headphones can be very useful problem-solvers in monitoring, but I don't recommend using them as a sole source of monitoring as the bass response and stereo imaging can sound quite different over loudspeakers. The way in which the headphone cushion seals around the ear affects the bass performance, which is why pushing the phones closer to your ears produces a noticeable increase in bass. This is a real problem in the context of monitoring, where one of the main aims is to achieve a proper tonal balance across the full audio spectrum.

Unlike loudspeakers, headphones are independent of the acoustics of the room in which they are used, and the sense of detail they convey makes it easier to pick out small noises or distortions that might go unnoticed on monitor speakers.

When a stereo mix is heard over loudspeakers, because the speakers are physically in front of us, our natural hearing mechanism perceives the soundstage as being in front of us. With headphones, because the 'speakers' are on either side of us, there's no real front-to-back information, which can make the stereo image seem as though it's passing through the head rather than being on a virtual stage in front of the listener. Furthermore, when listening to stereo from loudspeakers, some of the sound from the left loudspeaker is picked up by the right ear, and vice versa.

In contrast, headphones provide a very high degree of separation between the left and right channels, resulting in an artificially detailed stereo image. This characteristic is useful when checking the positions of various sounds in the stereo mix, or when checking for recording faults, but the same mix heard over speakers will seem to have a stereo spread that's not as wide or clearly focused.

Open-Phone Advantages

Open headphones are usually ventilated with slots or holes so that sound can pass in and out. In other words, they don't present the same kind of sealed environment as enclosed headphones, but the bass performance still varies from model to model and changes to some extent depending on how the phone fits over the ear. As a rule, the sound from an open phone is less coloured than that from an enclosed one, and the overall sound quality of open headphones can be surprisingly good. Their ability to resolve fine detail or small amounts of distortion makes them idea for double-checking a mix that already sounds balanced on loudspeakers, and in the case of the home-studio operator, it's possible to use headphones at times when noise might be a problem. Even so, the mix should also be checked on loudspeakers before being finally approved.

Headphone Impedance

Headphone come in a variety of impedances, ranging from eight ohms or so up to several hundred. Most headphone amplifiers will happily drive any impedance you're likely to encounter with no trouble, but if for any reason you want to split the output from a headphone socket to feed two sets of phones, you'd be just as well to pick phones of the same impedance. Otherwise, one set will be louder than the other.

Key Points

- Choose an accurate speaker rather than a flattering one, and don't go for a large system with an extended frequency response if you have only a modest-sized room.

- Set the speakers up on proper stands a little way behind the mixing console, ideally between four and six feet apart and between four and six feet from the listening position. Angle them inwards so their axes intersect either at or just behind the engineer's head position.

- Don't put the speakers in corners or too close to rear and side walls.

- Avoid mounting monitors on their sides unless they are designed for side mounting.

- Ensure that the power amplifier can drive the speakers at a reasonable listening level without going into clipping on the peaks. It's better to use an amplifier that's too powerful at a sensible level than it is to use an under-powered one flat out.

- Use heavy speaker cable, but don't feel obliged to buy anything too expensive.

- Make sure that the speakers are wired in phase with each other.

- Take a rest between recording and mixing to let your ears readjust. Play a few records to regain your sense of perspective.

- Check your mixes at both high and low levels, as well as at the sort of level at which the end user is likely to hear your material.

- Don't think that having good monitors means you don't need a good pair of headphones. Headphones can show up subtle distortions and minor clicks that you may never hear on loudspeakers.

- After setting a balance, listen to your mix from the next room, with the door open. This is more likely to show up any balance problems than sitting directly in front of the monitors.

Basic Acoustic Treatment

Few of us are in a position to fit our houses with false walls, suspended ceilings and floating floors, but it's still possible to create a reliable monitoring environment. Without a good monitoring room, the mix may sound great in the studio, but as soon as it's played back on another system, you may find the balance is all wrong, the bass is wildly out of control and what seemed like a masterpiece at the time in now just plain embarrassing.

There's more to monitoring than simply buying a good pair of loudspeakers – the room also has a great influence over what you hear. But what are the consequences of working in a room with poor acoustics? What are we actually listening to when we sit down in front of our consoles to mix?

Obviously, we hear the sound coming directly from the monitor speakers, but added to that is a significant amount of reflected sound, as our latest mix bounces off every reflective surface in the room. The reflected sound arrives later than the direct sound, and because some frequencies are absorbed more than others the reflected sound is also highly 'coloured'. An instinctive first response might be to suggest mixing in a totally dead or acoustically absorbent room which should remove all reflected sound, leaving us with just the pure sound of the speakers. In theory, this is fine, but in practice we can't ever create a completely absorbent room because of the need to have equipment in the studio, and all equipment has reflective surfaces, especially the mixing desk.

More significantly, we're used to living in a moderately reflective acoustic environment, and the vast majority of people find totally anechoic (non-reflective) rooms psychologically disturbing. On a more practical note, to create a truly anechoic room that absorbs energy right across the audio spectrum requires the walls to be lined with an absorbent material such as Rockwool to a depth of many feet,

which is impractical in most commercial installations, let alone home studios and MIDI suites. Even if it could be achieved, you'd need a very powerful monitoring system because the perceived sound level is much lower in a totally dead room.

Real-World Monitoring

I've left what I consider to be the most powerful argument against anechoic monitoring environments until last, and that is that most people listen to their music either in a domestic living room or in the car, neither of which are remotely anechoic. If music is going to be played back in a normal room, it makes some kind of sense to mix it in a room with similar characteristics. This argument breaks down if you need to use a very large monitoring system or one with an extended bass response, but for the person working from home with small or medium-sized monitors, a reasonable monitoring environment can be created with very little effort or expense.

Nearfield Advantages

In a room with imperfect acoustics, near-field monitoring offers the advantage – by virtue of its close proximity – that the listener hears a greater proportion of the direct sound from the loudspeaker compared to the sound reflected from the walls, floors and ceilings of the room. This is an important advantage because, in an untreated room, the reflected sound won't have the same characteristics of the direct sound; it will be 'EQ'd' in an unpredictable way by the physical properties of the room and any furnishings or equipment within the room.

It's also true that most untreated rooms perform least accurately at the low bass end of the spectrum, so using small or medium-sized monitors that don't generate very low bass neatly sidesteps that problem. That doesn't mean you have to put up with thin-sounding monitors; you can still use speakers that go down to 50Hz or so. Just don't expect to be able to reproduce 20Hz organ pedal notes with any degree of accuracy.

Solving Room Problems

So far we've got a pair of decent monitors and, hopefully, an amplifier capable of providing at least as much undistorted power as the speakers can handle. The monitors are sensibly positioned behind the console, away from corners, and the engineer's chair forms the apex of an equilateral triangle with the monitors. In a small room, this often means setting the speakers up against the longest wall simply to avoid getting the speakers too close to the corners (and by too close I mean ideally not closer than 18 inches), but we're not out of the woods yet because room reflections can still interfere with what we're hearing.

Flutter Echo

A common problem is flutter echo caused by sound bouncing back and forth between two parallel surfaces, the outcome being an audible ringing. Try clapping your hands in a room that has hard, parallel walls and you'll hear what I mean quite clearly. Professional studios are built with non-parallel walls, but in a typical house moving the walls is rarely an option. Fortunately, as you'll be spending most of your time in the engineer's chair, you only have to worry about curing flutter echo in that position.

The easiest solution is to fix a square metre of acoustic foam tile to the wall directly on each side of your normal listening position and centred at

It can sometimes help to put one or two acoustic tiles behind the monitors to prevent reflections from the front walls from confusing the direct sound of the speakers

Figure 5.2: Acoustic tiles used to damp out flutter echoes

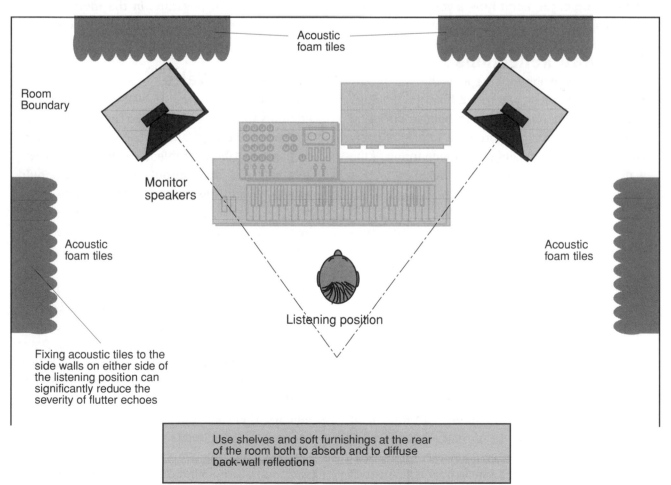

Acoustic foam tiles

Room Boundary

Monitor speakers

Acoustic foam tiles

Acoustic foam tiles

Listening position

Fixing acoustic tiles to the side walls on either side of the listening position can significantly reduce the severity of flutter echoes

Use shelves and soft furnishings at the rear of the room both to absorb and to diffuse back-wall reflections your (seated) head height. As well as reducing the flutter echo, this treatment should also clean up the stereo imaging quite noticeably. Low-cost two-inch foam tiles will work quite adequately, although a similar thickness of fire-proof, open-cell upholstery foam will do almost as well, and a thin fabric covering will make it look more appealing. (You can easily tell if the foam is the open-cell type. If it will soak up water, it's open cell.)

Wrong Things To Do

Don't be tempted to try carpeting all the walls instead, because most carpet absorbs only the very high end of the audio spectrum, leaving the bass and mid range to bounce around uncontrolled, resulting in a boomy, boxy-sounding room. A more practical approach for the project studio is to use small areas of acoustic tiles on problem surfaces but to leave the majority of the walls and ceiling reflective. Figure 5.2 shows a practical monitoring layout with sound-absorbing tiles used to damp out flutter echoes.

Rear-Wall Reflections

The remaining major trouble spot is the wall directly behind you, because any sound from the monitors that doesn't hit you is going to bounce off it and come back to you a short time later, seriously compromising the quality of your monitoring. If the wall is more than ten feet or so behind you, you don't really have to do very much. You could, for example, put a soft settee along the bottom of the wall and fix a heavy curtain folded into drapes above it, spaced two or three inches from the wall. Alternatively, you could break up the flat geometry of the wall by fitting it with shelves for your tapes, manuals, records, CDs and so on to help scatter the reflections, although some absorbent material (such as the settee) is still recommended.

If you have an even smaller room and the back wall is only a few feet behind you, the ideal solution is to make the wall 'disappear' as far as audio is concerned by covering it entirely with absorbent material. A six-inch depth of Rockwool slab fixed between battens should be adequate for use with near-field monitors, and a simple porous fabric such

as hessian is fine for covering the finished 'trap' However, if you don't want to go to these lengths, consider hanging a heavy curtain over most or all of the rear wall and then fixing a row of acoustic foam tiles to the wall, behind the curtain, at head height. In most instances, mixing shelving (which acts as a diffuser, scattering reflections) with areas of absorbent material will yield satisfactory results.

In rooms that are very nearly square, or where the height of the room is similar to one of the wall dimensions, peaks in the low-end frequency response are likely to occur because of the action of room modes. A full discussion of room modes is beyond the scope of this book, but in effect the room acts as a resonator, and the worst case is a cube-shaped room, where the resonances due to room width, room length and room height all occur at the same frequency. In such a room, use as much depth of absorbent material as you can along the back wall and, if possible, in the room corners. Choose nearfield monitors with a very modest bass response, and work as close to them as is practical.

Floors And Walls

If at all possible, a wall-to-wall carpet should be fitted, as this helps kill floor-to-ceiling reflections, at least at the high end of the spectrum, where ringing might be a problem. Heavy underfelt will also help with soundproofing. Symmetry should extend beyond the monitor placement, so try to match reflective surfaces on one side of the room by a similar area of reflective surface on the other. However, avoid having flat, reflective surfaces directly facing each other, as this re-introduces the danger of flutter echoes. If you have a window, try putting vertical blinds up. If left half open, these will reduce high-frequency reflections by a significant degree, and because glass isn't a particularly good isolator of low-frequency sound, you won't get much low-frequency reflection, either – it'll go straight through.

If you have equipment racks on one wall, balance them as much as possible by adding shelving to the opposite wall. If you have room for them, adding some more soft furnishings will help damp down room resonances. In this respect, putting absorbent furniture in the rear corners of the room probably has the most beneficial effect. It follows that a typical bedroom studio with the bed still in it will probably make quite a good mixing room with very little modification.

Get used to your monitoring system by playing your record and CD collection in the studio, and keep a few test CDs handy for comparison purposes when mixing. Also – I make no apology for repeating this – take a break after recording before you come to mix. If you give your ears a chance to recover, you're far more likely to come up with a good mix.

Why Not Equalise?

Why bother with acoustic treatment at all? Why not just put a graphic equaliser in the system and adjust it until the combination of direct and reflected sounds is OK? Well, that used to be an accepted way of working, and even today equalisation is used to compensate for minor room deficiencies, but realistically EQ is of little practical use in this context. For a start, our ears don't just average out the direct and reflected sound – they have the ability to 'focus in' on the direct sound and so take less account of the reflected room sound than you might think.

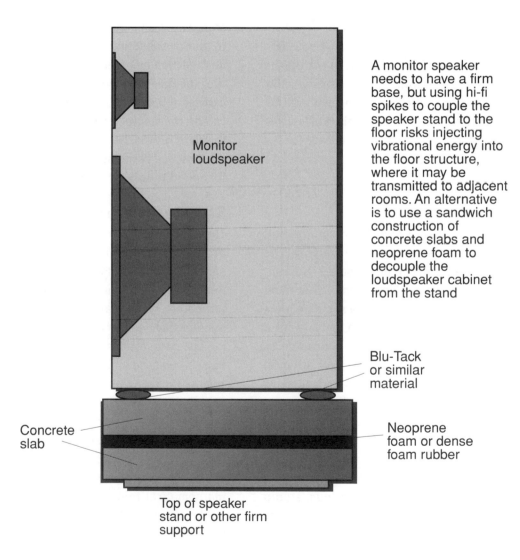

Monitor loudspeaker

A monitor speaker needs to have a firm base, but using hi-fi spikes to couple the speaker stand to the floor risks injecting vibrational energy into the floor structure, where it may be transmitted to adjacent rooms. An alternative is to use a sandwich construction of concrete slabs and neoprene foam to decouple the loudspeaker cabinet from the stand

Blu-Tack or similar material

Concrete slab

Neoprene foam or dense foam rubber

Top of speaker stand or other firm support

Figure 5.3: Isolating a speaker with Blu-Tack, concrete slabs and foam

Perhaps more importantly, a poor listening room sounds bad because its natural reverberation time is wildly different at different frequencies. Room reflections and re-reflections are time-domain problems, in that they occur after the original event, and no amount of EQ can change the reverberant characteristics of a room. Indeed, a room can be considered as a kind of mechanical equaliser, and the only way of adjusting that is by mechanical means – juggling with the area and type of reflective and absorbent surfaces until the reverberation time is more or less even over the whole audio band. Put simply, the situation as I see it is this: If you have good speakers in a bad room, at least the direct sound is correct, even though the reflected sound is wrong. If you then equalise the monitors in an attempt to correct the room, the direct sound from the monitors will now be wrong – and the reflected sound will still be wrong! The only real exception to this rule is using some bass-end adjustment to compensate for the boundary effect that occurs when speakers are located near a wall.

Sound Leakage

Not everyone can justify building a soundproof, acoustically treated studio, but with just a little effort and ingenuity you can often make significant improvements to the sound isolation of your room at very little cost. If you don't have a separate room to use as a studio, or if you're living in rented accommodation, you may not be in a position to build a dedicated studio, and if you have a typical bedroom studio, cutting down on noise leakage is probably one of your main priorities.

Unfortunately, there's no cheap-and-cheerful way to soundproof a room totally. The techniques discussed here can make a significant improvement, but there's no way you're going to be able to contain the sound of a drum kit or a serious studio monitoring system turned up full-bore without doing major structural work. Anything short of a custom designed studio is a compromise, and if you're working in a typical domestic room, this means taking measures to reduce the amount of noise you

actually produce as well as trying to reduce the amount of noise that leaks in and out.

Most home recording set-ups are based around MIDI systems and DI'd instruments, so most of the sound you generate will come from the monitor speakers. It's also true that floors and ceilings tend to be less solidly built than walls, and you'll find that most of your sound leakage gets out via floors, ceilings, windows and doors. Partition walls also leak sound badly, but unless you're prepared to build a heavy false wall in front of the existing one, any improvements in this area can be only minor.

As the monitor speakers are the source of the sound you're trying to contain, it makes sense to start with them. Obviously, speakers are designed to launch sound into the air, but what with action and reaction being equal and opposite, every time the speaker cone moves, so does the speaker cabinet. Although small, this vibrational movement can be transmitted through the speaker stand into the floor or wall, and once you have a vibration in the structure of the building, you have the potential for sound to leak into adjoining rooms.

Structural Vibrations

There are several things you can do to minimise the problem described above. For a start, don't use speakers with a massive bass response, because low frequencies are the hardest to contain. In a small or untreated room, bass frequencies behave very unpredictably, so by choosing a speaker with a more modest bass response, you'll actually end up with a more accurate sound, as well as reducing the amount of bass thumping through neighbouring walls.

Set up your monitors so that you're working in the near field – in other words, with the monitors around three or four feet away from you and just a little more than that apart. Because sound intensity works according to the inverse square law (a fancy mathematical term that explains why things are louder when they're closer), the closer you are to your monitors, the less power you'll need to hear the same sound level. A further advantage of working in the near field is that you hear more of the direct sound from the speakers and less of the sound reflected from the walls and objects in the room, so you gain an increase in accuracy without actually doing anything at all to the room.

Monitor Isolation

However, this still doesn't address the problem of structurally borne vibration originating from the speaker cabinets themselves. What's needed here is some way of isolating the loudspeakers from the surfaces on which they normally stand. You could simply stand the speaker cabs on a piece of two-

inch foam rubber, but the isolation may be improved even further by placing a small concrete slab on top of the foam and then standing each speaker on four lumps of Blu Tack on top of the slab, as shown in Figure 5.3. Even with nearfield monitors, a significant amount of low-frequency energy is generated, and this is radiated in all directions – not just in the direction in which the speaker is pointing. This being the case, if you're worried about sound passing through a wall and into the adjoining room, it's best not to put the speakers too close to the wall.

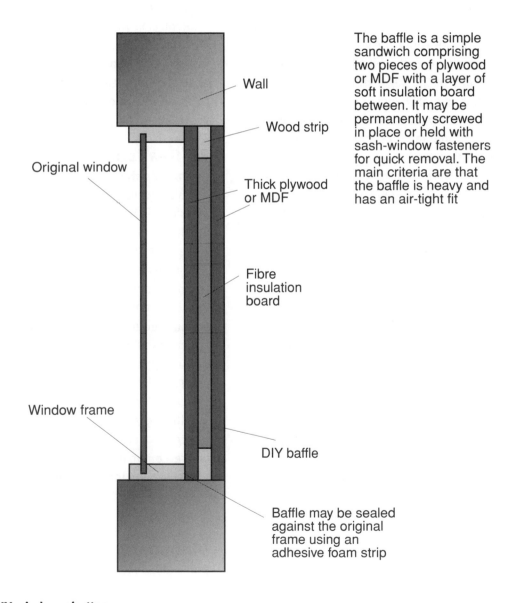

Wall

Wood strip

Original window

Thick plywood or MDF

Fibre insulation board

Window frame

DIY baffle

Baffle may be sealed against the original frame using an adhesive foam strip

The baffle is a simple sandwich comprising two pieces of plywood or MDF with a layer of soft insulation board between. It may be permanently screwed in place or held with sash-window fasteners for quick removal. The main criteria are that the baffle is heavy and has an air-tight fit

Figure 5.4: A DIY window shutter

Sound Absorption

Sound tends to leak through ceilings and floors, and the best low-cost remedy when dealing with floors is to fit thick hair underfelt in your studio room and, if possible, also beneath the carpet in the room above. The combined weight and thickness of the carpet and underfelt provides both absorption and damping, so buy the heaviest grade possible. Also, avoid tapping your feet to the music, as this is often more annoying to the people below than the sound of your monitors!

If your room is fitted with plenty of soft furniture, you probably won't have any serious acoustic problems, but if you've had to clear out a lot of the furniture to make room for your equipment, you might find the room just a bit too live. If you don't want to try any of the suggestions made earlier in the chapter, try simply hanging up an ordinary quilt on the wall facing your monitors. Another option is to buy two or three rag rugs and hang these on the back wall so that they're a couple of inches away from the wall's surface. It may also help to ensure that there are no hard, reflective surfaces directly on either side of your normal listening position. If there are, the ploy of fixing a couple of foam tiles on either side of this position usually does the trick. Use double-sided tape if you don't want to damage the walls.

Containment

This leaves just doors and windows, and in most cases these are the most vulnerable areas when it comes to sound leakage. If you don't have double-glazed windows and you have a problem with either sound getting in or sound getting out, fitting secondary double-glazing is highly recommended. There are DIY kits available for this at sensible prices. Because the space between the original window and the secondary glazing is quite large, you'll often find that the amount of sound reduction is better than you'd get from conventional double-glazing alone. If there's a choice of fitting different thicknesses of glass, use the thickest you can, because more mass equates to better low-frequency isolation.

If daylight isn't a major consideration, a cheaper

alternative is to build a heavy wooden shutter and screw it over the window, as shown in Figure 5.4. If you want to take it down between sessions, use sash-window fasteners to hold it in place.

Doors are rather less simple to deal with because their mass is much lower than that of the surrounding walls. Fitting good-quality draught-proof seals will prevent sound leaking around the edge of the door, but a typical lightweight domestic internal door provides only something like 15dB of sound attenuation, even when it fits properly. Fitting heavy curtains over the door helps a little, but don't expect miracles.

Replacing the door with a heavy fire door will yield some improvement, but it's not until you start fitting double doors that you make any real headway against serious leakage. In most rooms, it's possible to fit double doors with the thickness of the wall providing an air gap, as shown in Figure 5.5.

Be Realistic

As long as the room adjoining your studio isn't inhabited while you're working, just fitting door seals should be fine, but don't expect to be able to monitor at full volume without upsetting someone if the next room is occupied.

All the above measures are pretty straightforward to implement and all will bring about some improvement, but isolating loud, low-frequency sounds requires heavy walls and double-skinned structures with large air gaps. Using the methods discussed here, you won't get anything like the sound isolation you'd expect from a properly built studio, so you'll still have to keep an eye on your monitoring levels and stop work at a sensible time of night. It also helps to use headphones when you're composing or editing music – they aren't great for mixing, but as long as you have a comfortable pair, you can often use them in place of monitors.

Diplomacy

Don't underestimate diplomacy. Most people will put up with a little noise if they don't think you're being inconsiderate to them. Try to agree times when

**Figure 5.5: Double-door construction,
as viewed from above**

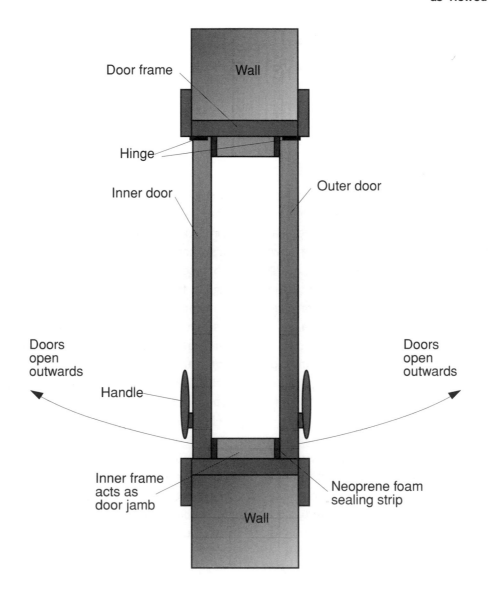

your neighbours will let you monitor more loudly, and in return agree not to make too much noise during the times when they want a bit of peace and quiet. Whatever else you may think of MIDI, it has at least made it possible for us to compose and record music without having to shake the house.

6 MIDI AND SEQUENCING

MIDI has proven to be a key technology in the way that music is made today, enabling equipment from different manufacturers to communicate. However, occasionally problems arise that have to be dealt with by applying a little logic. In tracking down MIDI problems, I find it very useful to have a MIDI analyser, as these devices provide a visual indication of the type of MIDI data being received and on what channel. (Note that, when I say something can be recorded 'to tape', this is intended as a generic term that applies to any type of audio recorder.)

MIDI Analysers

The simplest type of MIDI analyser is inexpensive and usually comprises a display of LEDs, next to which are marked the MIDI channels and the MIDI message types. MIDI In and Out connectors are fitted so that the device can be connected in line with an existing MIDI circuit. An even cheaper option comes in the form of a MIDI plug with a LED built into it which flashes whenever there's any MIDI activity. These are simple devices and can't tell you what data is being passed along the cable, but at least they show you something *is* getting through. For those more used to computers, various MIDI analyser utilities are available as software for both Mac and PC computers.

System problems can come in many forms, but the most common problems are probably instruments that don't play when you think they should, instruments that play when you think they shouldn't and stuck notes. If an instrument isn't responding to the messages you're sending it, first check with your MIDI analyser that the messages are being received. On several occasions, I've found that no MIDI data is being sent when my computer sequencer appears to be operating properly, and it's often down to the MIDI interface getting itself confused. Switching the interface off, then back on again, then quitting and reloading the sequencer software usually does the trick, and if you're a PC user, you need to check that you don't have another program loaded that's laid prior claim to the interface. Sometimes a program will refuse to relinquish control over the MIDI interface, even when you exit the program, in which case you'll need to reboot the computer.

The other thing to check is that the software is addressing the MIDI interface correctly. Mac users normally connect their MIDI interfaces via either the modem or printer port, so check that your software is actually addressing the port to which your interface is connected. It's no use plugging the interface into the modem port if the software has been told it's connected to the printer port.

PC users may have a choice of MIDI destinations, including the MIDI interface on a soundcard, external MIDI interfaces plugged into the serial port, the onboard synth section of a soundcard or a completely separate synth soundcard that's installed in addition to a multifunction soundcard. Providing that the correct drivers for these have been installed, and providing that these drivers are compatible with the sequencing program you're running, they should all be available as options from inside the sequencer. Make sure the right one is selected.

Before panicking, make sure all your MIDI cables and MIDI interface connection cables are pushed fully home. I've had a situation where my MIDI interface was registering the fact that it was receiving data but none of it was being passed on. The problem was that the interface-to-computer lead wasn't pushed in properly and only some pins were making contact. This was enough to light the status LEDs that said all was well, but nothing worked!

MIDI Instrument Modes

Assuming that MIDI data is now finding its way to your MIDI module and that the module is properly connected, switched on and turned up, the next step is to check that the MIDI Receive channel is set to the same as that on which the data being sent. If the module is multitimbral, make sure it's in the correct mode – some instruments have one mode for multitimbral operation and another for using layered sounds on a single MIDI channel. These modes may be referred to as Multi and Single, or something similar.

Instrument Check

Once the channels match and you can confirm data is being sent, check the instrument display to see if the MIDI Receive light is coming on. If it isn't, the instrument's microprocessor might have locked up, so switch off the power, wait ten seconds or so and then switch the power back on. Sometimes instruments get in such a mess that they have to be re-initialised, but this usually means that you lose all your user patches, so make sure these are backed up somewhere. Each machine has a different initialisation process that should be described in the manual, and it usually entails powering up the unit while holding down a couple of the front-panel buttons. If you're lucky, this will bring up a warning message, asking you to confirm that you really want to go through with it.

MIDI Volume

If the MIDI Receive light is flashing, it's possible that the MIDI volume has been turned down by a command from the sequencer. For example, you may have just played a song with a fade-out using Controller 7 data. Unless another message comes along telling the synth to turn up again, the volume will remain off, so if you're including volume changes in your sequence, remember to put the desired starting-volume values somewhere in the count-in bar.

Omni Present

Some instruments have an irritating habit of booting up in Omni mode, which means that they'll try to play everything coming out of the MIDI port to which they're connected. The resulting cacophony usually reminds you of what's happened, in which case you simply enter the MIDI Setup menu and select Poly mode. If you have synth for a master keyboard that defaults to Local On mode, you'll also notice that, whenever you try to play a module, it's accompanied by the sound of the master synth. Switching to Local Off should solve the problem.

Stuck Notes

Stuck notes are those that don't stop sounding when a key is released, and they can be caused by a number of things. The first thing to suspect is a MIDI loop. If your master keyboard synth has defaulted to Local On and you try to play it via the sequencer, you could find yourself sending the synth back its own MIDI data, and this circulates around the system in a MIDI equivalent of acoustic feedback, preventing any meaningful data from getting through. Switching to Local Off and then sending an All Notes Off message from the sequencer should clear the problem.

Another cause of stuck notes is Note Off messages getting lost of corrupted, usually because the MIDI chain is too long. If you have more than two instruments slaved onto a single MIDI output, you should consider getting a MIDI Thru box. These useful devices are quite inexpensive and split the MIDI signal into several buffered outputs so that no output needs to drive a long chain. Figure 6.1 shows a Thru box in use.

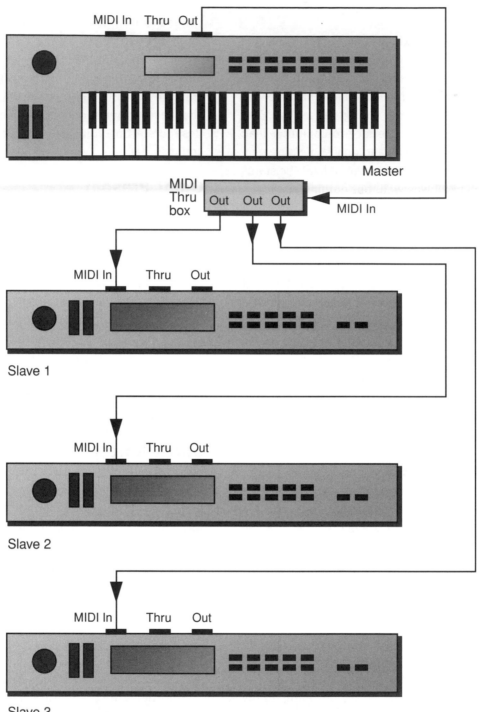

Slaves will respond only if set to the same MIDI channel as the data sent from the master device. The use of a Thru box prevents the MIDI signal from deteriorating as it passes from one device to the next. Such deterioration is often responsible for problems such as stuck notes, notes failing to play and so on

Figure 6.1: A MIDI Thru box in use

Notes can also get stuck if you edit a MIDI sequence in such a way that you miss out one of the Note Off commands. Note Offs can also be missed with some instruments if you try to instigate a patch change while a note is playing. Unfortunately, some PC soundcards occasionally throw up a stuck note for no obvious reason, and the only way to silence them may be to close down and then reboot the program. If this happens to you, remember to save the current state of your sequence before quitting.

Loss Of Memory?

What if everything is working perfectly, but when you come back to your system a few days later, all your synth patches have evaporated or reverted to their factory presets? This is a sure sign that the internal-memory backup battery has finally gone, although most last five years or more. If you haven't saved your patches by doing a sysex dump to your sequencer or to a librarian program, I'm afraid they've gone for good, so back up everything valuable before going any further.

Replacing the battery isn't always easy, as some are physically soldered to circuit boards. Unless you're handy with a soldering iron and know exactly what you're doing, you should have the battery changed by a qualified service centre. Shorting out or overheating these batteries can cause them to explode, or at least to become very hot. If you're the sort of organised person who can keep a log of things like when the battery was last changed, you might do well to have the batteries replaced every four years or so. Some repair shops will back up and replace your patches for you while changing the battery, but it's still best to keep a copy at home, just to be safe. The easiest way to back up your patches is simply to put the sequencer into Record and then initiate a sysex dump of all patches. Store the resulting few seconds of apparent nonsense as a song file and replay it back into the instrument when you need to restore the sounds.

Sync Methods And Problems

When synchronisation systems are working properly, they are wonderful, but when they go wrong, the results can be disastrous. This section covers the basics of the most common sync systems used in recording studios, before examining some common problems and possible solutions.

Synchronisation is an important concept in recording. Without it, we would have no way of making tracks on tape and tracks recorded onto a sequencer run together. Even if they were started at the right time, the timing would almost certainly drift due to small speed instabilities in the tape machine's speed. This is less of a problem with digital tape recorders, as these run at far more constant speed than analogue machines, but over a period of time they can still drift enough to cause problems. What is required to achieve synchronisation is some way of forcing the sequencer to change tempo to match any speed fluctuations in the tape machine, and that's where the various sync options come in.

FSK Sync

Probably the simplest sync system you'll encounter is based on FSK (Frequency Shift Keying), a series of electronic tones that are recorded onto a spare track of the tape machine. These tone patterns are derived from the drum machine or sequencer's MIDI clock, and there are 96 'ticks' per bar of music, so as the tempo is increased, the ticks on the electronic sync track are spaced closer together.

At one time, FSK sync was used quite extensively, but it has been largely superseded by more sophisticated options. However, it is still used in some drum machines, and of course there's a lot of second-hand gear around that still uses it.

To sync a drum machine to tape using FSK, you must first program your drum part, complete with any tempo changes. Now, when you play back the drum sequence, the sync code output from the drum machine can be recorded onto one track of your tape recorder. (Those using cassette multitrackers may find they have a dedicated sync in and out function, usually on the highest numbered track, but if not, always record the code with no EQ and no noise reduction.)

Note: Noise reduction – particularly dbx – can distort time-code signals to the extent that they cannot be read back reliably. You may also have to experiment with the recording level before you can get the code to play back correctly.

To play back the drum-machine part in sync with the tape machine, the tape output from the sync track you've just recorded must be plugged into the Sync In socket on the drum machine and the drum machine must be switched to Tape Sync. Once the tape is set playing from the start, the drum machine will automatically start at the right point and should stay in time with the tape until you stop the tape machine. You can add a sequencer to the system simply by setting the sequencer to External MIDI Sync and connecting the MIDI Out from your drum machine to the MIDI In of your sequencer, as shown in Figure 6.2

FSK Problems

FSK sync is very simple and usually reliable, but it has one big drawback: whenever you stop the tape, you have to wind it right back to the beginning again to establish sync. This is a limitation about which you can do nothing, other than move up to a more sophisticated sync system, such as Smart FSK, MTC or SMPTE, which will be covered shortly.

If you do experience problems with equipment that is synced via FSK, here are a few things you can check.

- If the drum machine or other MIDI device doesn't start when a sync code is received from tape, check that Tape Sync mode (sometimes called External Sync) has been selected.

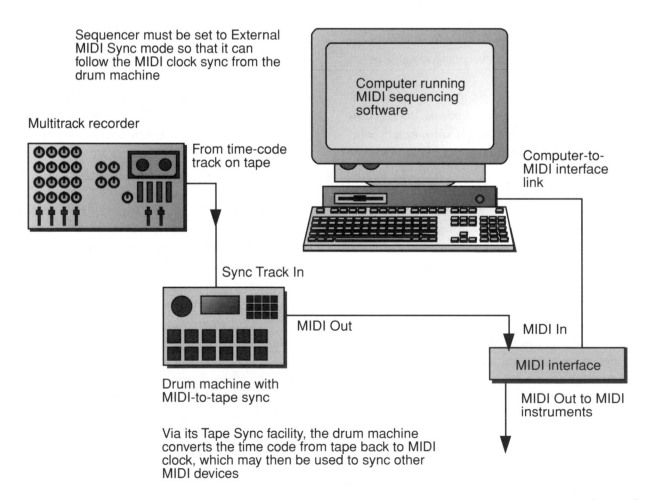

Sequencer must be set to External MIDI Sync mode so that it can follow the MIDI clock sync from the drum machine

Multitrack recorder

Computer running MIDI sequencing software

From time-code track on tape

Computer-to-MIDI interface link

Sync Track In

MIDI Out

MIDI In

MIDI interface

Drum machine with MIDI-to-tape sync

MIDI Out to MIDI instruments

Via its Tape Sync facility, the drum machine converts the time code from tape back to MIDI clock, which may then be used to sync other MIDI devices

Figure 6.2: Syncing a sequencer (to tape) via a MIDI drum machine

- If the device still doesn't recognise the code, check the code is actually there by plugging the cable carrying the code into a mixer line input and then monitoring the signal at a low level. You should hear a rasping tone not unlike that generated by a fax machine. If this isn't present, go right back to source by making sure that the code shows up on the tape machine's level meters and make sure you've plugged into the correct jack output. I know the latter sounds obvious, but you'll sometimes find a footswitch jack next to the sync jack, and it's easy to plug into that by mistake.

- If the code is being received but the timing still seems to drift out, the signal is most probably being corrupted in some way, and every time a tone pulse is missed, the sequencer will fall further behind. Recording level is very important, and too high a level can cause just as many problems as too low a level. Try recording the code at around −10dB on the VU meters and then adjust either side of that until you find the most reliable level. You may also have to adjust the level of the code being returned to the drum machine, and you may find that your tape machine has no level control on the sync output. In such cases, you usually have to improvise by finding something that can work as a variable-gain, line-level pre-amp. However, in most cases, the problem can be solved by recording the right level to tape.

- Another cause of unreliable code reading is crosstalk from loud percussion or drums recorded on the tape track adjacent to the time-code track. To get around this, ensure that the track next to the code track is reserved for non-percussive sounds, such as vocals or keyboard pads. You can also try re-recording the offending track at a lower level.

Smart FSK

Smart FSK is an improvement on the basic FSK system just described, but it still works by recording the code to tape in the form of tones that mimic the sprocket holes in cine film. The main difference is that it is designed to exploit MIDI SPPs (MIDI Song Position Pointers), the benefit being that the tape machine can be started anywhere in the song and the sequencer will always sync up in the right place. The code is still generated from the sequencer's MIDI clock, so any tempo changes will be reproduced accurately when the sequencer is synced to tape. As with basic FSK, however, it isn't possible to change the tempo of your sequence after the code has been recorded to tape, because as soon as you sync up, the time code will force the song back to its old tempo. The problems and solutions associated with this type of sync code are the same as for basic FSK.

Note: Smart FSK sync is built into some products, but it is more common to buy a separate unit, and the best type to go for is one that includes a MIDI merge facility. This is necessary if you want to be able to record new MIDI parts into the sequencer as the tape is running. Figure 6.3 shows how a system can be set up using a smart FSK sync box.

The sequencer must send and recognise SPPs for smart FSK to work, but unless you're using a very old or a very basic system, you're unlikely to find one that doesn't. SPPs are completely transparent to the user, so there's no new MIDI protocol or operations to learn.

SMPTE

SMPTE is the industry-standard, professional time code used for film, TV and audio alike, but unlike FSK, which is derived from MIDI clock, SMPTE has nothing to do with tempo. SMPTE is based on real time, measured in hours, minutes and seconds, with further subdivisions to accommodate individual frames of TV and film material. Several frame-rate options are included to accommodate US and European television and film, but in the context of music-only applications the actual frame rate isn't important, as long as you always stick with the same one. It is usual practice to set the SMPTE format to the local TV standard.

SMPTE stands for the Society of Motion Pictures and Television Engineers, and being pedantic, if we are to include European protocols, the code should

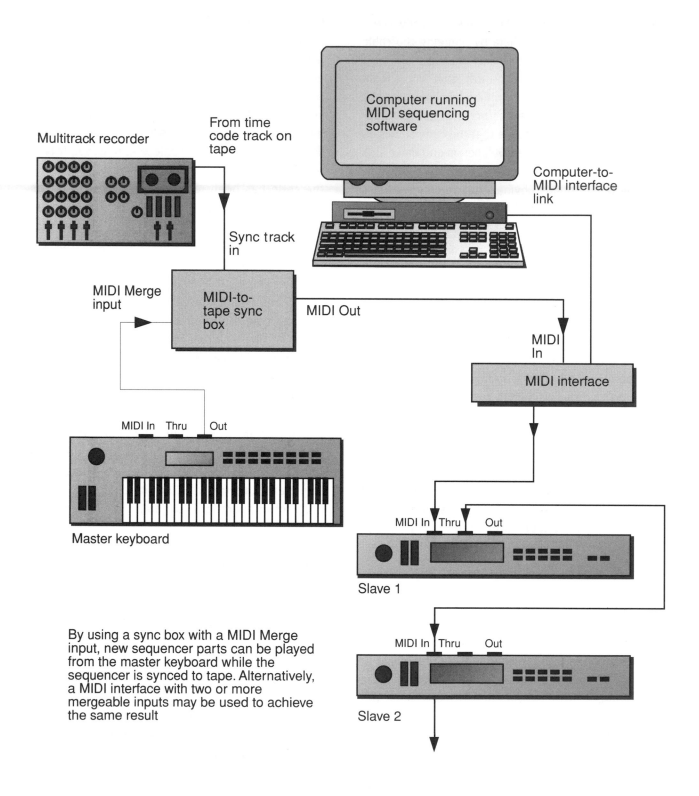

**Figure 6.3: Using a smart-FSK sync box
(merge during playback)**

By using a sync box with a MIDI Merge input, new sequencer parts can be played from the master keyboard while the sequencer is synced to tape. Alternatively, a MIDI interface with two or more mergeable inputs may be used to achieve the same result actually be called SMPTE/EBU. The American TV format is just under 30 frames per second (fps), film runs at 24fps and European TV has a frame rate of 25fps. Aside from the 24, 25 and 30fps formats, the standard also includes *drop frame*, which is used when converting film to TV. Drop Frame gets its name from the fact that whole frames of picture are periodically discarded to eliminate cumulative timing errors which would otherwise cause noticeable sync problems. Drop frame is not used in audio-only applications.

SMPTE time code also provides a useful way of synchronising one tape machine to another. Both machines carry a track of code and a synchroniser box then compares the time positions of the two codes. If the codes aren't identical, a control signal is derived which changes the speed of the slave tape machine, forcing it to move back into sync with the master machine.

Because SMPTE is independent of tempo, a whole tape can be recorded, or 'striped', with code before any recording or programming starts. In this respect, SMPTE is almost like a series of mile markers along an empty road. Of course, music is related to bars and beats, not to absolute time, so to use SMPTE in a musical application, a conversion has to be done somewhere along the line, usually by the computer used to run the sequencing software or by the SMPTE-to-MIDI sync box.

The way this works is that the SMPTE start point of the song is noted, and then the tempo is converted into time and stored in the form of a 'tempo map'. This tempo map also includes the location and degree of any tempo changes and must be referred back to by the sequencer every time the sequence is run against SMPTE. Most modern sequencers create a tempo map automatically and store it as part of the sequence file data, but with some older systems using external MIDI to SMPTE sync boxes, the user had to manually input the location and value of every tempo change. This is tedious and is to be avoided if at all possible.

Unless you're planning to work to picture, SMPTE is not essential, but the advantage it offers

over something like smart FSK is that, if a piece of code is misread, the sequencer won't fall behind the tape to which it is supposed to be synchronised. Because SMPTE behaves like a mile marker on a road, the precise location can be read off the next time a marker is encountered. In other words, if a piece of code goes missing, the position will be corrected the next time a valid piece of code is read. Other than that, both SMPTE and FSK offer ostensibly the same benefits – both allow you to start at any point in a song and both can accommodate tempo changes.

Key Differences Between SMPTE And Smart FSK

SMPTE allows you to stripe the tape before starting work, while smart FSK requires you to have previously programmed your sequence, at least as far as its length and tempo goes. SMPTE is also the standard sync reference for picture, so if you are anticipating any film or TV work, you need a SMPTE-based sync system. However, MTC is also compatible with SMPTE and is supported by the majority of current MIDI equipment.

MTC

MTC (MIDI Time Code) is a MIDI-specific equivalent of traditional SMPTE, complete with the same frame rate options and format. The main difference is that MTC can be transmitted along the MIDI cable along with other MIDI data. Again, MTC requires a tempo map to work, but any sequencer capable of working with MTC will almost certainly look after this for you.

Because MTC has to share the MIDI data highway with other information, its data is sent in short bursts – four to each SMPTE frame. It takes eight of these 'quarter frame' messages to carry enough data to make up one complete set of location data, which means that the receiving MIDI device must read two frames of code before it knows exactly where it's supposed to be.

For this reason, MTC can't pass on positional information as frequently as SMPTE, but for practical tape-to-MIDI sync applications, providing the sequencer software is intelligently written, there's really no practical difference. However, MTC's position in the MIDI data stream can get jostled about when a lot of data is being sent, so if you have a multiport MIDI interface, it's usually best to make sure the port carrying the MTC isn't clogged with other MIDI data.

If the MIDI data stream is running close to capacity, the MTC data may arrive a little behind schedule, which has the effect of introducing a small amount of timing jitter, and in really adverse situations this may be serious enough to be noticeable. Ideally, use a completely separate port for MTC.

Corrupted Time Code

If you find you have a time code track that won't play back reliably, there are a couple of tricks you can try to improve matters:

- Patch the time code track through a compressor before feeding it into the sync unit. The compressor's makeup gain control will allow you to adjust the code's level, and this may be all that's needed to get things working.

- If this doesn't do the trick, you can sometimes salvage the code by compressing it using the fastest attack and release times your compressor has. Set a ratio of around 5:1 and reduce the threshold so that some gain reduction is always registering on the gain-reduction meter. I've used this technique to rescue successfully an unreliable FSK type of code, and there's no reason why you shouldn't try it on SMPTE code.

- If none of the above remedies work, SMPTE codes can sometimes be cleaned up by being fed through a sync unit that includes a code-regeneration facility. Essentially, the code is read, then a brand new code is generated at the output. If successful, this can be recorded back to a spare tape track.

- Short gaps in the code may sometimes be repaired by using a so-called 'flywheel' sync

function, which means that, when you're using your sync unit to regenerate code, you can set it to carry on generating code for a short time, even when the original code has stopped or is unreadable. Most serious SMPTE sync boxes have this function, which will normally need to be set to only a few frames – a little longer than a typical tape dropout – and as soon as the original code becomes readable again, the output code reverts to following that.

Lost Time Code

If you're working to SMPTE or MTC and the time code track on tape is accidentally erased, you may have to do quite a bit of work to get your system back in sync. The first step is to record a new time-code track starting half a minute or so before the song itself starts. If you're using a digital tape machine, the speed is likely to be fairly consistent, so all you need do is go into the Sync page on your sequencer and enter an offset so that the tape tracks and sequencer tracks start together. If you have a visual SMPTE readout, you can note the value when the song starts and use that as your initial point. The chances are that it will still be slightly out, so then comes the tedious bit of adjusting a few frames either way until you're satisfied everything is tight again. This can take quite a bit of trial and error, followed by minor adjustments, but it is possible.

If, however, you're using an analogue tape machine, small speed fluctuations are likely to cause the MIDI and tape tracks to drift out of sync, even if you can find the right start time, so another ploy is needed.

Tap Tempo Sync

Fortunately, pretty much all of the serious sequencer packages have a facility that lets you create your own tempo map by tapping a key in time with the music. Providing you can tap evenly, the process involves simply running the sequencer in sync with the newly recorded time code (with the MIDI tracks muted for now) and then recording a series of MIDI notes from your keyboard, in time with the music on your tape machine. In other words, the two machines run in sync, then you record a sequencer 'metronome' part that is in time with the taped material. You can usually decide whether you want to tap one, two or four beats to the bar.

For songs that have no tempo changes, you may find that you have the facility to tap in the first beat of the song and the first beat of the last bar. Then you can tell the computer how many bars there should be between these points. The computer will then space the bar markers evenly between these two points to create a new tempo map.

Once the tape tempo track is in place, you need to find the appropriate sequencer function, which will have a name like 'Re-bar' or something similar. This essentially creates a new tempo map so that the previously recorded MIDI tracks line up with the tape track you've just created. As the tap track is in perfect time with your tape machine, the MIDI tracks will also end up in time. Tapping in perfect time isn't always easy, so it may take you a while to get this right, but persistence usually pays off. Don't forget to resave the song file with the new tempo map when you've finished!

If the music you're working on doesn't have a strong backbeat, it may be impossible to create a tap tempo track that is sufficiently accurate. You may also have a sequencer that doesn't have a tap tempo re-barring facility. If the project you're working on is for yourself, you can decide whether or not to start again by re-recording the taped parts, but if the project is a commercial job, you may not have the option. Fortunately, there is still a solution.

One way out is to load your MIDI files into a MIDI-plus-audio sequencer and then record your tape tracks onto the audio tracks of the system. The timing still won't be right, but most audio sequencers will allow you to drag the audio around so that at least the starting point of each track is in the right place. Run the sequence and you'll probably find that, after a minute or so, you can hear the audio drift away from the MIDI tracks. Don't worry about this because in an audio sequencer you can invariably divide the tracks up in to shorter regions, and if you make the regions short enough they'll stay in sync well enough until the next region starts.

Every time a region starts to play, its start point is synchronised to the sequencer, so once you've divided your tracks up into short regions, all you have to do is adjust the start position of each region so that it's in exactly the right place. In effect, you've turned your tape tracks into lots of short samples, and each one is being triggered at exactly the right point in the song. You could do the same thing with a sampler, providing you have enough sample memory, but doing the job within an audio sequencer is more straightforward.

If you don't have enough sequencer tracks, transfer as many tracks as you can, sync up an empty tape and then record the edited sequencer audio tracks back to tape. When you're done, load in the next lot of audio tracks, fix those up and transfer those back to tape. Because your new tape has a time code and is synced to your sequencer, you can transfer your tracks in as many goes as it takes.

Audio Sequencers And Tape

Leading nicely on from the last scenario is a problem commonly reported by people running audio sequencers in sync with tape machines. The audio/MIDI sequence runs fine on its own, but as soon as it's set to External Sync to run against the tape, the MIDI syncs up perfectly but the audio drifts. The problem is really the same as in the previous example, because most audio sequencers treat audio tracks as samples which are triggered at the right time and then left to their own devices. If the MIDI tracks are slowed down slightly by being synced to tape, the audio tracks will carry on as before and appear to be overtaking the MIDI tracks.

This is most likely to happen when you're running with an analogue tape recorder, and the solution is again to divide the tracks up in to shorter regions so that they don't have time to get out of sync before the next region takes over. Very often, breaking the tracks up into verses and choruses is enough, but in particularly difficult circumstances you may have to create a new region every bar or two. Try to separate the regions where there is a natural pause, and if you have to cut a sustained pad track or rhythm guitar part, try to do it on a drum beat so as to hide any slight discontinuities.

Note that some more advanced systems allow what is known as 'continuous resync' of the audio tracks, but this requires that a sync system capable of generating 'digital word clock' is employed. In such a system, the sample rate of the audio is also synchronised to the master machine so that, if the tape machine slows down slightly, the sequenced audio will slow down to match it. Obviously, if the audio is slowed down too much, it will sound flat, but the type of variations that happen in normal circumstances are only fractions of a percent.

Real And Virtual Tracks

Back when analogue tape was the normal medium with which to work, it was quite common to record everything onto tape prior to mixing. The concept of recording different chunks of music or audio onto adjacent tracks for later mixing was firmly established as the 'normal' way to work. However, now that we have hard-disk systems running on computers, there's a tendency to keep all audio and MIDI tracks separate, then mix them at the last minute. In fact, the ideal approach is often a mix of the old and new ideologies, so it may help to examine the pros and cons of both ways of working.

Track Mentality

With conventional multitrack tape, either analogue or digital, where the number of available tracks is limited, a conflict arises between the desire to keep everything separate until the last minute and the physical impracticality of having as many tape tracks as you have sound sources. This situation has become particularly acute now that virtually every studio includes a rack of MIDI sound-generating equipment, often with multiple outputs.

On the face of it, the introduction of low-cost MIDI-to-tape synchronisation should have solved the problem, because it eliminates the need to ever record MIDI-driven instruments to multitrack at all. Now the 'virtual' MIDI tracks can be mixed with the off-tape signals and committed directly to DAT, or whatever the mastering medium is. The only proviso

is that you need a mixer with enough inputs. So why is it that many professional engineers and producers still insist on recording their sequenced parts to tape? It can't simply be that they have tracks to burn, so what's the attraction?

In Support Of The Virtual

Running the virtual MIDI tracks directly into the mix is attractive because it means that fewer tape tracks are required, yet all the sounds may still be mixed and treated separately. Using SMPTE, MTC or smart FSK sync means that the sequencer locks to the tape machine very quickly, regardless of where in the song the tape is started. On conventional tape machines, a track is needed to record the time code, but with modern disk-based systems, which tend to generate MTC, there's no need even to lose a track. Here are some of the more obvious advantages of using so-called virtual tracks.

- **Quality Control** – Virtual tracks avoid one generation of quality loss. All tape recorders cause some deterioration in sound quality, and even the best digital models suffer some degradation because of the limitations of their A-to-D (Analogue-to-Digital) converters.

- **MIDI Automation** – Virtual tracks offer the greatest flexibility when it comes to the final mix because any of the sounds can be replaced at the last moment. Furthermore, real-time MIDI control from a sequencer means that a great deal of automation can be used in a mix: synth output levels and pan positions can be varied over MIDI, sound parameters may be varied in real time and MIDI effects-unit parameters may also be controlled.

OK. Now, having made the case for running MIDI parts live into the mix as virtual tracks, what does recording everything have to offer?

In Support Of The Reel!

If absolutely everything is recorded to tape, you may imagine there is no need to devote a track to time code. However, it may not be wise to dispense with time code entirely. For example, you may want to use a sampler to play more parts than it is capable of playing simultaneously, so the answer is to play fewer parts at a time and record these to tape. (See the section 'Limited Polyphony?' to see how this is done.)

One of the main benefits of recording to multitrack – particularly to a tape machine – is that you know it's always going to play back your stuff exactly how you recorded it. When a mix is undertaken using virtual tracks, there are many variables that may be impossible to duplicate exactly if a remix becomes necessary. Sounds may be edited or moved in the interim period or internal effects settings changed. There may also be one-off MIDI hook-ups that nobody bothered to write down, or you may change a sequencer part yet forget to save the change. You might even forget to back up your work and then find that the vital floppy has been eaten by the dog! At the very least, once something is on tape, you know you will be starting from exactly the same point every time you commence work.

While virtual tracks offer limitless opportunity for change, right up to the minute of the final mix, many professionals cite this as the very reason why they don't like it. It seems that they prefer the commitment of having something on tape and then moving on. If every option remains open right up to the last minute, you can waste hours changing things and end up with a worse result.

Sequencers are generally quite reliable, but when working synced to tape you can end up with unexpected problems, such as occasional stuck notes that defy explanation. You're also in trouble if the sync code on tape drops out or, worse still, if someone accidentally erases part of it. Once sounds are recorded on tape, you know that the various tracks are always going to remain in sync with each other.

Analogue Multitrack

Although relatively few analogue recorders are built nowadays, some engineers still record to analogue tape because they like the sound. A little analogue tape compression and second-harmonic distortion,

combined with minuscule amounts of wow and flutter, can warm up a cold digital synth sound quite considerably.

If you're one of those people who loves chopping up multitrack tape and then splicing the bits back together in a different order, the fact that everything is recorded on tape makes this a very straightforward process. However, the advent of hard-disk editing systems, combined with the rising costs of multitrack analogue tape, has probably reduced both the need and the desire to do this. Most simple editing tasks can be accomplished using the audio facilities of a typical sequencer.

Limited Polyphony?

If you're using a one of your multitimbral modules to produce most of the sounds in a song, you might well find that it runs out of polyphony and you end up with missing or truncated notes. You can get around this if you record to multitrack, as you can mute one or two of the busier parts on the sequencer before recording and then run through a second time after swapping the mute status, recording the remaining parts on another tape track. Even if you aren't short on polyphony, recording one part at a time to tape provides a means of separating the sounds from an instrument that may have only a single stereo output, enabling effects and EQ to be applied independently at the mixing stage.

Pros And Cons

Clearly, both virtual and real approaches have their strong points, and most people tend to adopt a mixture of the two methods. The simplest example of this is where one track is dedicated to time code, and all the MIDI instruments run into the mix as virtual tracks via a sequencer, but at the same time a stereo mix of just the MIDI parts plus their effects is also recorded onto two of the multitrack recorder. This way, the 'real' parts recorded onto tape can be remixed or updated without having to set up the whole MIDI system and any associated effects units. In the event that a major change does become necessary, at least the option of syncing up the sequencer and starting from the original virtual tracks remains open. Of course, working in this way means that you have to either leave the stereo mix of MIDI instruments exactly as you recorded it or go back to the sequencer and set up the whole thing again. The only non-destructive (ie non-permanent) possibility is to sync up the sequencer and maybe add one or two new parts over the top of what you already have.

Grouping

A rather more flexible approach is to break down the MIDI instruments into logical subgroups and record these onto pairs of tape tracks. The more tape tracks you have, the more you'll be able to break the MIDI parts down into sections, but a sensible split might be between stereo drums and percussion, stereo keyboard pads, and mono lead line and mono basslines. This leaves a reasonable degree of scope for rebalancing, and if you do want to change a sound or add a new part, you only have to worry about the instruments in the affected subgroup – the rest can be left as they are.

Ultimately, how you decide to work depends on how many tape tracks you have at your disposal and on which method or combination of methods makes you feel most comfortable. No one method alone has all the answers, but knowing the strengths and weaknesses of each approach, you'll be better placed to formulate your own optimum work strategy.

Streamline Your Sequencing

Most of us work with sequencers, and computer-based systems seem the most popular. However, while people seem keen to spend lots of money on equipment, they tend to take less care on making sure they're working comfortably. Sitting at a badly positioned computer for any length of time soon results in back ache, neck ache and wrist ache, none of which help the creative process of writing music. Even though you might think that you do most of your work using the computer's mouse, put the keyboard in a position where typing on it feels comfortable.

Computer Monitors

Even a high-resolution monitor can cause eyestrain, so position the screen so that it's two to three feet from your eyes, not right in front of you. You should also use adequate ambient lighting so that you don't get dazzled by the screen. An anti-glare filter might help, but as long as you follow the above guidelines and don't set the screen brightness to high, you shouldn't have any problems. If you do find that your eyes are getting sore, consider buying a pair of VDU operator's spectacles. These have the same effect as an anti-glare screen but work out rather cheaper, especially if you work with a large monitor.

Flat-panel screens take up less space, which in turn means less obstruction of the sound from your monitor speakers. They also eliminate 'scan coil' radiation, which causes hum when working with electric guitars in close proximity to the monitor screen.

Always use a mouse mat, not the tabletop or the back of a book. Apart from making the mouse run more smoothly, it will also extend its life by reducing the amount of dust and grime that accumulates on the ball and internal rollers. I currently use a mouse mat with a built-in wrist rest, which I find really helps to stop my wrist from aching after a long day at the computer. If you're really short of desk space, consider using a trackball. Even optical mice run more smoothly on mats.

Efficient Sequencing

Most sequencers have a host of inbuilt features to make your life easier, but it's surprising how often these go unused. Here are a few tips that have worked for me.

• Create your own metronome. Rather than use the default metronome when recording, program a simple drum part to play along to. As well as providing you with a better feel, you'll also find it easier to keep time to. Most modern rhythms are based on four beats to the bar, so if you're using a conventional metronome, you're playing directly over the top of it, which in turn makes it difficult to hear. By adding a suitable hi-hat pattern, you're much more likely to stay in time.

Rather than re-invent the wheel every time you start work, it pays to save your guide percussion parts either in a separate song or as a part of your default song. That way, they'll always be available whenever you start a new song.

- If your sequencer doesn't have the facility to create a default song, create your own and store it on a locked floppy or as a locked file on your hard drive so that it can't be overwritten by accident. These locked files may then be opened and saved under a new name (using the 'Save As' command) without changing the original. A typical default song contains the MIDI channel and track assignment for your favourite instruments, any user options the software might provide (such as length of count-in and tempo) and various MIDI-status functions, such as MIDI Thru, MIDI Clock and so on. To set this manually every time you start a new song is obviously a chore you can do without.

- Use your keyboard. Just because most jobs can be tackled with the mouse, some things are faster and easier from the keyboard – if you can remember the commands. A useful trick is to print out all the main keyboard commands and put the printout under a transparent-topped mouse mat. Failing that, take the low-tech approach and pin it to the wall.

- Copy key documentation. The trouble with most MIDI systems is that you end up with a stack of manuals a foot thick. It helps enormously to photocopy the preset patch lists for all your instruments and also to type out the names and descriptions of your user patches and memory-card contents. These sheets may then be put into plastic sleeves and clipped into a single binder (marked 'Voices' or something similar) or pinned to the wall.

- Use custom screens. Some programs, such as Emagic's Logic, have a system for saving and accessing various screen layouts. In a program

where several windows might need to be open at once, this can be a real time saver, because a single key can bring up a screen layout you have previously specified with all the windows properly sized and in exactly the right place. The smaller your monitor, the more you'll appreciate this function. Without it, you spend most of your time opening and closing windows, dragging them about the screen and resizing them so you can see everything you need to.

- Don't over-quantise. Those who criticise electronic music for its robotic feel have probably heard the result of too much quantisation. It's true that some forms of music demand a rigid, robotic approach to timing, but if you want to keep the feel of the original performance, it may be better not to quantise at all – just use the sequencer as you would a tape recorder. If you feel your playing needs tightening up but you don't want it to sound lifeless, try the Percentage Quantise function, if your sequencer has one; this will bring your playing closer to the nearest tick but will still leave some of the original feel intact. On a more practical point, it also helps if you don't rigidly quantise everything, because doing so makes the sequencer attempt to play lots of notes at the same time. This creates a MIDI bottleneck and may lead to MIDI timing errors in a busy mix.

- If you have a part that needs to be played 'free' (ie without any specific tempo reference), simply turn down the click track, turn off all quantisation and record the part just as if you were using a tape recorder. If you have to make this part match up to a more rigidly quantised section that follows, you could either move the whole free section backwards or forwards in time until it matches the start of the first bar of the next section, or you could insert a couple of radical tempo changes between the point where the first section ends and the next section starts. Putting in a fraction of a bar of very low tempo will create a longer gap, while speeding up the tempo for a while will reduce the amount of time between the two sections.

- Back up your work. In fact, be paranoid about backing up – computers have a habit of crashing or locking up when you least expect it, so save your work every few minutes. When working with a hard drive, back up important work to floppies or to a second drive at the end of each session. Modern drives are reliable, but they're not infallible.

- Keep a notebook. Paper may be low-tech, but when you come across a six-month-old disk filled with MIDI files named something like 'Ideas 1–99', a few notes are worth their weight in gold.

- Don't re-invent the wheel. If you create your own MIDI control data for cyclic panning, or if you have an assortment of killer drum fills, hoard it. You can create your own MIDI equivalent of clip art so that, instead of always working from scratch, you can copy and paste various useful odds and ends from a library song.

MIDI Realism

Having covered the mechanics of operating an organised sequencing environment, I'd like to pass on a few tricks I've learned over the years for making sequenced parts sound more realistic. MIDI creates the false illusion that all instruments are perfectly in tune and perfectly in time, but of course real life isn't like that. In fact, if you try to emulate an instrument like bagpipes by playing the bagpipe preset on your GM synth module, it'll sound nothing like the real thing, even if you play the appropriate drone and melody notes. While I'm not suggesting that bagpipes are going to make it big in pop music, the following techniques are useful when emulating any instrument that has a detuned element associated with it. The melody line on a bagpipe is played on a pipe that has finger holes and is fitted with a reed, known as the *chanter*, which has a range of around an octave. The

remaining pipes (there may be up to six) are fixed in pitch and are known as *drones*. Air is supplied to the pipes by the player blowing into a tube connected to an air bag, which may be compressed under the arm to maintain a flow of air while the player breathes.

Detuned Drones

To simulate something like the bagpipes, it is essential to set up the drones slightly out of tune with each other, and the easiest way to achieve this is to record each note on a separate track of the sequencer and assign it to a different voice of a multitimbral synth. Of course, all the voices used must be set to a suitable-sounding bagpipe patch. Pitch-bend information is used to provide the detuning and may be recorded afterwards on a separate track if you don't want to add it as you play. Only a small amount is needed to achieve a convincing effect. It may also help to vary the pitch bend slightly, in which case the bend data may be looped, in order to save time. If different loop lengths are used for each drone, the whole thing sounds more natural. The melody line is played on yet another voice and may be left nominally in tune, although pitch bend can be used to push high notes very slightly off pitch in order to emulate the organic nature of the real instrument.

Droning Strings

The sitar is in many ways similar to the bagpipe, in that it features drone notes which tend to beat with each other. I've found that the drone notes may be played as a slowly arpeggiating chord using a sitar sound with a long sustain, and if you can edit the patch to slow the attack of the sound, the simulation is even more realistic. The natural chorusing of the strings can be faked by duplicating this track on another voice of the synth (possibly delayed by a bar or two) and then adding subtle amounts of pitch bend to create the necessary detuning. The lead line should be played on a different voice, using generous amounts of pitch bend to create the necessary quarter-tone bends and flourishes.

Talking Drums

While the rock drumkit is the mainstay of modern pop music, I have to confess a liking for ethnic percussion, including African talking drums, Indian tablas and so on. In order to create the characteristic pitch-modulation effect, you'll need a sampler, and a good starting point is a conga sample. You might think that a drum machine would do the trick, but most drum machines don't respond to pitch-bend data in the same way as synths do – the sounds don't actually change in pitch as the wheel is moved. What tends to happen is that the pitch of the drum sound depends on where the pitch-bend wheel was set just before the drum sound was triggered.

If you need the sound of two drums – for example, a pair of tablas – record the two onto different sequencer tracks so that you can apply pitch bend independently. In the case of something like tablas, you'll also need to use two different sound sources: one sharp and ringing, the other deep and sustaining.

The Random Element

On a recent album project, I needed an African percussion sound, but the usual toms, woodblocks, congas, shakers and whatever else the drum machine had to offer didn't really hit the spot. As an experiment, I added a loop of pitch-bend information which affected the whole of the drum machine, and immediately the percussion took on more of an ethnic, carnival feel. However, I still wasn't quite happy with it and decided that a gospel-style tambourine might help. Of course, the tambourine was also affected by the pitch-bend data, which transformed it from a commonplace sound to a mystical tribal instrument that really made the track. It also supplied the much-needed something going on at the top end that the track seemed to lack.

Wind Chimes

Wind chimes are popular in new-age and relaxation music, and there's no argument that miking up the real thing produces the most satisfying result. Even so, there are advantages to faking your own wind chimes on a sequencer, simply because, working in this way, you aren't limited to any one musical scale or sequence of notes.

Most wind chimes are based on commonly used scales or modes and have either six or eight chimes. If you're not sure which notes to use, check out a wind-chime catalogue to see which notes the various models produce. The whole point of a wind chime is that it produces random music, so sequencing it might seem pretty contradictory, but by recording each note on a separate sequencer track and then setting up different lengths of repeating pattern on each track, you can end up with an overall pattern that repeats only every several hundred bars – which in most instances is as near to random as makes no difference.

Each sequencer track must be recorded with a random pattern of the same note, and it is imperative not to make the part too busy. Instead, spread the beats between one quarter and three seconds apart. The individual track-sequence lengths can be anything from four bars long to as long as you like, and the longer the loops, the more random the result will appear.

Finally, choose your favourite bell or chime patch and set the thing running. The tempo value is roughly equivalent to wind speed. You could even throw in a few tempo changes to simulate gusts!

Use Your Imagination

Most of the above examples – other than the wind chimes – rely on using more than one synth voice at a time to create a sound, but with so many inexpensive multitimbral modules around, this isn't really as extravagant as it might appear. These techniques really work, and once you're tried them out, other ideas spring to mind, such as simulating instruments that play the same notes in unison (such as the top two strings of a 12-string guitar) or even programming guitar power chords where the same note(s) often occur(s) twice. In fact, few real instruments are as clinically in tune as a digital synth, and it's surprising how often vitality can be added to a patch with a little contrived chorusing (applied by using pitch bend on duplicated tracks – chorus units are too regular to produce the same result).

Other tricks to try include adding loops of gentle vibrato-wheel data to a flute or other solo instrument track that's been played straight, or you can create complex percussion parts by using several tracks, all with different loop lengths, just as in the wind chimes simulation. It all goes to show that, even if you use only five per cent of the features in your sequencer, you can still do a lot of creative things with it using sound modules you already own.

Guitar Synths And Controllers

MIDI guitars have had a pretty chequered history, and it's probably fair to say that they still have their fair share of problems, but there are various strategies that can be adopted to make the best use of their unique capabilities. However, it's vital that players adapt their playing technique to meet them halfway. For those guitar players who don't feel comfortable with keyboards and who are prepared to adapt their playing technique where necessary, MIDI guitars provide a means with which to interact with sequencers.

Preparation

Getting to grips with different sounds is something that electronic-keyboard players have always had to do, but guitar players are conditioned to expect every sound they play to have an instant, percussive attack. Give a rock-guitar player a brass patch with a slow attack and he'll probably complain that the synth can't keep up with him. What he really should be saying is that the attack time of the instrument is too long to allow the notes to develop at the speed he's trying to play. A tuba player isn't likely to attempt double-time triplets, so why expect a tuba synth patch to be able to?

The most common MIDI guitar systems work on the principle of tracking the pitch of a regular guitar, and it is very important that any guitar you intend using with such a system is properly set up. To track the pitch of individual strings, pitch-to-MIDI systems for guitar are invariably based around a split pickup that has a separate pickup section for each string. This split pickup should be mounted as close to

the bridge of the guitar as possible, and the spacing between the pickup and the strings should be around 1mm when the string is fretted on the highest fret. This may differ slightly from model to model, so consult your handbook. It is important that the strings pass over the centre of each section of the divided pickup in order to avoid crosstalk between adjacent strings.

Fret buzz causes pitch-tracking problems, so if your action needs sorting out, you're best off paying to get it done properly if you can't do it yourself. In my experience, very low actions and guitar synths don't mix.

Technical Problems

Even when using a divided pickup to separate the strings, the action of picking a string creates a leading transient that is more noise than pitch, and until this has passed, there's little point in the circuitry trying to make sense of the signal. This results in a slight time delay between the string being plucked and the note being established; the string has to vibrate in a meaningful way before its frequency can be measured. The lower the frequency of the note, the longer its wavelength and the longer the delay. On a good system, the delay is virtually imperceptible, apart from on the bottom string or two, where it should be apparent only when you try to play very fast parts.

Even when the pitch has stabilised, there are other 'polluting' factors waiting to corrupt the pure tone, such as fret buzz or interference from other electrical equipment in the room, especially computer monitors. Although this interference isn't audible over MIDI, it can seriously affect the accuracy of tracking.

On most guitars, the level of the harmonics produced when a note is picked is comparable with the level of the fundamental pitch, which makes it harder for the tracking circuitry to lock onto the right frequency. Some instruments have rogue 'dead spots' at certain positions on the fingerboard, where the fundamental frequency dies away faster than the second harmonic, which can lead to certain notes jumping up by an octave as they decay.

Note On And Off

The start of a note is triggered by the action of picking a string, but the end of a note can be less easy to define. If the string is allowed simply to vibrate, the synth will continue to play until the note has decayed to a level that is too low to track reliably. Depending on the guitar and the model of guitar synth, this can be anything from a few seconds to tens of seconds. A note may also be terminated by damping a string with the right hand or by lifting the fingers of the left hand off the strings. In the case of synth voicings which have a long release time, damping the strings provides a more controlled way to end a note, since lifting the fingers from the strings in the usual fashion can cause the pitch of the sustained note to drop a little during the release period.

MIDI Guitar Playing Tips

• Many of the traditional techniques used to make guitars sound interesting are counter-productive when playing a guitar synth. For example, using the side of your thumb to dig in as you pick is great for producing squealing harmonics, but such harmonics can fool the tracking system of your synth into playing the wrong note. Plain picking may be boring, but it will produce the best results.

• Strumming chords, especially when damped, seldom works with guitar synths. These very valid playing techniques sound fine on guitar, but in reality they comprise a lot of unpitched noise, which will cause the guitar synth to mistrack in an embarrassingly unpredictable way. If you're using a piano sound, think what a piano player might do – try an arpeggio or a simple finger-picking pattern instead of strumming.

• Instruments like the piano have a rigidly fixed pitch. If you want your piano sound to be authentic, don't bend the notes or use the tremolo arm. If your guitar synth has a Bend Off function, this might produce better results when playing piano or organ lines.

• Don't think like a guitar player. Instead, think as if you are playing the instrument you're imitating. For example, if you're playing a solo flute patch, don't play chords as flutes are monophonic. Use note bends and the tremolo arm to simulate the way in which vibrato is applied to the instrument. Similarly, listen to the way your instrument is orchestrated. String parts can sound more convincing if you use just two or three notes at a time rather than six-note chords. If the sound you're using has a slow attack, play slow, uncomplicated parts in order to let the sound develop. If the slow attack throws your timing, listen to the sound of your pick on the guitar and take your timing cues from that.

• If your guitar synthesiser produces a noticeable delay on the bottom strings, try playing the part one or two octaves higher and then try using the Transpose function on the synth to bring the pitch of the synthesised sound back to where you want it. This will reduce the tracking delay considerably. Of course, the tracking delay doesn't matter at all on sounds that have particularly slow attacks, such as strings or atmospheric pads.

• Because you never know exactly how long a plucked note will sustain, use the hold pedal for long chords. This will also prevent any octave jumping if you happen to hit a rogue note.

• Some systems have the ability to transpose the synth sounds for each individual string on the guitar. This can be useful to create more authentic instrument sounds. For example, if you drop the bottom two strings by an octave, piano parts will sound more 'two-handed', while a string part can be made to appear like a combination of violins and basses. If your guitar synth doesn't have this feature, it is often possible to achieve the same result 'offline' by using your sequencer's Note Range, Track Copy and Transpose functions.

- Most people don't appreciate how much the amplified sound of a guitar affects the way in which the strings vibrate. When using a MIDI guitar patch that's, say, an octave above the regular guitar pitch, the sound from the monitors can affect the string vibrations so that they emphasise the second harmonic, which may consequently aggravate pitch jumping. The solution is to record while monitoring at a modest level, or to use headphones.

- Keep well away from computer monitors. Find a position in the room where the interference on the regular pickup is at a minimum and you should get the best possible tracking.

- Always ensure that your guitar synth and any expander modules are set to the same MIDI pitch-bend range.

- To record a guitar part using complex string bends, the sequencer must be set to record on all six MIDI channels simultaneously.

- Guitar synths tend to generate occasional spurious, low-velocity, short-duration notes due to handling noise while being played. These can often be cleaned up by using the 'Delete Notes Shorter Than...' function on your sequencer. Similarly, double-triggered notes can be removed by using the 'Check For Duplicated Notes' function.

- If the slow attack of the sound you're using is making it hard to play in time, pick an alternative sound with a more positive attack while recording the part. You can easily switch back to the original sound once the part has been recorded in your sequencer. Alternatively, monitor the conventional guitar sound as played through a practice amp.

- Make full use of any sustain- or hold-pedal functions available to help when playing sustained chords. Such functions as 'Note Length Quantise' and 'Force Legato' can also be used to good effect to recreate certain musical styles.

- Because the MIDI data from a guitar synth is always slightly late, timing-wise, try applying the 'Negative Delay Time' function on your sequencer to bring the existing sequencer tracks (especially the drum part) forward by a few tens of a millisecond while recording the guitar synth. This will fool you into playing a little early, and experimentation will determine what negative delay time is right to offset the inherent delay of the synth. You can then use quantisation if further precision is required, but over-quantisation can easily ruin the feel of a performance. If your sequencer has it, try using the 'Percentage Quantise' function. Don't forget to turn off the negative delay once the guitar part has been recorded.

Guitar Synths And MIDI

Some MIDI guitar systems come with their own sound modules, and these are often driven directly from the tracking circuitry rather than via MIDI. Although the sounds can also be accessed over MIDI, the outcome is that any parts played live using the synth's own internal voices are likely to track more accurately and with less delay than going via MIDI. If you're working with tape, it stands to reason that the more virtuoso parts of a composition might be best played live onto tape rather than recorded into a sequencer. You can still use a punch-in/out footswitch to help you replace any mistakes.

One way in which modern guitar-synth designers have found to improve note-tracking is to use MIDI pitch-bend controller information to correct the pitch of the tracked note on a continual basis. Hammer-ons tend to be implemented entirely by pitch-bend information, so if you're working with a sequencer, the notes you see on the Edit page may be a little different from what you actually played – for example, a hammer-on trill will be shown as a single picked note followed by a lot of pitch-bend controller data.

Mono Or Poly Mode?

To enable each string of a guitar to be used for independent note bends over MIDI, each guitar string must be handled by a different MIDI channel. The most guitar-like results are achieved via a synth that can work in MIDI mode 4; in effect, this puts each guitar string in control of its own monosynth. Even when there is no intention to bend notes, it is essential to stick with the one-channel/one-string approach if hammer-ons and slides are to be tracked accurately.

How well a guitar synth works with an external synth seems to vary depending on the model of synth expander being used. The tracking delay is usually increased slightly, but unless your MIDI instruments are very slow to respond, this need not be a major problem.

There are occasions when it can be advantageous simply to plug the guitar synth into a module set to Poly mode. Although bends, hammers and slides can't be used in this mode, it does provide a reasonably reliable way of triggering simple parts such as block chords or straight melody lines.

MIDI Guitar Strengths

One of the most powerful performance techniques at the guitar player's disposal is the ability to apply finger vibrato to individual strings with variable depth and rate, which makes things like 'cello emulation very realistic. Another strength is the way in which more conventional guitar sounds can be layered with synth voices to create a unique hybrid sound that still retains some of the organic characteristics of a 'real' instrument. In addition to providing guitarists with access to an almost unlimited range of sounds, working with a guitar synth seems to stimulate new ideas. You will almost certainly find yourself heading in new musical directions that might never have occurred to you while playing either a conventional guitar or a keyboard synth.

Quick And Easy Synth Sounds

Modern synthesisers are capable of producing a vast range of sounds, but in-depth sound design is a time-consuming process that requires a lot of skill and experience to do well. Most of the time, we'd rather get on with making music, but sticking with the factory presets can be very limiting, so here are a few things to try out which will give you lots of new sounds while having to spend very little time editing.

Sound Envelopes

Perhaps the simplest way to change the character of a sound is to change its attack and release settings – after all, how many times have you called up a string patch that's almost exactly what you want, but it hasn't quite got enough sustain, or the attack comes in too quickly? Rule 1 is to make sure that you know how to get directly to the envelope parameters, if nothing else. Some modern synthesisers have a Global Edit option which enables you to change the envelope characteristics of a complete patch rather than having to edit each of the individual elements that make up that particular patch.

Sound Layering

Layering two or more sounds to produce one new sound is a common trick, but there are a few techniques that can help to make it more effective. Layering lends itself best to ensemble sounds such as choirs, strings or pads, but it can also be used on drums or bass lines. I find that layering synth choirs with sampled vocals is particularly effective.

• Inject a sense of ensemble playing by copying a part played in real time (unquantised) to a new sequencer track and then quantising the copy. If you need to quantise the original part, try using the Randomise function to introduce small timing changes into the duplicate part.

• Use the sequencer Delay function to delay one track slightly with respect to the other. This also helps create a bigger ensemble effect.

• To liven up a layered string or choir sound, tune one part up by a couple of cents and the other part down. This creates a far more natural chorus effect than you'd get with a chorus processor.

- Try layering a digital string sound or sample with an analogue string pad. The analogue pad will help to warm up the digital sound and smoothe off some of the rough edges.

- Interesting results can sometimes be achieved by using sequencer edit functions to remove some of the notes in a copy part. For example, a busy string part could be copied and the copy stripped down to its simplest form, leaving out any fast runs or flourishes. The note lengths of the edited part could then be increased where required.

- In a sequencer which has a Force Legato function, a copied track may be transformed into something quite different to the original sound. When the two parts are layered, this can sound very effective, although the occasional discordance is possible, which will have to be edited out manually.

- When trying to create a natural choir sound, you may find you have several modules, all of which provide choir patches, but none of which sounds right in isolation. One problem is that such sounds can have obvious loop and keyboard split points. However, by layering two or more sounds from different instruments (or even from different parts of the same multitimbral instrument), these artifacts are disguised. Layer a male choir with a female choir that has a slower attack and you'll create the illusion that the singers are coming in at different times, giving a natural lift to the sound. It can also be effective if the female choir comes in one octave above the male choir. Setting different vibrato rates on the different layers also helps to open up the sound.

- Pan the different layers to different parts of the soundstage. This not only widens the sound but, if you've chosen patches with different attack times, it will add a welcome degree of movement to the sound.

- Marimba and vibe parts can be made more interesting by copying the track and then both transposing and delaying the copy. The delay time should be just enough to create a mild 'flam' effect. Although octaves work well, try transposing by fifths as well, if the music allows it, and adjust the relative balance of the two parts if necessary. Also consider using two different marimba patches or layering a marimba with a vibe patch or some other form of tuned percussion.

- Never forget that old and obsolete synth that's lying in the corner, even if it sounds a bit weak in isolation. Using a short, percussive bass sound on one synth and a more sustained sound on the other can also create dramatic new sounds that are far better than might be expected from either of the original patches.

- Never be restricted by the name of a patch. A piano sound with a slow attack sounds almost sitar-like, while a bass sound pushed up a couple of octaves becomes a new lead instrument. Flutes or pipes can be dropped a couple of octaves to provide a demonic backdrop to a choir, while percussive sounds such as cow bells, tambourines and ethnic drums can be layered with conventional synth-bass sounds to provide an interesting attack.

Mix The Unexpected

When layering, you aren't restricted to sounds from the same instrument family, nor do they have to be complementary instruments, as exemplified by the innumerable piano-and-string layers you come across. To create a new-sounding picked instrument, for example, you can combine virtually any sounds, providing they have suitably fast attacks, and you'll find that sounds such as harpsichords, guitars, hammer dulcimers, bass guitars tuned up by an octave or two, pianos and so on all work well together. The result is often an instrument that has some of the characteristics of its component sounds but, at the same time, has a distinctive character of its own. One example of this type of layering that works exceptionally well is the addition of a short, percussive sound such as a stick click or noise burst to the start of a conventional synth-bass sound. This really adds attack and definition to the note without robbing it of any of its depth.

You can still create radically new sounds from familiar patches by making use of just two simple facts: firstly, the brain relies heavily on the attack characteristics of an instrument in order to recognise it, and secondly, familiar sounds can seem quite different when transposed up or down from their normal range. Take a GM piano sound – give it a slow attack and straight away you lose the identity of the piano and end up with an abstract, bowed sound. Similarly, take a mandolin – drop it by a couple of octaves and notice how much more pronounced the attack part of the sound becomes. High flutes can be dropped in pitch to provide deep pipe sounds while a bass sound can be raised a couple of octaves to provide a new lead instrument. Slow brass can be given a fast percussive attack, church bells can be given a slow attack to create a haunting quality – in fact there's little limit to what you can achieve simply by experimenting with the Level Envelope and Voice Transpose parameters of your synth.

After experimenting for a little while, you'll start to realise that even the most apparently pedestrian patches can be given a new meaning, and it often helps to forget about the original patch name and concentrate solely on the sounds you can wring out of it.

Real Meets Abstract

Another approach to creating your own sounds through layering is to try combining one recognisable sound with one abstract sound. Simple filter-sweep pads sit alongside string samples quite happily, but you might also find that layering the attack part of a distorted guitar with a piano provides you with a less predictable alternative to your existing piano or clav patches. More exotic results still can be achieved by layering unpitched sounds such as water bells with tuned percussive noises such as woodblocks or marimbas.

Pseudo-Morphing

Another of my favourite techniques is to find two sounds or instruments that have some tonal element in common and then crossfade from one to the other as the note evolves. This can be achieved simply by adjusting the envelopes of the two sounds so that the second is building up as the first is dying away. Human voices are similar in many ways to reed instruments, flutes and violins, and if you choose the right crossfade rate (simply by using the normal level envelope parameters for each sound), you can create quite an eerie morphing effect that sounds far more subtle than the crossfade it really is. Brass pads merge nicely into strings, different types of wind instrument can be merged one into the other, and choirs can be merged into just about any smooth pad sound. My current favourite is a patch that starts out as a clarinet and then moves into a slightly electronic-sounding voice created from a voice waveform rather than from a full vocal sample. There's just something very evocative about these crossfades, but you never know if the combination has the necessary magic until you try it. The secret is to match the fade-out rate of the first sound to the fade-in rate of the second sound so that the patch level remains nominally constant during the changeover.

Hybrid Sounds

Crossfading can also be used to graft the attack of one sound onto the sustain of another, which can yield some musically interesting hybrids. Earlier on I mentioned that the attack of an instrument provides strong clues as to what that instrument is, so if you take something like a plucked attack and then quickly merge into a wind or string sustain sound, you surprise the hearing system and make it pay attention.

Synth Effects

Effects are part of the sound-creation process and not just something to dress up an existing sound. If a string preset has too short a release time and you can't change it easily, add a long reverb instead. This will at least get you by until the song is complete, after which you can worry about creating a more suitable patch.

- To create an novel layered effect, use a pitch shifter to add one octave up to the original sound and then use reverb to smoothe out the shifted sound. If this is used at a low enough level in the mix, it can sound quite natural.

- Instead of simply adding reverb to a sound, try using just the reverbed sound with none of the dry sound present at all. This works well when you're layering similar sounds but can also be useful in creating a brand new texture. Try patching chorus or flanging before the reverb to add more movement and interest to the result.

- Drum sounds can be beefed up by being fed through a guitar pre-amp with a hint of overdrive, and the same is true of synth-pad and organ sounds. Even without overdrive, the speaker-simulator section of a guitar pre-amp or studio multi-effects unit can add warmth to a hard digital sound.

- If you're layering sounds, try applying different effects to the different parts to add further variety. For example, try flanging one part of a choir layer while adding delay or reverb to the other. Light flanging is immensely useful for adding movement to choir, string and pad patches without sounding overdone.

- Don't be afraid to abuse effects. Deliberately overdriving a reverb unit might sound disastrous on vocals but can work magic on a snare-drum sound.

- Use a triggered gate to chop up a sustained sound rhythmically. This is an easy way to create a driving bass for a dance track, and again a percussive sound may be layered over the chopped sound for that added weight.

- Don't be afraid to go low-tech. Borrow the guitar player's wah-wah pedal and try your synth through that. Even if you don't want to reproduce the clichéd wah-wah sound, you can always park it in one position and use it as a very selective equaliser.

This is just a small selection of the things you can do to broaden your range of sounds without spending too much time editing. Third-party soundcards and disks can also be a useful source of variety, and there's nothing defeatist in using these – after all, the violin player doesn't feel guilty that Stradivarius, and not he, built the instrument he's playing. You don't have to use these sounds just as they are – they can be twisted and manipulated in all the ways described in this article – and once you start to experiment, you're certain to come up with other techniques that work for you. When it comes to music, the end always justifies the means.

Transferring Sequencer Files

If you need to transfer a file from one sequencer to another, unless a specific file-translation facility exists between the sequencers you intend to work with, you'll need to save the sequence as a Standard MIDI File. However, as with most standards, things aren't quite as cut and dried as they might seem, as there are actually three different versions of Standard MIDI File.

- **Format 0** – In this format, the entire song is saved as just one sequencer track, which means some unravelling is needed in order to separate the tracks.

- **Format 1** – In this format, the tracks are kept separate but any pattern information is lost, so the whole song is effectively transferred as a single pattern.

- **Format 2** – This is similar to format 1, but pattern information is also retained.

Format 1 is the most commonly encountered

Standard MIDI File type, but even then, you may find the tracks don't load into the sequencer with their original MIDI channel numbers, and sometimes they lose their names, too. This isn't a fault of the file structure itself but rather depends on how the sequencer creating the file deals with Standard MIDI Files. Restoring the original order is usually fairly straightforward, providing you've kept a note as to what instruments are supposed to be playing on what MIDI channels.

Unfortunately, Standard MIDI Files only cater for standard 16-channel MIDI data – they don't yet convey MIDI port information (although some progress in this area seems imminent), so if you're using a multiport interface you may have to save the channels allocated to each port as separate SMFs and then load these into the destination sequencer one file at a time, resetting the MIDI port data before loading in the next set of channels. This is tedious, but at least it's possible.

Atari disks are compatible with PC machines, and vice versa, but you have to keep in mind that an Atari can't read a high-density floppy; double-density disks are fine, but HDs can't be read. Apple Macs can also read PC-format disks, as long as either System 7.5 or above is in use or a file-exchange utility program (such as AccessPC) is installed. However, some hardware sequencers have their own file formats, so they can't read disks from desktop computers.

Non-Disk Transfer

Even if you find you're working on machines with incompatible disk formats, it should still be possible to transfer files over MIDI by playing them out of one sequencer while at the same time recording them into the other. However, there is a potential problem in that most sequencers are better at outputting lots of MIDI data than they are at inputting it, so you could end up with a MIDI traffic jam which will corrupt the note timing. In order to avoid this problem, the receiving sequencer needs to be set up as master and the sending sequencer as the slave. The following steps outline the procedure.

- Connect the two sequencers together with MIDI leads so that the MIDI Out of each machine feeds the MIDI In of the other, as shown in Figure 6.4

- Set the source sequencer to External Sync mode. It must be clocked by the destination sequencer to ensure optimum timing accuracy. The destination sequencer must be set to Internal Sync mode. If the destination sequencer has a Soft MIDI Thru function, switch this off to minimise the amount of data sharing the MIDI Out with the timing clock, making the timing of the transfer more accurate.

- Set the destination sequencer to record MIDI data, but set a slow tempo in order to give the best possible timing accuracy. (The original tempo can be restored once the transfer has been made.) A tempo of around 50bpm should be OK, but if the track is particularly busy, you could go even lower.

- Start the destination sequencer recording and the transmitting sequencer will automatically start in sync with it. Let the sequencers run until the data transfer is complete.

Note: If you're still getting timing problems, the only option is to transfer a few tracks at a time, maybe even just one track at a time. Repeat the procedure exactly as before, selecting a suitable destination track but with all the source sequencer's tracks muted except for the one you want to transfer. Record the track as before and then, when the recording is complete, select a new source track and a new destination track and repeat the procedure. Continue until all the tracks have been transmitted. Any tempo changes will need to be entered manually into the new sequence file.

If you're using a multiport MIDI interface and you have more than 16 tracks to transfer, you should transfer the data from one port at a time and then reroute the tracks once they've been safely received.

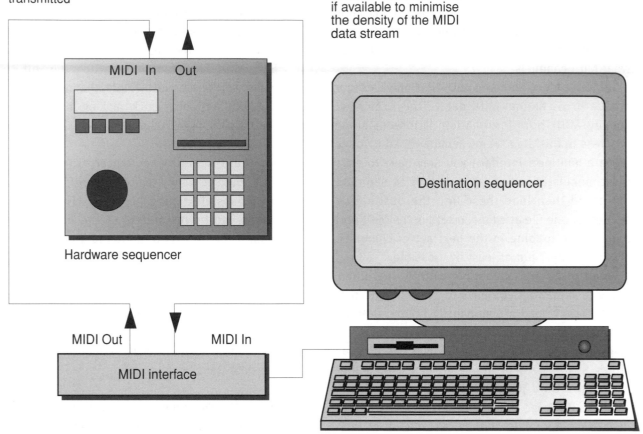

Source sequencer set to External MIDI Sync so that the destination sequencer can control how fast the data is transmitted

Turn off Soft MIDI Thru if available to minimise the density of the MIDI data stream

MIDI In   Out

Destination sequencer

Hardware sequencer

MIDI Out   MIDI In

MIDI interface

Destination sequencer set to Internal MIDI Sync so that it acts as the timing master. If timing problems arise, reduce the tempo of the destination sequencer until the transfer is accurate. In extreme cases, it may be necessary to mute some source tracks, then transmit just a few tracks at a time. Once the data has been transferred, tempo data and tempo changes (where used) must be entered manually. It will also be necessary to separate the transferred data by MIDI channel, as most sequencers will record it as a single composite track

Figure 6.4: Transferring songs between sequencers

Tidying Up

If you successfully transferred all of your song data in one pass, you'll find that your whole song now occupies a single track in the destination sequencer. Fortunately, most sequencers have a 'Separate By MIDI Channel' function that automatically places the data into new tracks based on MIDI channel. If you don't have such a function, you'll have to sort through the data manually, in which case it may actually be quicker to transfer the song a track at a time.

MIDI INSTRUMENT QUICK FIXES
Low-Output Synths

A number of the synths and sound modules that have found favour in home recording produce very low-level outputs designed to interface with hi-fi equipment rather than serious mixing consoles. The outcome is that you have to turn the mixer's line gain to maximum in order to get enough level, which also tends to increase the level of background noise. But is there a better way?

One solution is to feed the output from the instrument into one of your console's mic inputs (or pair of inputs in the case of a stereo instrument). Mic inputs have far more gain available than line inputs, which means that shortage of gain is no longer a problem, but there are a couple of points to watch:

- You'll need the right kind of lead – synths have mainly unbalanced jack or phono outputs, whereas mic inputs are balanced and on XLRs. You'll need to buy or make up a cable with an unbalanced jack at one end and an XLR plug at the other. The hot signal from the tip of the jack should be connected to pin 2 of the XLR plug while the screen should be connected to both pins 1 and 3 of the XLR.

- IMPORTANT: Make sure that phantom power isn't applied to the mic input to which your synth is

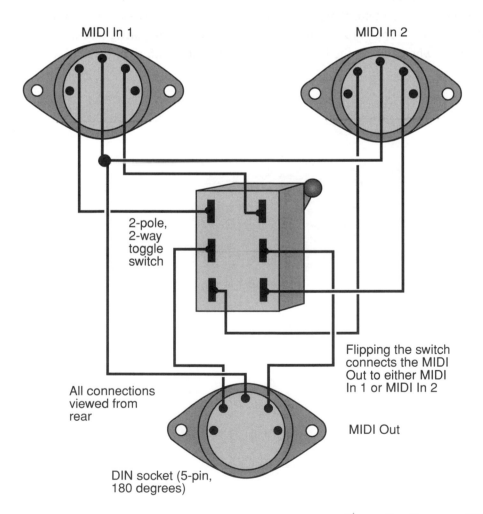

Figure 6.5: Two-way MIDI switch box

connected. If it is, there's a very real possibility that the synth's output stage will sustain damage.

Synth Impedance Problems

Very occasionally you'll come across a synth module that has both a low-level output and a higher than normal output impedance. In this case, the mic input of the mixer will present a load impedance that's just too low and may compromise the sound. The best option in this case is to use an active DI box with a high-input impedance. Most of these may be phantom powered and they simply connect between the instrument and a console line input. For a stereo instrument, you'll either need a two-channel DI box or two mono DI boxes.

Simple MIDI Switch

Even in the simplest MIDI system, there's often a need to switch between one MIDI source and another. For example, when editing, the input to the computer often needs to be taken from the output of the instrument in question, while the multi-instrumentalist might need to switch between a master keyboard, a MIDI guitar and a set of MIDI drum pads. A programmable MIDI patchbay can take all this in its stride, but if you don't have one, you can still get the job done by making your own hardware MIDI switcher.

The diagram in Figure 6.5 shows a simple two-in/one-out MIDI switch box based around a two-pole, two-way toggle switch. However, multiple inputs can be accommodated just as easily by using a rotary two-pole wafer switch. Wafer switches are available with various numbers of positions – I use a four-position switch in my own studio to give me four possible MIDI Ins – and suitable switches are available from most good electronics component suppliers. They should also be able to supply you with suitable plastic cases, which have the benefits of being both cheap and easy to drill.

7 MEDIA AND EQUIPMENT MAINTENANCE

While analogue multitrack machines are now something of a novelty everywhere except second-hand markets or the studios of analogue devotees, there are still significant numbers of older open-reel machines in service, who knows how many cassette multitracker and countless millions of stereo cassette decks worldwide. What all these machines have in common is that, in order to function properly, they must be cleaned and serviced on a regular basis – and proper cleaning means more than running a dry head-cleaning tape once every six months.

Analogue Recorders

There are several factors that can cause a cassette or open-reel analogue machine to perform at less than its best, but by far the most common is inadequate cleaning. Indeed, some people admit to never cleaning their machines! Forget all about head-cleaning tapes – they don't work well enough. To do the job properly, you'll need a pack of ordinary cotton buds – ideally those with wooden stalks – and a bottle of pure isopropyl alcohol.

Head Access

Cleaning open-reel machines is essentially the same as cleaning cassette decks and cassette multitrackers, the main difference being that the heads and guides on cassette decks aren't as easy to get at as they are on open-reel recorders. If your cassette deck has a removable door, this will provide better access, but even without this you should be able to reach the heads, capstan shaft and tape guides using your cotton buds. Dislodged particles of tape oxide build up to form a hard, dark-brown layer on the heads,

causing a loss of top end or even dropouts, but oxide also builds up on the tape guides, where it can interfere with the smooth passage of the tape over the heads. Audible effects include wow and flutter (a dithering of pitch) and a phasey kind of sound as the tape snakes across the heads in an uneven way.

Cleaning Method

Using a cotton bud soaked in the alcohol, clean the record and playback heads, the capstan and all the guides, then repeat the process using a new cotton bud. You may have to rub quite hard if the heads haven't been cleaned for some time, and keep on cleaning until the cotton bud comes away clean and no more oxide can be seen on the heads. Repeat the process for any parts touched by the tape, including the guides and capstan, but try not to let alcohol run into the capstan bearings as it could dissolve the grease, resulting in accelerated bearing wear.

If the deck is left switched on, you might find that the capstan rotates obligingly, which means that cleaning it is simply a case of holding a moistened cotton bud against it for a while. Ensure that no cotton fibres get wrapped around the capstan – if they do, you'll need to remove them.

Once everything is clean, swab off any excess alcohol with a dry cotton bud and wait a couple of minutes for any remaining alcohol to evaporate before putting a tape into the machine, or you might find the tape sticks to the capstan and gets jammed in the machine. Figure 7.1 shows a typical cassette-deck head and tape-guide layout. The layout for an open-reel machine is very similar – it's just that all the parts are bigger and so may take longer to get clean.

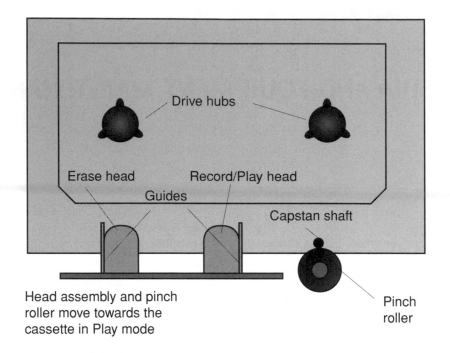

Head assembly and pinch roller move towards the cassette in Play mode

Use alcohol to clean:
Heads
Metal guides
Capstan shaft

Use detergent solution to clean:
Pinch roller and any other plastic or rubber parts

Note: Take care not to let alcohol run into the capstan or other bearings as it may dissolve the grease, compromising lubrication and causing accelerated bearing wear

Figure 7.1: Layout of a typical cassette-deck head

Rubber Pinch Rollers

The rubber pinch roller also tends to collect oxide, which eventually causes the surface to become slippy, resulting in tape slippage and speed instability. Although alcohol will remove the oxide, it may also damage the rubber, so a different cleaning agent is required. Proprietary rubber-cleaning fluids are available, but most of these are simply weak solutions of detergent in water. A drop of washing-up liquid in a cup of water works fine, and as with heads, the aim is to keep cleaning until no more brown oxide comes off on the cotton bud.

Make sure you clean the heads thoroughly before every important recording project and, in any event, at least once a week. Inspect the pinch roller regularly and clean it whenever you see signs of oxide build-up.

Demagnetisation

Analogue tape recorders of both cassette and open-reel varieties contain many ferrous metal parts, and if any of these are allowed to become magnetised, not only will the quality of your recordings suffer but previously OK tapes played back on the machine may start to lose their high frequencies. To prevent this from happening, all of the heads and guides should be demagnetised once a month or so as a routine precaution.

For open-reel machines, you'll need a hand-held demagnetiser, and it's important to follow the instructions very carefully. The device must be switched on well away from the tape machine (which MUST be switched off), then brought towards the machine quite slowly so as to allow the demagnetising field to build up slowly. The demagnetiser is then passed slowly over the heads and guides before being slowly withdrawn to a safe distance (about the length of the mains cable is OK) prior to switching off. A slow withdrawal is necessary as it is the gradual reduction of the alternating demagnetising field that neutralises the magnetic charge held by the tape-machine parts.

Cassette Demagnetisers

Although a conventional open-reel tape demagnetiser may be used on a cassette deck, the battery-powered, automatic types that come built into dummy cassette shells are easier to use and seem to work OK. If you don't already own a demagnetiser, I'd recommend that you buy one of the cassette types, which are available from most hi-fi stores. Because there's no easy way to measure the magnetic charge build-up, routine preventative demagnetising is the only practical measure you can take.

Tape-Machine Alignment

Like open-reel machines, cassette decks have to be aligned, a job which is done at the factory and, in most cases, never gets done again unless the machine is sent in for a major service. Because most cassette decks use the same head to both play and record, they'll often play back their own tapes without too many problems, even if the head is quite severally out of alignment. However, play that same tape on another cassette deck that is aligned properly (or differently) and the result will be a noticeable lack of brightness, clarity and possibly level. You may even end up with one track significantly louder than the other, and if you're using noise reduction, the audible effects of any alignment problems will be exaggerated. For this reason, it's worthwhile having the alignment of your studio cassette deck checked and adjusted if necessary, a task that any

reputable hi-fi service department will be able to carry out. This still doesn't guarantee that you won't have any incompatibility problems if people try to play back your tapes on other poorly aligned machines, but at least your copies will be correct.

All of these problems can also occur on open-reel machines, and while it is possible to carry out your own alignment with the aid of a test tape and a CD of test tones, it's advisable to have somebody take you through the process before you try it for the first time. Alternatively, have your machine checked over every few months by a service centre.

Speed Check

All standard cassette decks are supposed to run at a standard speed of 17/8 inches per second (some cassette multitrackers run at twice this speed), but not all machines are set up accurately at the factory, and even if they were, the settings can drift over time. If you don't want your clients complaining about tapes having the wrong tempo or pitch, you should get the speed of your cassette deck checked by a service technician. Again, this problem won't affect tapes recorded and played back on the same machine, but as soon as you put the tape in a different machine, the tempo and pitch will be different.

Noise-Reduction Alignment

Noise-reduction systems are also a source of incompatibility between different cassette machines, not only because of the different types available but also because they are subject to misalignment problems. Mechanical head misalignment will cause the noise reduction to work improperly, but there are also electrical adjustments that can further compromise the performance of the noise-reduction system. These types of adjustment are beyond the means of most end users and so should be entrusted to a service centre.

Dolby B is still the standard noise-reduction system for mass-duplicated tapes, but as many car cassette machines aren't equipped with Dolby my preference is to record cassettes without noise reduction at all. As long as the brand and type of cassette is good, and as long as you record at as high a signal level as possible, noise is unlikely to be unduly obtrusive unless you're recording classical music with a wide dynamic range. In any event, a little hiss is less of a problem than a wrong tonal balance. Even if your machine is set up perfectly, consumer machines are notorious for their poor standard of set-up, so it's still best to leave the noise reduction switched off when recording and evaluating cassette demos.

Mechanics

Analogue tape recorders are machines, with lots of moving parts, and like all machines, they need maintenance. Other than head and tape-guide alignment, a tape recorder needs lubrication, and every once in a while parts subject to excessive wear, such as rubber drive belts and brake pads, will need to be replaced. Eventually, the heads will also need to be replaced, and although there are no hard-and-fast figures for head life, it is usually reckoned that analogue heads will last for something over 1,000 hours of normal use. Their precise life expectancy depends on the design of the head itself, the abrasive properties of the tape being used and how regularly the heads are cleaned. On more professional machines, worn heads can be relapped to restore the correct profile.

Failure of any of mechanical parts or heads will be picked up during a routine service, but be warned that open-reel multitrack heads can be surprisingly expensive. Take this into account when considering buying a second-hand machine.

Analogue Tape

All analogue machines are delivered set up for a certain type and brand of tape – all tapes have different magnetic characteristics, so it's impossible to make a machine that works equally well with all of them. For example, the bias, record and playback circuits of the machine have to be set up to give a flat frequency response with a specific type of tape. Having said that, some types of tapes have similar enough characteristics to be interchangeable, and it's not at all uncommon to find that a machine performs better with a brand other than that recommended.

If you can afford it, use type II (chrome type) tapes in cassette decks rather than ferric, and as well as the tape recommended for your machine, try out a selection of equivalents from other top manufacturers to see if one or more of them performs better. To do this, record a selection of pieces of music from DAT or CD, then listen carefully for overall tonal balance. Quite often, the bass end or overall tonal balance will sound wrong if the cassette type is unsuitable.

At the top end, listen for over-brightness, dullness or sibilant distortion on bright sounds such as hi-hats. Finally, listen to the overall sound and try to judge whether it sounds as clear as the original or whether it sounds in any way muddled or cloudy. If you find a brand that passes all the tests aside from sounding a touch too bright, you might find this more acceptable than one that sounds a little dull.

Once you find a brand and type that works, stick with it and run a few more tests to determine how much level you can put on it before it distorts. Cassette-deck metering is notoriously inaccurate, so decide on the maximum recording level by ear, then make a note of what the meters were reading when audible distortion became evident. If you record your peaks a decibel or two below this figure, you should get the best signal-to-noise performance. Avoid budget tapes as many of these shed oxide rather too readily and exhibit poor sound quality.

Open-reel tape doesn't come in a choice of ferric, type II or metal, but different makes still have different characteristics. If you intend to use a brand of tape other than that for which your machine was set up, it is recommended that you have your machine realigned to suite the new tape.

Analogue Tape Care

Tape doesn't respond well to extremes of temperature, dust or humidity, and if left wound part of the way through, the cassette may eventually become too stiff to play properly. Tapes should be wound back to the start before storage and should be returned to their library cases so as to help keep out dust. Normal room temperature is fine for storage, but try to pick a dry place where the temperature stays stable. Make sure that your tapes are never in direct sunlight, too, as this can cause serious damage through overheating. For more details, see the section on tape storage and labelling later in this chapter.

Cassette Copies

If you want to make multiple copies from a master cassette, don't use the original, as repeated playing will cause it to deteriorate; instead, make the best-quality copy you can and then make your copies from that. If you can copy your cassettes from DAT, DCC or MiniDisc, you're likely to end up with a better-sounding result than if you copy from one cassette to another.

Cleaning Digital Tape Machines

Most digital tape machines, including DATs, use a rotating-head system, rather like a video recorder. Dry cleaning tapes are available for these, and they help to some extent, but wet cleaning is far more

effective. Isopropyl alcohol may be used, but there are specialised cleaners that work more thoroughly. Head access is usually a matter of taking off the top cover, but when you're doing this, make sure the machine is disconnected from the mains first.

Cotton buds must never be used on digital machines as the fibres become jammed in the head gaps. Instead, use a purpose-designed cleaning cloth (it looks a little like heavy silk), moisten a piece with the cleaning fluid and then hold it gently against the head drum while you rotate the head by hand one way and then the other. When no more dirt comes off, use a clean piece of cloth and repeat the process. Clean the tape guides and rollers the same way, but don't use excessive pressure or you could bend something and put the machine out of alignment. Never try to adjust any of the screws holding the tape guides as these adjust the tape-path alignment and require very specialised equipment to set up. Figure 7.2 shows a typical head drum assembly, including the position of the heads themselves.

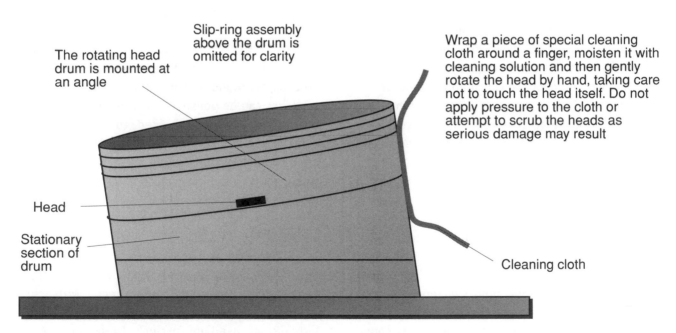

The rotating head drum is mounted at an angle

Slip-ring assembly above the drum is omitted for clarity

Wrap a piece of special cleaning cloth around a finger, moisten it with cleaning solution and then gently rotate the head by hand, taking care not to touch the head itself. Do not apply pressure to the cloth or attempt to scrub the heads as serious damage may result

Head

Stationary section of drum

Cleaning cloth

Heads are small but clearly visible around the periphery of the drum. Some systems have two heads per drum while others have four

Figure 7.2: MDM head drum assembly showing the heads

Notice how small they are compared with analogue tape heads. If in any doubt as to your ability to do this, get somebody to take you through the process first. It's very easy, but you can't afford to be careless. DAT machines are more fragile than VHS-format ADAT machines, so it is important to get proper instruction before tacking these for the first time.

Drying-Off Time

Once the transport is clean, allow it to dry out thoroughly before you attempt to thread a new tape or you may find it wrapped around the capstan. If your machine has an Error Readout mode, format a tape and then play it back, checking the error rate. Ideally, this should remain in single figures for a machine in reasonable condition.

Equipment Valeting

The outside of your equipment will benefit from the occasional clean, but what cleaner is safe to use? Open any equipment manual and one of the first things you'll come across is a warning not to clean with petroleum spirits, thinners, paint stripper and various other things you'd never dream of cleaning it with anyway. Then it will usually suggest that you use a damp cloth. But have you ever tried cleaning a greasy front panel with a damp cloth?

Spray furniture polish is just about the best way to clean studio equipment – it works on both plastic and painted metal, it doesn't appear to attack anything other than the grime it's intended to and it also cleans perspex display windows. However, there are one or two things to bear in mind. Firstly, don't spray it into faders or jack sockets; spray it onto your cleaning cloth first. Secondly, if you're in the habit of sticking masking tape and labels over everything and you find your gear covered in sticky patches of encrusted adhesive from long-forgotten bits of sticky paper, spray polish will once again do the job for you. This time, spray directly onto the affected area and allow the dried adhesive to soften for a minute or two before you try to wipe it off. Stubborn patches may need two or three treatments, but it'll come off in the end. The same trick applies to residue left by double-sided sticky pads or tape.

Touching Up

Once you've got your machine clean, you might find yourself seeing scratches in the paintwork or anodising which you never noticed were there before. If the equipment is black – and so much of it still is – a fine indelible black felt marker pen can be used to touch up minor scratches. Even the best-cared-for equipment usually ends up marked along the edges of the front panel or around the rack-mounting holes, and although the colour and finish of a typical permanent felt pen differs slightly from the paintwork you're patching up, the improvements that can be made are quite significant.

For non-black equipment, pay a visit to your local car-spares shop and try to find a matching touch-up paint – the type that comes in a narrow cylinder with its own brush. You'll probably need to buy a fine artist's brush to apply it, though, and don't expect a completely invisible mend as car paint tends to be more glossy than that used on music equipment. It's also advisable to try a little paint on the underside of the unit first, not only to check the colour match but also to make sure that the car paint doesn't attack the paint beneath it.

Scratched Windows?

While you're in a renovating mood, how do all the little display windows look? A trifle scratched? Minor scratches can be polished out with metal polish or the cutting compound used to restoring car paintwork, although toothpaste also works well on minor scratches. After you've finished polishing, a wipe-over with furniture polish is recommended to wipe away any greasy marks.

Tape Etiquette

The result of all your studio efforts is likely to end up on tape or CD-R, yet recording media is often treated with a casual disrespect. With the introduction of small-format tapes such as DAT and Video-8, as used in Tascam's DA88 and DA38 machines, there's a tendency to treat valuable recordings in rather too casual a fashion, and with physically small tapes, labelling becomes particularly important. There's an old studio saying that an unlabelled tape is free to be used. With DAT tapes and similarly compact formats, there isn't room on the tape for more than minimal information, so it may be wise to devise a system of codes so that tape cassettes may be matched with their notes or insert sleeves.

Tape Labels

Tackling the issue of labelling first (on the basis that you should always label a tape before storing it), there is a simple tape-labelling system devised by the APRS (Association of Professional Recording Studios) which has been introduced as an industry standard. This encompasses both multitrack and stereo master tapes, any copies or clones and, of course, DAT. Colour-coded labels are available from the APRS, but in the case of DAT tapes, many brands now come with a set of APRS colour-coded labels included. Even if you don't have the 'official' labels, writing the correct description on the box will suffice.

It seems self-evident that any tape should include details of the format, such as how many tracks there are, the speed at which they were recorded, what noise reduction (if any) was used and so on, but it still surprises me that tapes come in to my studio without any of this information. Analogue recordings should always include information on the tape speed, track format, noise reduction and record EQ (NAB/IEC), as well as the title, time and recording date of the material on the tape.

Open-Reel Tapes

Analogue, open-reel tapes are usually stored 'tail out', to reduce print-through, which means that the tapes must be rewound before playing. If noise reduction is being used, print-through is unlikely to be a problem, but it's still good form to adhere to this convention. Because the tape tends to pack unevenly for the first few turns on the hub, it is advisable to leave half a minute or so of blank tape or leader before recording starts and also to leave a little blank tape or leader at the end of the reel.

Before storing a tape, it should be wound back to the beginning and then spooled through to the end at normal speed rather than fast wind so that it packs evenly on the reel. Some machines have a special spooling mode for this purpose which is rather faster than real time.

Digital Cassettes

Digital tapes, both stereo DAT and multitrack (such as Alesis ADAT or Tascam DA88), should display the recording's sample rate and the type of recording machine used. One of the worst things you can do is to mix 48kHz and 44.1kHz sample rates on the same DAT tape, as this can create havoc if the tape is subsequently sent for digital editing.

Digital tapes – and analogue cassettes, for that matter – perform better if they are wound through to the end and then back to the start before being used for the first time. This helps loosen up any binding of the tape in the cassette shell and may reduce the number of record errors. It is also recommended that the first minute or so of any digital tape should be recorded with silence before the recording proper starts (although ADAT looks after this automatically when the tape is formatted). This is because the first few turns of the tape onto the take-up hub may wind less than perfectly evenly, increasing the risk of record errors which, if serious, may even cause audible drop-outs.

After a session using digital tape, it helps to wind the tape right through to the end and then fast-wind it back to the start before starting it again. Print-through is not a problem you have to worry about with digital tape.

Standard Tape Labelling

The following descriptions are condensed versions of the APRS labelling conventions.

Session Tapes

Usually a multitrack tape (analogue or digital), the *session tape* is used to make the original recordings, often containing both out-takes and wanted material. An album project may comprise several session tapes. Where the recording has been made 'direct-to-stereo', the original recording is still known as the session tape.

The tape format and the recorded contents

should be detailed on the tape box or inlay card and the tape itself should be titled to match the box details.

Label: blue with the words SESSION TAPE.

Original Master

When a multitrack tape is first mixed to stereo, the result is the *original master* tape, but this isn't the tape used for final production as it hasn't been edited. Furthermore, it would be unwise to send the only master tape away for duplication. In most cases, the mixed material will need to be assembled in the correct running order, the gaps between tracks will almost need editing and, in some circumstances, tracks may need to be faded in or out or crossfaded. Further processing, such as compression or EQ, is often applied at the mastering stage.

Label: red with the words ORIGINAL MASTER.

Production Master

The *production master* is a copy of the selected material from the original master tape or tapes presented in the correct running order with any gaps adjusted to the desired time. EQ and other signal processing may also be used to modify individual tracks, and some tracks may be compiled from different sections drawn from several takes or mixes. Effectively, the production master recording is exactly as it will appear on the final record or CD, although further adjustments may be made at the mastering stage. It helps if the DAT track IDs are correctly edited to mark the beginnings of each track.

For cassette duplication, it is normal to leave several minutes' gap between sides 1 and 2 to accommodate the turning over of the cassettes.

The type of release medium should also be noted on the tape data sheet as different master tapes are often required for record, cassette and CD production. For example, the tracks on a CD run continuously whereas the tracks on a vinyl or cassette album are arranged as two sides, and vinyl records may need special EQ or other processing. For cassette production, side 1 is usually made

slightly longer than side 2 so that, when the tape is turned over at the end of side 1, side 2 is ready to be played.

For DAT tapes destined for CD release, a sampling rate of 44.1kHz is preferred, although any CD-mastering house should be able to work from a 48kHz tape made on a semi-pro DAT machine. The most important thing is that the sample rate is clearly labelled and that under no circumstances is a tape sent off for CD duplication with mixed sample rates. No unrecorded blank tape should be left between tracks, and if the DAT recorder has an Absolute Time mode, this is probably the best mode to select when creating the production master. For more details on mastering, see Chapter 4, 'Post-Production Considerations'.

The production master DAT tape should ideally be recorded in a single take to eliminate the likelihood of glitches at the edit points. Some CD recorders are able to extract PQ information from DAT track IDs, so it is advisable to move these manually to just before the start of each track. Unwanted track IDs should be erased and the IDs renumbered on completion. Virtually all DAT machines have the facility to renumber IDs automatically.

A full listing of the songs by title, start time (Start IDs) and playing time should accompany the production master, including full details of the recording format and the type and model of machine that was used. This latter point is important, because masters made on some older DAT recorders – particularly Teac or Casio portables – are pre-emphasised during recording. Pre-emphasis is also covered in Chapter 4.

Label: green with the words PRODUCTION MASTER.

Production Master Copy/Clone

This is a copy (or clone, in the case of DAT) of the production master made in order to allow distribution of the tape for manufacturing without risking damage to or loss of the original. A tape made by analogue copying is known as a *copy* whereas a tape made by digitally transferring the data from one digital recorder to another is known as a *clone*. In theory, a clone should be identical to the original in all ways, although data errors requiring error-concealment can mean that the data isn't absolutely identical. An analogue copy will always undergo some slight degeneration and the recorded data may be quite different to the original as the signal has to pass via the analogue domain. When making analogue copies, take great care to ensure that the playback and record levels match as closely as possible.

Label: orange with the words PRODUCTION MASTER COPY CLONE. The appropriate 'Copy' or 'Clone' checkbox should be ticked and the information from the actual production master should be included.

Safety Copy/Clone

This is a backup copy or clone of any another tape, ideally made by digital cloning in the case of digital tapes, but the term 'safety copy' also describes analogue copies. All details from the original tape should be included.

Label: pink with the words SAFETY COPY CLONE. The appropriate 'Copy' or 'Clone' check box should be ticked.

Not-For-Production Tape

Any tape which must not be used as a source for media manufacture.

Label: yellow with the words NOT FOR PRODUCTION.

PQ-Encoded Master Tape

The manufacture of CDs is usually done from a U-matic master tape that includes coded data enabling the CD player to find individual tracks and to display the total number of tracks, the time remaining and so on. It may also be possible to insert other information at this point relating to track titles and automatic MCPS billing. Software is available for both Macintosh and PC computers that will allow the production of PQ-encoded write-once CDs or CD-Rs from which conventional CDs may then be mass-produced. CD-R is becoming very popular as

an alternative to U-matic for mastering. See Chapter 4, 'Post-Production Considerations', for more details.

Label: grey with the words PQ-ENCODED TAPE MASTER.

Checkboxes are provided to indicate the various release-media formats and whether the tape is an original or a clone. In most cases, the release medium will be CD, and different U-matic masters are needed for MiniDisc and DCC production. When having a batch of CDs made from a production master tape, insist on receiving a one-off copy for verification purposes before the batch is manufactured. Check this for correct playback speed, glitches, clicks and other problems, and ensure that the running order and times match those on your sleeve artwork.

Media Version

This is a copy or clone of original material made for radio broadcast, film/video soundtrack or similar purposes. If the tape is recorded with time code, details of the format and track start times should be included on the documentation.

Label: yellow and marked MEDIA VERSION.

Checkboxes are provided for 'Radio', 'TV', 'Film' or 'Video'.

Tape Test Tones

It isn't enough to know what's on a tape; we also need to know how high the signal level gets when the music is at its loudest. To this end, analogue recordings are normally preceded by test tones, although these don't give an accurate picture of peak signal levels because different engineers tend to push the record level into the red by different degree. To ensure that the left and right channels haven't been mixed up anywhere along the line, the tones should start with a burst in the left channel only.

There should be five seconds of 1kHz tone on the left channel followed by 30 seconds of the same tone recorded on both channels and recorded at

0VU. To assist in optimising the alignment of the replay tape machine to the tape, a 100Hz, 0VU tone should be recorded, followed by a 10kHz tone at around −10dB. All tone levels should be recorded on the box or label.

One exception is the production master intended for CD (or other digital format) manufacture. This can include no tones, or they might end up on the album, which would be disastrous. If it is necessary to check the peak level, the material will have to be played manually and the peaks noted.

DAT Tapes

Because DAT tapes can't be recorded above their maximum levels, it's usual for them to be recorded so that the maximum peak level falls around 1–2dB short of the maximum meter reading so as to build in a small safety margin. Record between one and two minutes of silence onto the start of the tape, and if test tones are required, a −14dB, 1kHz tone (14dB below the full-scale meter reading) will suffice. The level should be noted on the label or accompanying paperwork.

At the end of the recording, the machine should be allowed to run on in Record mode for at least half a minute before the tape is stopped. When recording DAT production masters, set the Auto ID function to On. However, Auto ID must sense the presence of the programme material before writing the ID, so there's a chance that the first fraction of a second of the track will be missed. To get around this, manually move all IDs back by half a second or so after recording. Renumber if any IDs are added or removed.

Running Time

Something that has to be decided upon fairly early in the proceedings is the running time of your material and how that relates to the medium on which you're going to release it. The running time of a cassette can be significantly longer than that of a CD; it's limited only by the maximum length of tape that you can get into a cassette shell, while the maximum CD recording time on a standard CD is 74 minutes. In the case of vinyl, it's best to discuss the recording length with the company handling the cutting, as the type of material can affect the maximum playing time.

Never send off an original master tape, and if you've paid to have a production DAT master made up, it makes sense to get at least one clone made at the same time so that you don't risk losing or damaging the original. Store the original tape in a safe place.

Long-Term Tape Storage

It is well known that analogue tapes deteriorate in storage, and many master tapes over ten years old are virtually unplayable unless they are first 'baked' at a controlled temperature of around 50°C for several hours to drive off the moisture they've absorbed over the years. Even this cure is only temporary, and it is advisable that digital copies of all valuable old material are made as soon as possible. (See the section on 'Sticky Shed Syndrome' for more details.) There's no guarantee that digital tape won't degenerate over time in some way, so the regular cloning of important material every few years is a wise precaution.

No tape will last forever, but storing it properly can make a huge difference to how long it does survive. The main enemies of tape are magnetism, moisture and heat, and even short terms of exposure to an excess of any of these factors can cause irreversible damage. Tapes also need to be kept clean, so storage in a dust-tight case is a good idea. Open-reel tapes should be boxed and sealed against dust.

Obviously, you shouldn't leave valuable tapes on top of a speaker cabinet, but other sources of magnetic fields include computer monitors and mains cables, especially those carrying large currents. Store your tapes at least a couple of feet from any of these. Contrary to some stories, transporting a tape on an electric railway or underground system shouldn't cause problems.

Most modern houses aren't excessively damp, but if you have a garage studio, store your tapes in the house. In this case, use a bedroom rather than a basement room, as bedrooms are less likely to be damp. If you do have to leave the tapes in the studio building, consider buying a dehumidifier to prevent moisture from building up. This will also help protect your gear.

Storage Conditions

Tapes are best stored at a constant temperature, and a bedroom cupboard is usually fine for project-studio tapes. Tapes should never be left in direct sunlight, not even for short periods, and if you have to transport them by car, take extra care as sunlight coming through glass can create a lot of heat.

Wind all cassette tapes back to the start before storage and put open-reel tapes tail-out in plastic bags before putting them in their boxes as an added precaution against dust. DAT tapes should be kept in their library cases. By treating your tapes with a little respect, the likelihood of encountering problems is much diminished.

CD-R For Archiving

Recordable CD, or CD-R, is now an affordable way of recording production masters, digital audio data and computer files, or archiving stereo audio, but the discs tend to be a little less rugged than conventional CDs (which should also be treated with more respect than they seem to be afforded). Keep the discs out of light when they're not being used, and protect the recording surface from scratches and dirt. Store discs in their library cases and always handle them by the edges so as not to leave fingermarks on the recorded surface. Special pens are available for marking the label side of the disc, while for more sophisticated applications small-run labelling systems are available based on adhesive labels that can be printed in a standard computer printer.

Sticky-Shed Syndrome

Sticky-shed syndrome is a problem that affects some older or poorly stored tapes, but it's not until you try to play back a tape afflicted by this condition that you realise how serious it is. Oxide sheds at an alarming rate, and what's more, it sticks like glue to the heads and tape guides. The first thing you

notice is a physical screeching noise as the moving tape is 'bowed' by the contaminated heads or guides, and this physical modulation transfers itself to the audio. The top end is usually dramatically reduced, and after just a few minutes of play the friction may cause the machine to grind to a halt. On occasions, the tape actually sticks to the heads and pulling it off can dislodge more oxide, increasing the risk of irrecoverable dropouts.

Apparently, the problem lies in the fact that, years ago, some manufacturers used a certain type of binder (the material used to fix the tiny particles of magnetic oxide to the flexible backing tape). Over time, the binders appear to undergo some form of chemical breakdown and, at the same time, absorb moisture from the air. The problem was later identified and improved formulations were substituted to clear the problem, but that still left thousands of reels of tape around the world that were literally rotting away. But what, if anything, can you do to recover material archived in this way?

Half-Baked?

A few years ago, several articles and papers were published on the subject and the general outcome was that baking the tape at a precisely regulated temperature for between 12 and 24 hours would drive the water from the binder, making it stable enough to play. Unfortunately, the cure is only temporary, and the tape will eventually return to its damaged state, so it needs to be transferred to DAT or some other suitable storage medium as soon as is practical. The baking temperature quoted is in the order of 50°C, and an agricultural incubator is idea for the job. Baked tapes often play back surprisingly well with no trace of sticking, although the heads should be cleaned regularly.

With the benefit of hindsight, there are a few rules you should follow if you find one of your tapes suffering from sticky shed syndrome. Most importantly, don't continue trying to play an affected tape once you realise there's a problem – you could cause more damage than the sticky shed syndrome itself. For example, if you pull large chunks of oxide off the tape, you're bound to get dropouts. If the recording is commercially valuable, you should contact the manufacturer's technical department for advice.

The incubator seems the ideal way of heating tape, but it is important that no part of the tape is in direct contact with any metalwork or any part of the heater. The wire-mesh shelf fitted to most incubators is ideal as it allows for even heating via the warm air in the box and not via conduction. Check the temperature of the baking system to ensure that it stays stable within a couple of degrees either side of 50ºC and bake for 24 hours. Don't attempt this using a domestic oven or a microwave!

After baking, play the tape as soon as it is cool and take this opportunity to replace any faulty splices that may have dried out over the years. Once you're happy that the tape plays OK, clean the machine again and transfer your recording to DAT or other suitable medium, ensuring you get as high a recording level as possible without running into clipping. If you have the time, make two copies, because it isn't certain how well the baking procedure works if you have to repeat it.

DCC Considerations

DCC tape recorders use a form of data compression to reduce the amount of data that needs to be recorded to tape. Although the sound quality can be very good, copying a DCC tape to another DCC machine will introduce another stage of data compression, and this is true even if the tape is copied in the digital domain. Progressive stages of data compression will reduce the quality of the recording, so it is advised that first-generation copies be used whenever the application is important. DCC recordings may be digitally cloned to DAT machines with no further loss of quality.

Digital Data Integrity

Digital audio and MIDI sequencing involves data storage to a number of different media, including floppy disks, fixed hard drives, removable hard drives, removable magneto-optical drives, tapes, RAM cartridges and even recordable CDs (CD-Rs). Patch data is also held in battery-powered RAM inside your synths and effects processors. If any of

this data becomes corrupted to the point where it can't be recovered, you may lose a huge amount of work. The purpose of this section is to examine the more common forms of digital data storage, to explore their weaknesses and to see what, if anything, can be done if the worst happens.

Safe Computing

Computers are designed to be tolerant of small variations in mains voltage, but high-voltage spikes in the mains may cause data held in RAM to be corrupted, and in extreme cases the hardware itself may be damaged. For this reason, it is advisable to buy a mains filter that includes a surge suppressor. Under normal circumstances, these should offer adequate protection, although you should still get into the habit of saving your work to disk every few minutes, as computer crashes can occur for all kinds of reasons and, if you haven't saved your work, it will be lost.

Lightning Strikes

One kind of power surge that your mains filter is unlikely to be able to protect you from is a nearby lightning strike. When lightning strikes the ground, it can generate surges of many thousands of volts in the mains and telephone wiring, often completely destroying any electronic equipment that is plugged in, even if it is switched off. The obvious precaution is to unplug all your recording and computer equipment from the mains during nearby thunderstorms, and also to make sure that your modem is disconnected from the phone socket, or a surge might get into your system that way, destroying not only the modem but possibly the computer too and any equipment attached to the computer, such as MIDI interfaces, sound modules and other parts of your audio system.

Fortunately, power surges of this magnitude are rare, but I have known it happen, and the damage has been catastrophic. Furthermore, unless you have categoric proof that a power surge existed, the electricity company will refuse to accept liability. You may also find that your insurance company views lightning damage as an 'act of God', and the terms of your policy may mean that they don't have to pay out. If in doubt, read the policy small print *before* you need to make a claim, not afterwards.

Backing Up Data

Unless your digital data is backed up, you can't consider it to be safe, no matter how wonderful the reliability figures claimed by the hard drive's manufacturer. It looks reassuring when you see a MTBF (Mean Time Between Failures) figure of five years (60 months), but these very same figures indicate that, in any group of 60 of these drives, on average one will fail per month!

This sobering thought doesn't even take into account data lost through user error, physically dropped drives, PSU failure or as a result of power surges and other unforeseen horrors, so any data that you may need to use again should be backed up on another drive. Similarly, data stored on floppies should be backed up, recordings made on digital tapes should be backed up (cloned) and important patch data stored in synths, effects units or RAM cards should be backed up to a MIDI sequencer or other data-archiving system. I know that backing up is boring, but when you consider that a single hard drive may have enough capacity to store a writer's entire life's work, it all gets a little scary.

When backing up to CD-R or DVD-R, use high-quality media and only write on the disk using a proper CD marker. Store the disk in a sleeve or jewel case away from the light.

Hard Drives

Fixed hard drives tend to be reasonably reliable, but in any organisation that uses a large number of computers or multi-drive systems, faulty drives are commonplace. Failure may be due either to data corruption or to mechanical problems, and if it is the latter, it is both difficult and very expensive to recover any data that may still be intact on the drive platters. In effect, a specialist company will need to rebuild the drive in clean-room conditions and then attempt to read off the data. If your life's work is at stake, this option may be worthwhile, but the cost can run into thousands of pounds.

Large corporations often use RAID arrays of multiple drives where a data-redundancy system is used to store the contents of, say, eight drives across an array of nine drives. If any one drive in the array fails, its data can be recreated from the redundant data stored on the remaining drives, but even with this level of security, I've heard of RAID arrays where two drives have failed almost at the same time, and in that case, there's no way to recover the data. The moral is that, no matter how secure the system appears to be, if you can't afford to lose the data, you must back it up.

Don't move a hard drive while it is switched on, and never plug in or unplug SCSI connections unless the pieces of equipment at either end are switched off. Failure to observe these precautions may result in serious damage and data loss.

Implications Of Data Corruption

A hard disk is rather like a book, where each file of information can be considered as being a separate chapter. However, unlike a book, a file may be split into several non-contiguous (ie non-consecutive) sections if the space remaining on the drive is limited or fragmented. Keeping track of all these files and bits of files is an electronic directory, which can be considered as the contents page of this digital book. If the contents page gets damaged, all your work is still on the drive, but you have no way of locating it.

In fact, data is never actually erased from a drive – when you delete a file, all that really happens is that you delete its entry in the contents page, leaving that disk space free to be overwritten. Once the data belonging to the deleted file is overwritten by new data, it is lost forever, but until that point, it is still there, even though it doesn't appear in your list of files. Even when a disk is reformatted, the data remains until overwritten, as several criminals have found to their cost when the police have recovered their supposedly deleted files as evidence!

Data Recovery

Although there are specialist companies that can recover data from seriously corrupted or physically damaged disk drives, there are utility programs that the average user can employ to fix minor disk problems or to rescue the remaining intact data from disks that can't be fixed. One of the most popular is Norton Utilities, but numerous packages exist that work on similar principles. Essentially, these programs can scan a faulty drive (hard, floppy or removable), looking for problems, and in many cases they can fix the problems automatically.

File Rescue

If the disk can't be repaired, it may still be possible to retrieve some of the files using a rescue utility – again, part of a program like Norton Utilities. These programs sort through the data on the disk and identify complete or partial files that seem to be intact, and although copying the individual files to a spare drive is a long and tedious job, it at least gives you a chance to recover much of your work.

How successfully this works depends on the nature of the damage and the type of file you're trying to rescue. For example, if you have a word-processor document and a few lines of text are missing, you can probably rewrite the missing lines, but if you have an incomplete program file, MIDI file or audio file, the missing data may render the whole thing useless. In such cases, only complete files are of any real value.

Enhanced File Recovery

Another trick provided by some diagnostic utilities is the ability to create their file-tracking system, to which they can refer if the disk directory is corrupted, but for this to work, the relevant utility software must be installed on the hard drive *before* you have problems, not after. By making use of such a feature, the chance of recovering files intact is rather better than using a basic file-rescue utility.

Reformatting Drives

If the problem is severe, or if the disk is so badly corrupted that the diagnostic software can't even access it to read it, there may be no choice but to accept that the data is lost and then try reformatting the disk. If no physical damage has occurred to the drive, reformatting it should make it useable again,

but all data will be lost (actually, it will still be there, but you won't be able to locate it). If the drive is physically damaged, there's nothing you can do other than replace it, unless the lost data is so important that you feel it worth the considerable cost of employing a specialist to attempt to recover it for you.

If the failure is in the drive motor, there's a good chance that all the data can be recovered intact by a specialist, but if the fault is due to the head physically crashing into the disk surface, some data is almost certain to be lost, and it's possible that the entire drive contents may have to be abandoned.

Drive Fragmentation

A typical hard drive contains hundreds or even thousands of files, and when you delete a file, the newly freed space may not be large enough for the next file you save to fit in once piece, so the file gets split into two or more parts. This is known as *file fragmentation*, and the fuller your drive gets, the more fragmentation is likely to occur. Computers are designed to cope with file fragmentation so that, as far as the user is concerned, nothing has really changed, but in reality file access takes longer because the disk head has to move around a lot more to track the various file fragments. While this might not matter in a word-processor file, it can cause trouble for audio files, where data needs to be read off the disk in a virtually uninterrupted stream. RAM memory buffers the data to prevent the data being interrupted by normal disk operation, but in a multitrack audio system a situation may be reached where data can't be read from the drive fast enough, and that results in audible glitching.

Defragmentation

The solution to fragmented drives is to defragment them, and on PCs running Windows 95 or later, a defragmentation routine is built into the operating system. This sorts through the data on disk and rewrites all the files in contiguous (ie unbroken) blocks, leaving all the free space on the drive in one place, rather than scattered throughout the files. Figure 7.3 shows a screen shot of a fragmented drive as reported by a utility program.

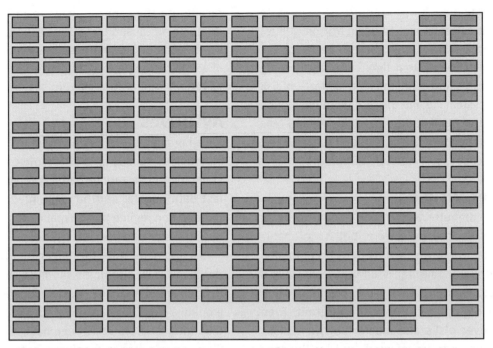

A fragmented drive has its free space scattered all over the disk in non-contiguous blocks

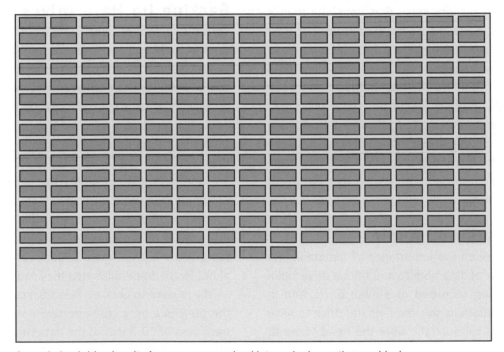

Represents a block of stored data

An optimised drive has its free space organised into a single contiguous block

Figure 7.3: A fragmented drive as viewed by a utility program

Apple Mac machines require a separate defragmentation program, and again Norton Utilities provides one. However, this can't defragment the drive on which the system files currently running are stored, so it's necessary to create a start-up disk with a basic system file and the disk defragmentation utility on it. Defragmentation can take several tens of minutes, depending on the size of the hard drive, but the processes is completely automatic.

Computer Viruses

Fortunately, computer viruses don't seem to be as popular now as they once were, but it's probably fair to say that not having a virus-detection program installed on your computer is unwise, especially if you are very tempted to try out public-domain software or files picked up on the Internet. Even magazine cover disks and master software disks have been known to be infected, and for the sake of a check that takes only a few seconds it's foolhardy to risk losing everything on your hard drive – which is possible, if you're really unlucky. You should also check music files from your friends and associates, as there's no guarantee that their data hasn't been exposed to a virus at some time, as viruses are designed to copy themselves onto any disk inserted into the host machine.

Take advantage of magazine cover disks and manufacturers' websites to upgrade public-domain virus-checker programs so that you always have the latest version. If you don't, you may find that some of the more up-to-date viruses can get past your current defences.

Hard Disks And Audio

Earlier, I stressed the importance of maintaining a constant flow of data both to and from a drive when audio is being recorded or played back, and in multitrack situations this requires the drive to have a fast access time (ie the time the head takes to locate the required data) and it must also have a high sustained data-transfer rate.

On their own, these figures don't guarantee trouble-free operation, because most conventional drives take a short break every once in a while to recalibrate their mechanisms in order to prevent errors being caused by thermal expansion. Although the periods of thermal recalibration are short, they may still be long enough to interrupt the data flow, especially in multitrack audio systems.

AV Drives

It's a far safer bet to use an AV drive for audio, and although these may be a little more costly than their general-purpose counterparts, they are designed for fast data transfer and have an intelligent thermal-recalibration regime that suspends calibration during data-transfer operations.

As a general rule, the larger the drive capacity, the faster it is, although you must still ensure it is defragmented regularly. Most serious audio systems employ a separate hard drive for the audio data so that, after a session has been backed up, the entire file can be deleted in readiness for the next session. This gets around the need to defragment the drive and ensures the fastest operation at all times.

Backing Up Hard Drives

With the advent of multi-gigabyte hard drives, the days of backing up all your crucial files on floppies is over, although I still use floppies to keep backup copies of things like MIDI song files, word-processor documents, small software applications and so forth. Audio files are a very different story, though, as each track of 44.1kHz audio takes around 5MB of hard-drive space.

Tape backup is probably the cheapest current option, and various tape drives are available that connect to your system exactly like another hard drive. Most of the cheaper systems use data DAT tape, which makes media costs very reasonable, although the trade-off is that they can be quite slow.

If you need to back up files from completed jobs, the CD-R is a very cost-effective option. The main weakness of CD-R is that the data can't be rewritten once it is stored – writing data to disk is strictly a once-only operation – but as a CD-R can hold around 700MB of data for around the cost of a DAT tape, it's still a cheap way to back up, and with the most modern drives backup can be carried out at many times normal speed. Data is stored in such a way that the CD-R shows up in your CD-ROM drive in much the same way as any other CD-ROM, so the system is simple as well as cheap. For those involved in digital audio, owning a CD-R recorder also provides a means to create one-off audio CDs from DAT masters.

Removable-Media Drives

Removable-media drives are exactly what they sound like, drives from which the media can be removed, usually in the form of a cartridge. The storage media may be a hard magnetic disk cartridge, a magneto-optical disk cartridge, a CD-R or a tape, such as data DAT. Different manufactures build disk cartridges operating on slightly different principles, and some are noticeably faster than others. At the time of writing, removable media drives tend to be slower than their fixed counterparts, but some of the faster ones are able to handle multitrack digital audio at a sampling frequency of 44.1kHz. Magneto-optical drives have the potential to be more rugged than purely magnetic drives, but they tend to be slower. Again, speed advances are being made all the time, and the faster MO drives will cope with direct-to-disk audio. Tape is the slowest format, but the low media costs make it attractive in some applications.

Medium-capacity hard-drive cartridges of between 100MB and 500MB capacity are particularly useful for storing audio-sample files for MIDI samplers, and although it is possible to use a single, large-capacity hard drive, splitting your sound library amongst several disks offers more security against data loss in the event of a failure. The faster medium-capacity drives are also useful for storing the audio files used within an audio-plus-MIDI sequencer, where the amount of audio needed might total only a few track-minutes per song.

The main point of this section is not to go into detail about how the various drives work but to suggest ways in which the data saved on removable media might best be protected. No matter how rugged a disk or tape cartridge might look, take great care never to drop it – the small physical size and consequent portability invites accidents, but

you must treat them as the precision mechanical devices they are.

In addition to protecting removable media from physical shocks, it is also vital to keep them away from extremes of heat, moisture, magnetic fields and dust. CD-Rs in particular shouldn't be left exposed to sunlight, as the sensitive surface can be damaged. Also, avoid scratching CD-Rs because, as with audio CDs, surface damage can prevent them from being read correctly.

Always be meticulous in following the manufacturer's instructions on how to mount and dismount the media. For example, cartridges can be damaged by attempts to remove them from the drive while the drive motor is running.

WARNING: At the time of writing, new removable drives seem to appear on the market every few weeks, and many of these are made obsolete within six months of their launch. If compatibility is important, find out what your clients or composing partners are using. In any event, it's worth securing a stock of media just in case availability becomes a problem.

Floppy Disks

Floppy disks also qualify as removable media, but they've been around for so long that we rather take them for granted. They come stuck to the covers of magazines, they lie around unprotected on your desk and they gather fluff in your shirt pocket – and most of the time they work fine. However, they can and do go wrong, so in addition to backing them up, you should treat them with the care due to other forms of removable media. In particular, try to keep them clean, as their ability to exclude dust isn't always as good as for other media.

Protected Software

It seems that more and more music software is delivered in a form that offers the manufacturer a degree of protection against piracy, and this protection may come as a plug-in key (dongle) or as an uncopyable master floppy disk providing a limited number of installs. Some newer programs come on CD-ROM, and every once in a while the user has to re-insert the original CD-ROM to revalidate the program.

Plug-in dongles are generally reliable, but some may cause conflicts with other hardware and peripherals in your system. If this occurs, all you can do is remove the conflicting item. However, some dongles also suffer from intermittent contacts, which shows up as the computer not being able to recognise the dongle and hence refusing to run the program. Such problems can be minimised if the dongle contacts are cleaned with a soft eraser, and if the dongle protrudes from the side or rear of the machine then it may also help to support it in some way so that the contacts don't take all the weight. Most modern dongles plug into the computer's USB port and should work fine in a USB hub.

Protected Disks

Protected disk installs usually work fine. The master disk has the capacity to install the program on your hard drive once, or sometimes twice, and once installed, the number of remaining installs on the master disk is decremented by one. This procedure authorises your hard drive to run the program you've installed. If you need to move the program to a different drive or reformat the drive, you'll need to uninstall it first to increment the count on your master disk. Failure to do this means that your install will be lost, and if the master disk only comes with one install, you won't be able to reinstall your software.

Often, you can still run the software if the master disk is left in the floppy drive as a key, but I find this whole system of protection exceedingly inconvenient and would encourage as many people as possible to complain about it. If your hard drive crashes, you may have no choice but to reformat it without having the opportunity to deinstall the protected software, in which case your installs will be lost. Furthermore, you may have a large number of protected programs on your drive, especially if you use software plug-ins for an audio program that are protected in this way, and when you come to change your drive, you have to remember to deinstall each and every one – which means locating

the correct version of each master disk, and spending a great deal of time going through the deinstallation routine.

As there's little I can do about this system other than complain about it, I suggest that, as you install software, you should log the fact in a notepad file, including the version number, so that, if it becomes necessary to remove your installs, at least you'll have a document reminding you of what's on there. Fortunately, the phasing out of floppy drives is helping to kill off this annoying system.

MDM

MDM (Modular Digital Multitrack) machines such as the Alesis ADAT or Tascam DA88 series use videotape cartridges as their storage media, although it's important to follow the manufacturer's recommendations as regards the best type of tape to use as not all physically compatible tapes will perform as well in a digital audio application. One of the beauties of MDM is that, in systems comprising two or more machines, data can be cloned from one tape to another, and because machines can occasionally damage tapes, backing up is vitally important.

In my own studio, I prefer to back up clients' tape as soon as they come in so that I can overdub and mix using the clones rather than the originals. Not only does this guard against a technical problem causing data loss but it also protects the original data from somebody putting the wrong track into Record during an overdub!

In the event that you suffer a chewed tape and you don't have a backup, it is sometimes possible to render the section playable again by holding the damaged section of tape out flat and pressing it between the pages of a heavy book. This involves defeating the brakes in the tape cassette (by pushing a matchstick into the appropriate orifice in the cassette), opening the tape cover (which again involves pushing release tabs), pulling out a loop of tape containing the damaged section and then using stickytape to hold the tape cover open so that it doesn't wreak further damage on your tape as you try to flatten it.

The success of this process depends on the type of MDM you have and on the degree of tape damage. I've managed to make a damaged ADAT tape playable using this method, and the error correction is so tough that there were no audible glitches. Of course, a tape rescued in this way should be cloned straight away. Obviously, if the tape is stretched or torn, you won't be able to play it, and indeed any attempt to do so may damage or clog your tape heads. If you're careful, you may be able to copy the work either side of the damaged section, but the damaged section itself will be lost.

TIP

Digital tape cassettes tend to shed the most oxide when they are first run through the machine, and the rotating head will also polish the tape slightly, which ostensibly reduces the error rate. ADAT users can usefully employ an old VHS video recorder in the studio in which new tapes can be wound through in Fast Play mode and then rewound before being formatted in the normal way. Doing this should help keep your recorder clean for longer and may reduce the incidence of recording errors.

TIP

MDMs are quite slow to lock up when you want to do drop-ins, so to speed up the proceedings, and to reduce tape wear, make a rough mix of the backing tracks onto a new tape and then record the vocals and any solo overdubs onto the remaining tracks. This way, you can overdub using just one tape machine and then, when you're ready to mix, bring the MDMs carrying the original backing tracks back online.

DAT

DAT tapes are normally quite rugged, but I've still experienced the occasional tape getting tangled inside the machine, and when this happens, there will invariably be a dropout at the point where the damaged section passes over the head. As with other digital tapes, you shouldn't attempt to play the damaged section unless you can flatten it and ensure that there are no tears in the tape itself.

DAT tapes can be cloned by connecting the S/PDIF or AES/EBU digital output of one machine to the corresponding input of another and then setting the second machine to Digital input mode. Although you can usually get away with using a short audio RCA phono jack lead to link S/PDIF sockets, it is far better to use a lead supplied for the purpose as the cable needs to be of a specific impedance. If you're unlucky, using an audio cable may result in increased recording errors or even audible glitches and clicks.

Severely damaged tapes may still be cloned on either side of the damaged area, as long as the tape isn't actually tangled inside the cassette shell. If it is, the shell may need to be dismantled in order to rescue the remaining tape. Although you shouldn't touch tape with your bare hands, this is unavoidable during salvage operations, so make sure your hands are clean, dry and free from grease before you start work.

WARNING: Never try to splice DAT or MDM video tapes, as the splice will almost certainly contaminate the head as it passes over it and may damage it.

If a tape has broken and you need to rescue the material on both sides of the break, you may need to load each half of the tape into the cassette shell in turn, fixing the broken end (after trimming away any torn tape) directly to the cassette hub. The data may then be cloned to a fresh tape in a second machine. Attempting this operation requires only a little persistence, but you must have at least one cassette shell that can be unscrewed to allow you access to the inside. Tape can be removed from welded cassette shells either by winding it out or by breaking the shell, but you must have a shell that can be unscrewed in which to reload the tape for playback.

To help ensure reliability from MDM digital tape cassettes, treat them as you would any other type of tape, but also take care not to drop them, as the mechanisms can easily sustain damage.

CD-Rs

CD-Rs are useful for backing up data that doesn't need to be subsequently changed or updated, and they tend to be reasonably robust, as long as they're shielded from sunlight and not subjected to scratching. Nobody knows for sure how long the data on a CD-R will last, but some manufacturers suggest that ten years may be a conservative estimate. To ensure a long life for CD-Rs, keep them in a disk-storage unit or jewel case when not in use and exclude any unnecessary light.

Because of the low expense and high capacity of CD-R, it is a useful medium for backing up MIDI sequences along with their audio files once a composition has been completed. DVD-R has a much higher capacity, and as prices of both drives and disks continue to fall, it's becoming increasingly attractive as a backup medium.

Patch Memory

Most electronic instruments, effects units, synth modules and rewritable patchcards use battery-backed-up RAM for storage, but the batteries will eventually fail, and then all the data will be lost. ROM read-only patchcards don't need batteries and so should, with care, last indefinitely.

The batteries used for RAM backup are similar to those used in calculators and personal organisers and may last up to five years. If you simply wait until the battery fails, all your user patches will be lost, and if you take out the battery to fit a new one, it is still probable that any stored data will be lost, so the sensible approach is to back up the memory to a MIDI sequencer or MIDI data filer. This

is done simply by initiating a sysex dump of all the user memory after setting the sequencer or data filer to Record, and a typical memory dump will take only a few seconds.

Restoring the memory entails playing back the MIDI file into the MIDI In port of the device. For precise details on how to do this for your equipment, consult the section of the manual that deals with sysex dumps or bulk dumps.

Patch Cards

Patch-card data will normally have to be transferred to the user memory of your instrument or effects unit before it can be backed up, so make sure your existing user patches are backed up first. Most cards can be backed up to a sequencer by performing a sysex dump. Also, because data storage is fallible, keep copies of the backed-up data both on floppies and on your hard drive.

Normally, patch cards lose their data when you change their batteries, although some are designed to retain the data without batteries for a minute or two in order to allow you to fit new batteries. Always assume that all data will be lost and create a backup. Then make sure that the new battery is to hand before you remove the old one. If you're lucky, your patches may stay intact, but don't ever rely on it.

8 TECHNICAL FACTS AND PROBLEMS

This chapter provides basic information relating to impedance matching, gain structure and mains wiring, as well as offering practical methods of dealing with problems relating to equipment installation and limitations.

Impedance

When you come across the term *impedance*, do you nod your head sagely or quickly turn to the next page? While impedance-matching may have a long way to go in order to qualify as fun, it is nevertheless an essential part of making a recording system work, and it helps to have a grasp of the fundamentals, at least.

Electrical resistance is something for which most of us can feel an affinity. Even those who don't know the maths can relate to the idea that the higher the resistance of a circuit or component, the more effort it takes to push current through it. That 'effort' is known as *voltage*, and the relationship between voltage, current and resistance is very succinctly encapsulated by Ohm's law, which states that R = V/I ohms, where V is the voltage across the circuit and I is the current (in amps) flowing through the circuit.

Impedance – Just AC Resistance?

Understanding impedance is just one more stage beyond Ohm's law. While resistance relates to the behaviour of circuits under DC conditions, impedance is essentially a means of expressing a circuit's resistance to an alternating current. Both audio signals and the 50/60Hz mains are examples of alternating currents, and to keep things simple, impedance is also expressed in ohms. Why do we need both resistance and impedance if both are expressed in ohms? Well, most real-life circuits have different impedance values depending on the frequencies at which they're measured, whereas a purely resistive circuit will always measure the same, regardless of frequency.

In the case of audio equipment, the circuitry is designed so that, wherever possible, the impedance is kept reasonably constant over the entire audio range. However, this *isn't* always possible – for example, loudspeakers in particular show a significant increase in impedance at their resonant frequencies.

Input And Output Impedance

Input Impedance is a measure of the load that a device presents to the signal driving it. For example, if a line input has a 50kohms impedance, the device feeding it needs to be able to drive a signal into a 50kohm load without running out of current. Although the impedance will vary slightly with frequency, it's common practice to quote impedances at a single frequency (often 1kHz).

Output impedance is slightly less intuitive but is essentially a way to define the load impedance that the circuit is capable of driving. In other words, input impedance is related to how much electrical current is soaked up by a circuit while output impedance is related to how much current an output can supply. This is a necessarily simplified definition, but in order to get a better mental picture, consider the following analogy.

Imagine a person pedalling a bicycle up a slope: the cyclist has an output impedance related to his ability to turn the pedals, whereas the pedals themselves present a load impedance in that they put up resistance to being turned. As the hill gets steeper, the load impedance will increase, and eventually a point will be reached at which the cyclist is no longer able to supply the necessary effort to continue. Progress can occur only when the input impedance is equal to or greater than the source impedance. In electrical terms, the larger the load impedance, the less current is required to maintain a specified voltage across that load, so the higher the load impedance, the easier it is to drive. As far as the source is concerned, the lower its impedance, the more current it is capable of delivering.

Impedance Matching

The bicycle analogy leads neatly onto the concept of impedance matching. When we're dealing with transferring the maximum amount of power from one circuit to another, an circuit matched to its optimum is one where a circuit with a given output impedance is feeding a load which has the same value input impedance. In other words, a 600-ohm output feeding a 600-ohm input is perfectly matched. Referring back to the cyclist, this situation is roughly analogous to the bike being geared so that the cyclist can achieve the maximum speed without having to work so hard as to become exhausted. If the wrong gears are chosen, the cyclist either pedals too quickly but makes little process or, at the other extreme, the pedals are so hard to turn that it becomes impossible to continue. Either situation is a mismatch between the energy provider (the cyclist) and the energy receiver (the pedals).

This kind of matching is important between things like batteries and lightbulbs, but with most audio signals we're not concerned about transferring lots of energy – we just want to get the signal voltage from equipment A to equipment B with as little loss as possible. In other words, we want our bike geared so as to be easy to pedal – we don't care if it doesn't get anywhere as long as the pedals go around. To achieve this, the source impedance needs to be significantly lower than the load impedance, and in most audio systems output impedances are at least five or ten times lower than

input impedances, and often much more. Not only does this prevent the signal from being unduly loaded but it also enables one source to drive two or three loads simultaneously, if required – for example, by means of a splitter lead. Here the analogy of one man pedalling three easy-to-pedal bicycles at the same time becomes rather messy and so will be abandoned!

Typical Audio Impedances

Console mic amps have an input impedance of around 1 kohm while a low-impedance dynamic microphone might have an impedance of between 150 ohms and 250 ohms. This satisfies the criteria for a good match. If, however, you were to plug a high-impedance mic with a 47 kohm output impedance into the mic input of a desk (1 kohm), the signal from the mic would be severely loaded by the mixer, resulting in a drastic loss in level and possible distortion. In cycling terms, this relates to extreme fatigue and loss of performance!

Line inputs have an impedance of around 50 kohms, whereas most line-level equipment has an output impedance of no higher than 10 kohms and often as little as a few tens of ohms in the case of really well-specified equipment.

A loudspeaker is one device for which you do have to be fairly precise about matching. Although power amplifiers have extremely low output impedances, they are designed to operate with a specified impedance of loudspeaker. If the loudspeaker impedance is lower than that specified, the amplifier may overheat and even sustain damage, while a speaker with too high an impedance will result in less audio power. For example, if an amplifier is rated at 100W with a 4-ohm speaker, it is likely to produce only around 50W with an 8-ohm speaker.

Impedance-Matching Rules

- When matching amplifiers to loudspeakers, the rated impedance of the amplifier should be equal to the input impedance of the loudspeakers. If the rated amplifier impedance is lower than that of the speaker, the system will still work but the maximum power available will be lower.

- When matching mic- or line-level signals, the source impedance should be significantly lower than the load impedance, ideally by a factor of ten or greater.

- Provided that the load impedance is considerably less than the source impedance, it should be possible to split the signal to drive two or more loads. However, *never* join two outputs together in order to feed one input. This must be done only via a mixer circuit. Directly connecting two outputs may cause circuit damage as well as signal degradation.

Gain Structure

You've plugged a perfectly good mic into a perfectly good mixer and ended up with a noisy recording. In all probability, it isn't the equipment that's at fault but the way in which the various gain controls are set. To understand why this is so, it's necessary to learn a little about the nature of electronic circuitry and the dynamic range of sound.

Sound covers a vast dynamic range, from the dropping of a pin to a hard snare-drum beat, and to reproduce this electronically means the signal levels we have to deal with might vary from just a few microvolts (millionths of a volt) up to 10V or more. In a typical studio, the signal from a microphone is amplified to bring it up to *line level* (a vague term meaning closer to a volt than a millivolt) and then the signal is passed through a whole chain of circuitry where it is equalised, routed, mixed and effected before being recorded onto the final medium.

All Circuitry Adds Noise

The main problem when processing electrical signals is that each piece of circuitry adds noise to the signal – there's no such thing as noise-free circuitry. This noise is actually due to the random movement of electrons, and until we find some way around the limitations set by quantum mechanics, we're stuck with it. However, a well-designed circuit adds only a tiny amount of noise, and this is nominally constant in level and largely independent of the

signal level being fed through the circuit. This being the case, it's pretty obvious that, if you feed a very low-level signal through the circuit, the ratio of the noise to the wanted signal is going to be worse than if you feed a strong signal through the circuit. To minimise noise contamination, make sure that you're passing as high a signal level as possible through the circuit. However, there's a limit to how hot your signal can be, because if it's too high in level, it will exceed the maximum level that the circuit can handle. If this happens, the circuitry will clip and you'll hear distortion. (Distortion is defined as any difference – other than in level – between what you put into a circuit and what you get out of it, and clipping distortion is about as severe as it gets.)

Optimum Level

Getting the best signal level is a compromise – the signal level must be high enough so that it overpowers the circuit noise but not so as high that it causes the circuitry to clip and distort. You also need to leave a little safety margin or headroom to accommodate any unexpected signal peaks.

If you visualise the VU meters on an analogue tape recorder such as a cassette deck, this whole concept makes more sense. The nominal operating level is where the signal peaks at around the 0VU mark (where the red area starts) and the safety headroom is how far you can push the level into the red before you hear distortion.

Gain And Digits

Most analogue circuits don't suddenly clip when the level gets too high – instead, the amount of distortion rises gradually as the last few decibels of headroom are used up and then hard clipping occurs. Digital circuits have very similar limitations to analogue ones – if the signal is too high in level, it will still clip as the maximum numerical value that the system can handle is exceeded. However, there's no safety margin or area of progressive distortion as there is with analogue – once the maximum level is reached, the signal clips. For this reason, the nominal operating level for digital equipment is usually chosen around 12–15dB below the actual 0VU or clipping point.

Digital circuits also suffer from noise in a similar way to analogue circuits. If too small a signal is fed into a digital system, it is represented by fewer bits, which in practical terms means that the signal suffers from quantisation distortion, which sounds very much like noise. In other words, digital circuitry doesn't mean that you don't have to worry about noise; you still have too feed it the right level.

Correct Gain Structure

To obtain the best sound quality and the lowest noise, you need to optimise the gain settings of each piece of equipment connected to your mixer. In other words, everything should be set so that the input signal is as high as possible without running into clipping. When it comes to the inside of your mixer, you don't have too much control over what goes on, but the designers will have done their best to ensure that the internal gain structure is right. However, this carefully planned gain structure can be compromised if you plug something into a channel insert point that significantly reduces the level of the signal passing through it, for example and a compressor with the output gain set too low would be a good example of this. Here, the signal fed back into the mixer is lower than it was, so you have to restore the level by turning up a gain control somewhere further on in the signal path. Unfortunately, when you turn up the level, up comes the level of any background noise that's present, too. The golden rule when using insert points is that your peak signal level should stay the same whether the external piece of gear is connected or not.

Note: Semi-professional audio equipment is designed to work with a nominal signal level of −10dBV, whereas professional equipment is usually designed to run at +4dBu. It's usually possible to combine both types of equipment within the same system, but there may be some compromise either in noise performance or available headroom.

The Start Of The Chain

Perhaps the most important place to get the gain structure right is at the start of the audio chain, especially if you're using microphones. Make a habit of using the PFL buttons on your mixer to help you set the input gain-trim control so that the peak signal is just going into the red on the console PFL meters. It takes a few minutes to do this for all of your mics individually, but it's something that you really have to do religiously if you're to stand any chance of making a clean recording.

Other Noise Sources

Don't have anything that's not being used feeding noise into your system. For example, if you have an effects unit patched in that isn't being used, make sure the appropriate mixer inputs or returns are turned right down, and similarly, if you're a MIDI user, don't forget to turn down any channels handling synths that aren't being used – some synths put out far more background noise than is decent for a well-designed piece of audio equipment.

Disconnecting unwanted items of equipment also applies to bits of your mixer that aren't being used, so if you have unused channels, don't just mute them; make sure they're not routed anywhere, either, as even a muted channel can contribute mix-buss noise.

External Effects

Another potential source of trouble is the external effects unit. If you have your console effects-send controls turned nearly right down and then turn up the input stage of your effects unit to compensate, you'll end up with more noise than if you had the console levels set higher and the effects input level set lower. The best scenario, where line-level signals are concerned, is to maintain a unity-gain situation wherever possible – in other words, the signal stays at nominally the same level instead of being constantly built up and then knocked down again. On most mixers, a channel aux send setting of around seven corresponds to unity gain, and the same is true of the master send control. If you make sure that the channel with the highest effect-send setting has a send setting of around seven, you won't go too far wrong. Of course, it helps if the unity-gain setting is marked on the mixer controls. Some manufacturers actually do this for you.

If your effects unit has an output-level control, this should also be set at around seven, or to the unity-gain position. If you set your gain structure first and then use the effects return to fine-tune the amount of effect on the most heavily effected channel, you'll end up with the best possible signal-to-noise ratio.

Effects And Buss Noise

Mix-buss noise build-up also affects your aux sends, and the more channels you have, the greater the level of background hiss. Quite often an effects unit gets blamed for being noisy when the problem was aux mix-buss noise all along. Unfortunately, except on high-end studio consoles, there's usually no way of turning aux sends off. Even so, on some desks you can route the aux sends to different busses, often in pairs, and this can help. For example, aux 1,2 may be switchable to aux busses 1,2 or 3,4. If your effects are connected to busses 1,2 you could route any unused sends to 3,4, thus reducing the noise on busses 1,2.

This is fine as long as you don't need sends 3,4 for anything, but if you need all your sends or have no routing options like the ones described, you can still help to keep the noise down by paying proper attention to gain structure. This means setting the channel aux-send levels as high as possible, enabling you to use a lower setting on the aux-send master control to get the same level of effect in the mix. In effect, by doing this you've optimised the signal-to-noise ratio of the signal being fed into the effects unit.

If you have an effect that you only need to add to one channel, consider feeding the effects unit from either the insert-send point or the direct channel output, or patch the effect directly between the recorder output and the mixer-channel input. You'll be surprised at how much cleaner it sounds.

The Importance Of Gain Matching

Just as you'd never dream of making a tape recording without setting up the input level on the recorder itself, you should apply just as much care to matching the signal levels when two or more pieces of audio-processing equipment are connected together. Once noise is added to a signal, it's amplified by circuits further along the line in exactly the same way as the wanted signal, so there's no way to get rid of it. For this reason, it's important not to have any unused equipment (or mixer channels) adding noise to your mix.

The most vulnerable level-matching stage is the mic amplifier, because it's here that the tiny signal from the microphone is brought up to line level before its journey through the rest of the mixer. When it comes to effects and processors, try where possible to use unity-gain settings, because every time a signal level is changed, it has to be changed back again later on in the system, leading to a build-up of noise. If you take the time to optimise not only your mic levels but also your effects-send and -return levels, you're far more likely to end up with a professional-quality recording.

Balanced Wiring

Analogue audio signal connections can be either balanced or unbalanced. An unbalanced connection relies on a two-conductor cable, and in the case of screened audio cable this comprises a central core surrounded by woven or foil conductive screen. Although the screen (which is generally connected to ground) offers a degree of protection against electromagnetic interference, it is still possible for traces of outside interference to become superimposed on the wanted signal.

Balanced systems were developed to provide increased immunity to electromagnetic interference, and the principle is very simple. Instead of a two-conductor system, balancing involves using three conductors, one of which is still an outer screen, the other two being inner wires used to carry the signal. The reason for having two signal cables is that one has to be fed with a phase-inverted version of the signal, and if you look at the wiring details for a balanced connector (usually an XLR or stereo jack), you'll see that the normal signal connection is usually referred to as 'plus' while the inverted signal is 'minus'.

At the receiving piece of equipment, the 'minus' signal is inverted once again to bring it back into phase with the 'plus' signal and the two are added together. Why does this help? As the two signal wires are physically very close to each other, it's reasonable to assume that any interference will affect both conductors pretty much equally. When the 'minus' signal is re-inverted at the receiving end, any interference on that line will also be inverted, so when the 'plus' and 'minus' signals are added, the overall result is that the two interference signals cancel each other out, while the wanted signals combine. Even this isn't quite perfect, however, as you don't get exactly the same interference signal on each conductor, and the phase-inverting circuits at either end of the line aren't 100 per cent accurate, either, but even so, the amount of interference

remaining on the final signal is a tiny fraction of what it would be on an unbalanced connection in similar conditions. Figure 8.1 shows a balanced signal connection.

Matching Digital Recording Levels

The process of matching digital recording levels is covered at the beginning of Chapter 4 in the section 'Digital Recording Levels'. Following on from this description, because most DAT masters destined for album release are re-compiled on some form of editing system, it is generally safer to leave level matching until that stage. Aim to set your programme peaks at two or three decibels below the level at which clipping occurs. A number of hard-disk editing

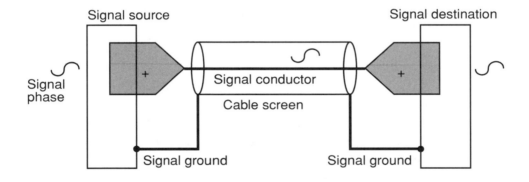

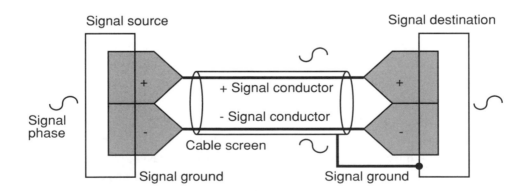

Note that, in a balanced system, the screen may be left disconnected at one end to assist in the prevention of ground loops

Figure 8.1: Balanced signal connection

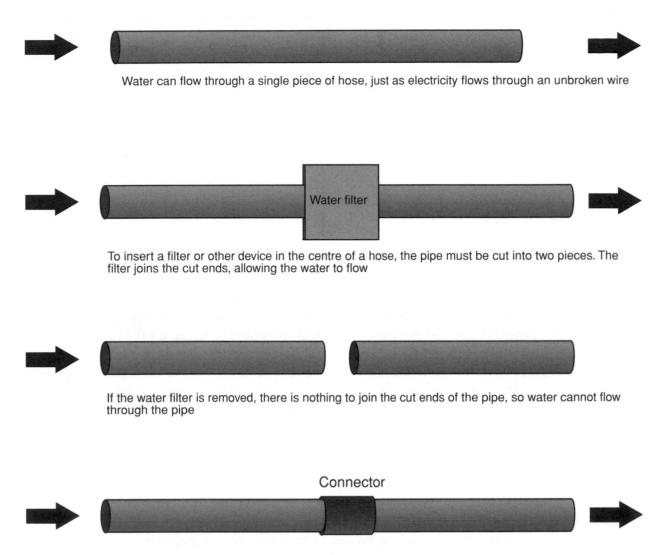

Water can flow through a single piece of hose, just as electricity flows through an unbroken wire

To insert a filter or other device in the centre of a hose, the pipe must be cut into two pieces. The filter joins the cut ends, allowing the water to flow

If the water filter is removed, there is nothing to join the cut ends of the pipe, so water cannot flow through the pipe

Connector

By using a connector piece between the cut ends, water can again be made to flow through the pipe. In the same way, a console insert send and return must be joined in some way when there is no external device connected to complete the circuit. You could use a simple patch cable, but the normalising contacts in a patchbay jack socket do the job automatically

Figure 8.2: Hose analogy of an insert point

packages include very good limiters for mastering purposes, so it's probably best to accept that your DAT recordings won't always match up in level and instead to record each song at the highest level possible without processing of any kind and without allowing the peaks to clip. Not only does this produce the lowest background noise level, but it also ensures the lowest possible distortion and the best signal resolution during quiet passages or fades.

Max Headroom

When recording a live performance, it's particularly important to leave sufficient headroom to cope with unexpected rises in level. In effect, headroom is the safety margin between the level you think you'll need and the point at which the signal level hits the end stops. Because you can't always predict the level of the highest peak, you have to decide how much headroom to leave, but this may vary depending on the type of music you are recording. For example, a dance track may have a very limited dynamic range, so you could get away with something like 12dB of headroom above the average signal level, but there's no way to guarantee this. Alternatively, ignore the average level and just concentrate on the peaks, then leave 6–10dB of safety margin. It's the peaks that matter, as far as the DAT machine is concerned, so keep a close eye on them.

More dynamic forms of music may need to be recorded with even greater headroom, but even if you've done a trial run, the chances are that the levels will change significantly during the actual performance. In this case, you might want to set your nominal recording level at around 20dB below clipping and your peaks at 12dB or so below, just to be on the safe side. Theoretically, this will compromise the signal quality to some extent, but because of the wide dynamic range of DAT, this is unlikely to be serious and, in any event, is far better than audible clipping. To make doubly sure, consider using a good stereo limiter when recording, just to provide a safety net, with the limiter threshold set 1dB or so below clipping. Although limiting isn't favoured by purists, it sounds a lot better than accidental clipping.

Effects, Inserts And Patching

Inexperienced users can encounter problems when patching in effects and processors, but a little understanding goes a long way to avoiding setbacks. The ability to patch signal processors and effects units into different signal paths is the key to the flexibility of traditional recording systems, and even in all-digital workstations, the analogue metaphor of the console insert point and aux/sent return is almost universally employed. Although the concepts of console insert points and aux sends are fairly straightforward, they're often confused by inexperienced users, so in this section I'm going to describe exactly how they work and what they can be used for.

Insert Points

If electrical signal flow can be thought of as analogous to pumping water through a garden hose, an insert point can be thought of as a break in the hose which allows a device, such as a sediment filter, to be fitted. The cut ends of the pipe clip onto the input and output of the filter, and all the water passes through the filter on its way to the end of the hose, as shown in Figure 8.2

This is straightforward enough, but what happens if you want to remove the filter from the hose? You can unfasten the clips, but then you're left with a break in the pipe. The answer is to find some way of joining the cut ends when the filter isn't being used, and that's almost exactly the same thing that happens at a mixing console insert point.

On a typical analogue mixing console, the insert socket is actually a stereo jack, but it isn't wired to carry stereo signals. Instead, the socket is arranged so that it can handle both the send and return routes of a mono signal – rather like the cut garden hose.

A stereo jack has three sets of contacts, as can be seen in Figure 8.3, and when used as an insert point the screen connection is common for both the send and return cable – the ring connector is the insert send and the tip is the insert return. Some manufactures have been known to wire the send and return connections the other way around, so check your mixer manual if you're unsure.

To prevent the signal flow from being broken when nothing is plugged in, special sprung contacts within the socket join the send and return connections when no plug is inserted. This is known as *normalising* and can be though of as automatically fitting a junction to our cut garden hose.

The Insert Socket

The adoption of a stereo socket, as an insert point isn't particularly convenient as either a special lead must be made up (or you can use an adaptor) before you can connect an effects unit or processor to the insert point, but it does conserve space. What's needed is known as a *Y-lead* because it has a stereo jack plug at one end and a pair of mono jack plugs at the other, although you can use a 'stereo-to-two-monos' adaptor plus a couple of straight mono leads if you prefer.

The most convenient way to use insert points is to wire them to a patchbay so that you have

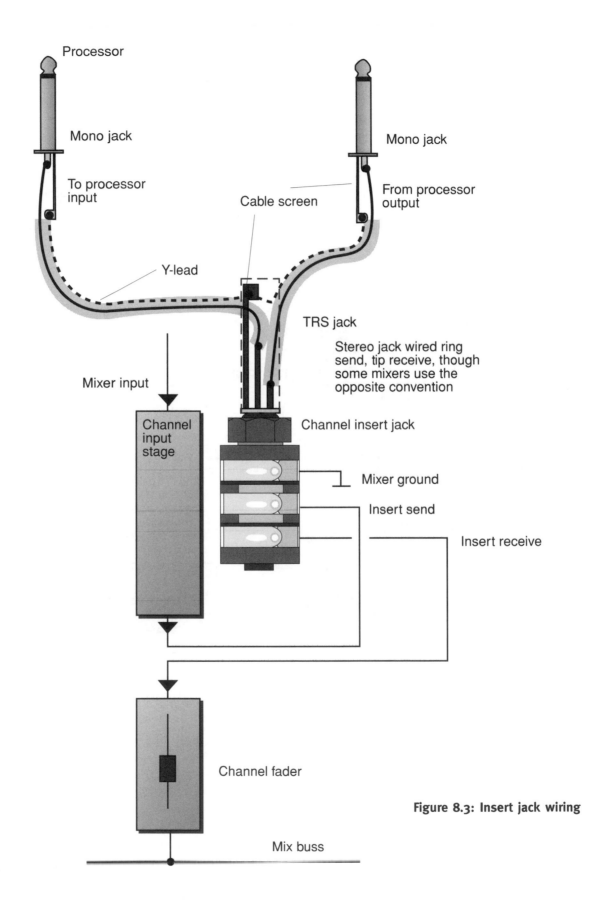

Processor

Mono jack

To processor
input

Cable screen

Mono jack

From processor
output

Y-lead

TRS jack

Stereo jack wired ring
send, tip receive, though
some mixers use the
opposite convention

Mixer input

Channel
input
stage

Channel insert jack

Mixer ground

Insert send

Insert receive

Channel fader

Mix buss

Figure 8.3: Insert jack wiring

separate mono sockets for the insert send and return. The patchbay connections must be normalised to maintain the signal flow when nothing is plugged in.

Figure 8.4 shows how the channel signal is routed via an external processor patched into the insert point. In the case of an effects unit which works with a mix of the original signal and an effected version of that signal, such as a reverb or delay unit, the balance between the effected and dry sound must be set up using the Mix or Balance control on the unit itself.

Effect Or Processor?

To avoid confusion, I like to separate external processing devices into two categories: effects and processors. This distinction is carried throughout other books in this series, but I'll recap briefly. Devices categorised as effects generally include some form of delay circuitry and include echo, reverb, chorus, pitch-shifting units and so on. Invariably, effects provide the option to mix some of the original untreated signal with the effected signal, so some form of dry/effect balance control is provided for this purpose.

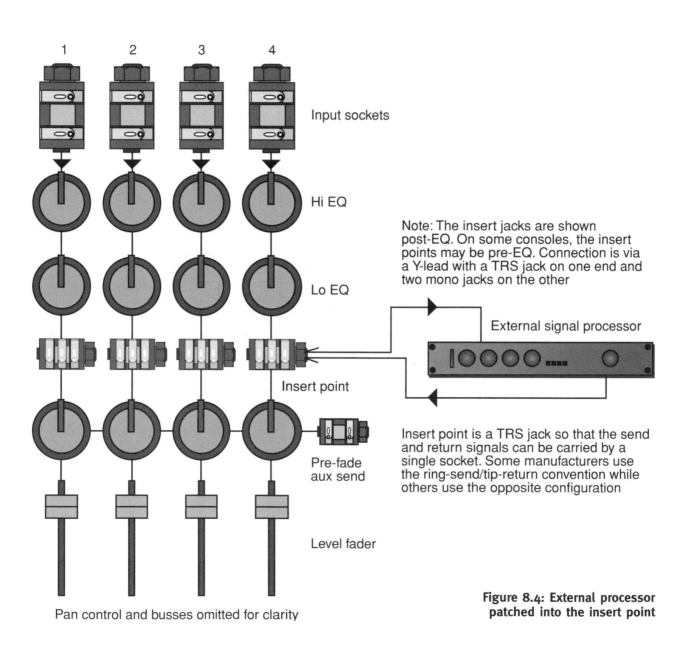

Input sockets

Hi EQ

Note: The insert jacks are shown post-EQ. On some consoles, the insert points may be pre-EQ. Connection is via a Y-lead with a TRS jack on one end and two mono jacks on the other

Lo EQ

External signal processor

Insert point

Insert point is a TRS jack so that the send and return signals can be carried by a single socket. Some manufacturers use the ring-send/tip-return convention while others use the opposite configuration

Pre-fade aux send

Level fader

Pan control and busses omitted for clarity

Figure 8.4: External processor patched into the insert point

Processors don't mix the treated and untreated signals together but instead change the signal passing through them in some way, usually by affecting the signal level or spectral content. Processors include such devices as gates, expanders, equalisers, compressors and limiters.

So why the distinction between effects and processors? The main reason for this is to determine how external devices may and may not be connected. Effects may be connected via an insert point (in which case the dry/effect balance is set on the effects unit itself), but it must be realised that a device plugged into a channel insert point cannot be shared with other channels.

If, on the other hand, the effect unit is connected to the aux-send/return system, the effect may be used on any number of channels, the amount of effect added being controlled by the relevant aux-send knob on each channel. If an effect is being used via the aux-send/return system, the dry portion of the signal passes through the channel as normal, so the effect device is required to supply only the effected signal. To achieve this, the dry/effects mix control should be set to 100 per cent effect, zero per cent dry. Aux sends are described a little later in this chapter.

Processors, on the other hand, can be used only via insert points or by being connected directly between the output of one piece of equipment and the input of another. This is because they don't work on a 'dry plus effect' basis but rather are designed to process the entire signal. For this reason, they should not normally be connected via the aux-send/return system, although advanced users may occasionally use an aux send to feed a signal out of the mixer, via a processor, to some other destination, such as directly to a tape-machine input. So, both processors and effects may be used at the insert points, but only effects may be connected via the aux-send/return system. This is an important point, so I make no apology for coming back to it from time to time.

Group And Master Inserts

Most multitrack mixing consoles also have insert points on their groups and main stereo outputs, providing the ability to pass an entire subgroup or even the entire stereo mix through an external processor. Group inserts also allow all the elements routed to a particular track to be passed through an external processor during recording. For example, you may want to pass the signal through a limiter to prevent a digital multitrack machine from overloading during unexpected signal peaks. It is unusual to add effects (reverb, delay and so on) to a finished stereo mix, but it is common practice to use processes such as equalisation, enhancement or compression to fine-tune what is an otherwise complete mix.

Aux Sends

Aux sends come in two types: pre-fade, for use with foldback or monitoring systems, and post-fade, for use with effects. Figure 8.5 shows an effects unit connected via the post-fade effects-send system of a mixer. The post-fade aux-send controls come after the fader, in terms of signal flow, so that, whenever the channel level is changed, the level of the signal fed to the effects unit varies accordingly. This maintains a consistent balance between the dry and effected part of the signal, regardless of the channel fader's setting. If you use a pre-fade send to drive the effect, the effect level will remain independent of the channel fader. For example, if you fade out a track that has had reverb added to it via a pre-fade send, the reverb will remain. This is sometimes useful as a special effect, but it is the exception rather than the rule.

Aux Returns

The outputs of the effects unit (these are nearly always stereo devices) are fed back into the mix via the aux-return inputs, which are really just additional mixer channels with simplified controls. As stipulated earlier, it is essential that the balance control on the effects unit is set so that only the effect is present at the output, not the dry signal. The dry or uneffected component of the signal is fed to the mix through the input channels, allowing the aux-send controls on the different channels to determine exactly how much effect is added to that specific channel.

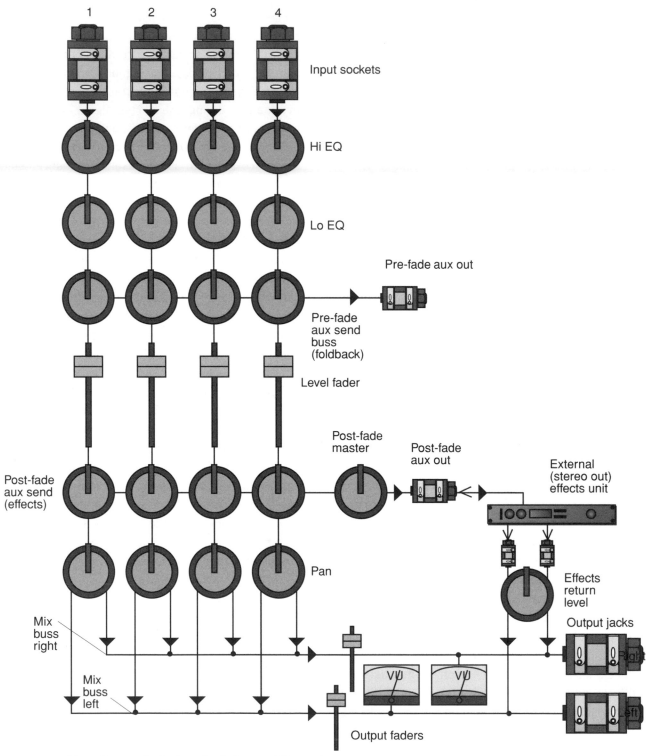

Note: On a typical mixer, the fader would be at the bottom of the channel strip. For convenience, the control layout is shown here in the order of signal flow

Figure 8.5: Effects unit connected via the post-fade aux send

Effects And Groups

Does this problem sound familiar? You've assigned several mixer channels to a group (thus forming a subgroup) to make mixing easier. However, when you change the group fader setting, the effects you've added don't vary in level. What's wrong?

We've all fallen for this one at some time or another, but if you're assigning channels to groups when mixing, if you want to create a subgroup it's important to realise that any effects used on those channels won't change in level when you move the group fader if you just feed the effects returns straight into the stereo mix. The aux-send level is dependent only on the channel-fader settings, so if these are left in one position, the effect level will also be constant.

The right way to add effects to subgroups is to route the effects returns back to the same group as the channels being effected so that now, when you turn down the subgroup fader, both the dry submix and its effects change in level together. Better multitrack mixers have signal routing on the aux returns, but if you're working with a mixer that doesn't, simply feed the effect unit into the mixer via one or two spare input channels and route those to the desired subgroup (or pair of subgroups, in the case of stereo).

Important: Whichever aux send is driving the effects unit should be turned right down on the channels that are being used as effects returns. If you don't do this, you'll end up feeding the effects unit output back to its own input, resulting in a howl of feedback.

Patchbays

While it's possible to plug effects and processors directly into your mixing console, it's hardly convenient, especially if the relevant sockets are around the back, where you can't get at them easily. For this reason, most studio installations include patchbays,

EFFECTS

Delay
Echo
Pitch Shift
Chorus
Flange
Phase
Reverb

PROCESSORS

Equalisers
Compressors
Limiters
Gates
Expanders
Enhancers
Single-Ended
  Noise-Reduction Units

which bring the most commonly used connections out to a central, easily accessible point. Although a large patching system can look daunting, the underlying concept is quite simple. In reality, all a patchbay does is get all the inputs and outputs that you might need to access out to a patch panel, where they can be linked or routed as necessary using short patch cables.

In professional studio installations, patchbays are generally wired for balanced operation and use miniature stereo jacks called *bantams*. However, in the private studio, the common currency of audio connection is the quarter-inch jack, so it makes more sense to use a standard jack patchbay. These are available in both balanced and unbalanced versions, depending on your needs. While line inputs and tape-recorder feeds should be kept balanced, if at all possible, most budget and mid-priced mixers have unbalanced insert points, so the insert patchbays need not be balanced.

Figure 8.6 shows a typical patchbay, and a modern 1U version will offer 24 pairs of sockets, usually with some means of labelling the various inputs and outputs. In addition to the front-panel sockets, there are further sockets at the rear that facilitate the connection of the patchbay to the rest of the system. Alternative versions are sometimes available with solder or clip connections on the rear. Convention is that the bottom row of sockets is used for signal inputs while the top row is used for outputs.

Non-Normalised Connections

Most patchbays can be configured to work normalised or non-normalised, with non-normalised sockets used purely to connect equipment inputs and outputs to a centrally accessible point. A typical application of a non-normalised patchbay is to bring out the signal connections for outboard effects

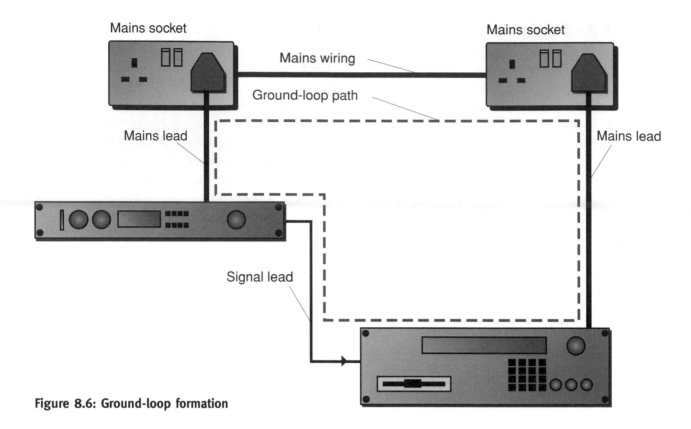

Figure 8.6: Ground-loop formation

and processors and to make certain mixer connections – such as aux sends and returns – and line inputs more accessible.

Normalised Connections

As explained earlier, insert points need to be normalised, or the signal flow would be broken if nothing was plugged into the insert jack. For example, if we were to connect the insert-send and -return points (the ring and tip of the stereo jack plug) to a non-normalised patchbay, there would be no problem if an effect or processor was plugged into the patchbay, but if no device was connected, the insert point would remain open and the signal path would be broken.

The solution is to use a patchbay incorporating sockets with built-in normalising contacts so that, when no plugs are inserted into the front of the panel, the top and bottom jacks are connected together automatically. In fact, a more correct term for the type of system used in conventional patchbays would be *semi-normalised*. Here, plugging

a jack into the lowermost socket breaks the circuit, allowing an external signal processor to be inserted into the signal path, but pushing a plug only into the upper socket leaves the normalising intact. There is a very good reason for this – it allows you to use the top socket to take a feed from an insert point without affecting the normal mixer operation. This provides a convenient way to split a signal, and in a typical studio an output may be split to feed several destinations simultaneously without problem. However, you can't mix outputs by simply combining them together; to do this, you need to use a mixer of some kind.

Patching Practicalities

Most patchbays can be configured for normalised or semi-normalised use, and if necessary some socket pairs may be normalised and others non-normalised within the same patchbay. Figure 8.6 shows a normalising link which may be made either with a short length of wire or by running a blob of solder between two printed circuit 'pads', although some manufacturers now make it even easier by mounting the sockets on a reversible circuit board. One way around, the sockets operate in a normalised fashion, while inverted they operate non-normalised. Consult the instructions that came with your patchbay to see how to convert between normalised and non-normalised operation.

Patchbays should be wired using high-quality screened cable, and most professional installations use foil-screened cable, which is easy to wire up, reasonably thin and offers good electrical screening. Most of the interconnections will be between the mixer and the patchbay, so locating the patchbay close to the mixer helps to keep the cable runs short. The cable run from the effects rack should also be kept as short as possible.

Patchbay Pragmatics

Some form of patching system is essential if a studio is to run smoothly, but there is an argument in favour of making as many permanent connections as possible in order to minimise the number of plugs and sockets in the signal path. Normalised patchbays tend to cause the most problems, so buy the best ones you can afford. If you must save money, do so on the non-normalised patchbays. Even so, you should buy or make decent-quality patch cables rather than use budget moulded types, and take care to clean the plugs regularly.

Patchbay Reliability

No matter how much you spend, any form of socket is prone eventually to become unreliable through contamination of the contacts, and normalised contacts are particularly bad in this respect as they don't wipe themselves clean whenever a plug is pushed in or taken out.

Smokers, please note that cigarette smoke is particularly bad for causing contact problems, shortening fader life and contaminating recording heads. It has also been known to affect the reliability of people!

If you unplug an effects unit to find that the mixer channel doesn't come back on properly, or if the signal is intermittent or distorted, then the chances

are that a dirty contact is to blame. Specialised contact-enhancing fluids can extend contact life, and deoxidising solutions are available for contact cleaning, but occasionally, you may have to replace a socket, especially on budget patchbays using basic moulded jack sockets. If fitting a new patchbay, it may be worth treating the contacts with a commercial contact enhancer before installation. These materials are expensive, but they help prevent oxidisation while at the same time ensuring a more consistent, low-resistance contact between mating surfaces. To minimise problems, check the following points.

- Clean your patch lead plugs regularly with a cloth moistened with a proprietary contact cleaner or isopropyl alcohol.

- Non-normalised sockets aren't so much of a problem, as the contacts are 'wiped' to some extent whenever a jack is inserted or removed. Sockets with gold-plated contacts tend to be more reliable than the cheaper types, but even these may need occasional cleaning. This means disassembling the patchbay and physically cleaning the contacts with cotton buds dipped in isopropyl alcohol or a proprietary deoxidising solution.

- A dirty contact can cause a significant degradation in signal quality without causing the signal to disappear altogether. Distortion, intermittent changes in level and background noise can all be introduced by dirty contacts, so if you experience any of these, investigate further. Dirty ground contacts can also result in an increase in radio-frequency interference problems from radio stations, taxis and so on. Even if the RF interference isn't directly audible, it can sometimes degrade the quality of the audio you can hear.

- Vertically mounted patchbays will accumulate less dust and debris than horizontal ones. If you need to use a horizontal bay, cover it with a clean cloth when it's not in use. The same applies to mixers, which should be covered up between sessions.

Ground Loops

Most studio users are aware of *ground loops*, which can cause problems with hum, but how do you know if you've got one, and what can you do about it if you do?

Individually, most mixers, recorder, synths, effects units and all the other studio bits and pieces will work OK. It's only when you start to hook them all together that the problems start. Sometimes things will be fine, but on other occasions the system will start to hum. It may not even be a very loud hum, but it'll be enough to compromise the quality of your work.

The hum is generally caused by ground loops, and there's no instant cure, but once you understand what causes them, it's not too difficult to track them down and eliminate them. A note of caution, however: although some hum problems can be cured by disconnecting the ground lead from the plug of the offending item, this is potentially a very unsafe thing to do. The ground connection is there for your safety, so leave it intact and instead deal with ground-loop hums by ensuring that the signal connections are made correctly.

Audio Connections

Most home studios rely on a mixture of balanced and unbalanced connections, a situation that in itself is potentially problematic. In an unbalanced system, line-level signals travel along cables comprising a single insulated core surrounded by a screen. The screen is grounded by being connected to the mains ground at some point, the idea being to 'earth' any electrical interference before it reaches the signal on the centre conductor, but this isn't a foolproof arrangement. If the entire screen was all held at ground potential, this would work, but in practice, the impedance of a typical cable screen isn't infinitely low.

In an unbalanced system, the audio signal is effectively the voltage difference between the centre (hot) conductor and the outer screen, so if the screen

isn't held firmly at 0V, any audio-frequency voltages that find their way onto the screen will end up superimposed on the audio signal. So, what's the relationship between connecting cables and hum?

Cable Impedance

All cable has an electrical resistance, and although this may be fairly low, it is nonetheless finite. If you pass an electrical current through any material that has an electrical resistance, a voltage will be developed between the two points of contact, the magnitude of which will depend on the strength of the current and the resistance of the material, as predicted by Ohm's law. If you pass a current through the screen of an unbalanced cable, there will be a difference in voltage between one end of the screen and the other. All problems connected with ground-loop hum stem from this simple fact.

The Ground Loop

A typical project studio includes numerous mains-powered pieces of equipment, some of which are interconnected via unbalanced screened cables. All the screens and mains grounds interconnect to form one large network of grounds, and because cable does have a finite resistance, there's a real danger that induced hum signals will cause small but significant alternating current to flow in the cable screens. The result is audible hum.

While most interfering signals – such as signals from distant radio transmitters – are pretty feeble, the 50/60Hz mains supply feeding your studio is a different matter. If you were to place a closed loop of wire inside a studio, sensitive measuring equipment would be able to detect a 50/60Hz current flow in the wire, because the loop acts exactly like a transformer, picking up any radiated signal. Admittedly, a single loop of wire makes a pretty inefficient transformer, but the principle is valid. As audio signals are measured in millivolts rather than volts, even the most inefficient coupling of the mains supply into the wire loop will produce enough current to generate a voltage across its impedance, which, when added to a typical audio signal, will be audible as hum.

Real-Life Loops

Far from being hypothetical, the ground wiring of a typical studio is likely to comprise several such loops, all connected to ground at some point, either directly or via other loops, and Figure 8.6 clearly illustrates how the ground and screen connections between just two pieces of equipment can form a closed loop. In reality, studio wiring has the potential to create multiple, interacting ground loops.

In Figure 8.6, the circuit is completed by the mains-lead grounds and the signal cable screens to form what is in effect a single-turn transformer. Any voltage resulting from circulating mains frequency currents within this loop will, effectively, be in series with the signal path, and that's why it is sometimes known as *series-mode interference*. Whatever the technicalities, the outcome, to a greater or lesser degree, is hum.

Fighting The Hum

The best way to make sure that there's no ground-loop hum is to make sure that there is no ground loop. The loop must be broken at some point, and to do this, you must ensure that each piece of equipment has only one ground-current path between it and the rest of the system to which it is connected. It's also important that your studio has a good earth, which means a very low impedance connection to ground. If in doubt, get an electrician to check this for you, and have a new grounding spike fitted if necessary.

This creates a dilemma: you must either disconnect a signal screen at some point in order to break the loop, or you must remove the mains ground and keep the signal screens connected. The latter usually works, but then there's no protective ground, other than via the signal leads (which won't stand the kinds of currents that occur during serious fault conditions), and if the signal lead is unplugged, the ground protection is completely removed. From a safety point of view, removing mains grounds is not recommended.

Note that equipment operating from external mains adaptors or fed via captive two-core mains cables is designed to be used unearthed and so may be less susceptible to ground-loop problems (although some authorities on the subject suggest that you ground their cases anyway and then treat them in the same way as other grounded equipment). Other outboard equipment may be fitted with a ground-lift switch, which means that it has a mains earth, but as far as ground loops are concerned, it behaves as though it has no mains ground.

A possible ground path overlooked by many people may occur when a ground-lifted or ungrounded unit is bolted to a metal rack. In this case, a ground loop may be created via the casework of the unit, connecting via the rack metalwork to other grounded units. If this is suspected, the unit should be mounted with plastic screws and insulating washers. It may also be necessary to use insulation tape to make sure the unit is isolated from the metalwork of the units directly above and below it.

Important note: AES (Audio Engineering Society) recommendations state that any balanced piece of outboard equipment should be wired pin 1 ground, pin 2 hot and pin 3 return, with pin 1 grounded to the chassis directly inside the socket. Not all outboard equipment follows AES grounding practice, however, and the variations you may encounter include equipment where a deliberate 'ground lift' resistor of a few hundred ohms has been placed between the electrical ground and the signal ground and, in rare cases, devices where the signal ground is completely isolated from the mains/chassis ground. These techniques were originally adopted to reduce the risk of ground loops, and often they do, but the downside is that the equipment may be more susceptible to RF (Radio Frequency) interference.

Wiring Remedies

Balanced systems are designed to cancel out interference by employing not one but two centre conductors, one of which carries a signal opposite in phase to the other. (The principles of balancing are more fully described earlier in this chapter.) In a balanced system, the screen isn't part of the signal path; it is merely there to ground interference, so it can quite safely be disconnected at one end of the cable in order to avoid ground loops.

In an unbalanced system, you could still disconnect one end of a screened cable, but only if the devices at both ends of the cable are electrically grounded by some other means. If they're not, you've broken your signal-return path and you'll be greeted by a monitor-numbing hum!

Even if the two pieces of equipment are grounded via the mains, disconnecting one end of a screen can still cause problems, because then you're relying on the mains-cable ground to act as return path for the audio signal – a role it was never designed to fulfil. This can lead to RF interference problems, usually in the form of radio breakthrough or high-pitched whines and whistles.

Unfortunately, unbalanced systems can't easily be sorted out in any clean or simple way, but a simple and usually effective technique is to connect a small resistor in series with the screen at one end of the cable, as shown in Figure 8.7. In a typical audio system, a resistor of around 100 ohms will be large enough to reduce significantly the magnitude of any induced hum currents while still being low enough not to compromise the level of the signal passing through the cable. However, using a resistor alone doesn't address the problem of RF interference, so a 100pF capacitor should be connected in parallel with the resistor to maintain a low-impedance path to ground for any high-frequency interference. Because signal currents are very small, low-wattage resistors may be used, and a quarter (or even eighth) -watt metal-oxide film resistor can, with care, be mounted inside most plastic-bodied jack plugs. Figure 8.7 also shows how the capacitor is wired, and again the component size is very small. Now, if a crucial ground lead is removed, the 'cold' signal still has a path via the screen and the resistor.

In theory, this method of tackling ground loops is a compromise, because the induced current isn't eliminated but merely reduced by the added impedance of the resistor. Nevertheless, it is a relatively simple solution to implement, and using

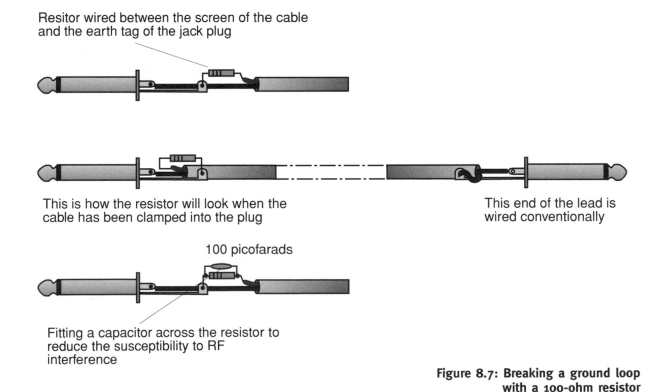

Resitor wired between the screen of the cable and the earth tag of the jack plug

This is how the resistor will look when the cable has been clamped into the plug

This end of the lead is wired conventionally

100 picofarads

Fitting a capacitor across the resistor to reduce the susceptibility to RF interference

Figure 8.7: Breaking a ground loop with a 100-ohm resistor

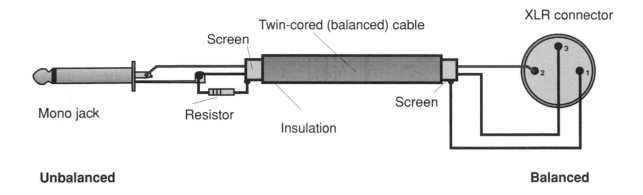

XLR connector

Twin-cored (balanced) cable

Screen

3

2

1

Mono jack

Resistor

Screen

Insulation

Unbalanced

Balanced

Figure 8.8: Unbalanced signal into balanced input

these simple loop-busting leads can bring about a dramatic improvement, reducing hum levels by orders of magnitude.

Connecting Unbalanced To Balanced

If you have a desk with balanced line inputs but your outboard gear is unbalanced, the most effective form of connection is outlined in Figure 8.8. A balanced input only 'sees' the difference between the positive and negative input lines, so if both carry identical interference signals, the interference cancels out, as described earlier. This concept is known as *common-mode rejection* and can be exploited when connecting unbalanced sources to balanced inputs. To prevent significant ground currents flowing in the cable screen, (which in extreme conditions could compromise the common-mode rejection of the input stage, allowing hum to reappear), a series resistor of around 100 ohms is connected in series with the screen connection. This is more satisfactory than putting a resistor in series with the screen in a completely unbalanced circuit because we're not relying on the screen to act as a signal return path – it works purely as a protective screen. In my experience, the resistor can be omitted completely in most situations.

Pseudo-Balancing

Some mixing consoles use a pseudo-balancing system, alternatively referred to as *ground compensation*. Details of how to connect both balanced and unbalanced signals to these mixers should be included in their handbooks, and in most instances the additional effort involved in making or adapting cables to take advantage of these inputs is well worthwhile.

Patchbays And Grounds

Project studios invariably use unbalanced jack patchbays to handle signal connections, and although this doesn't present any great problem, there are one or two points to bear in mind. For a start, in the interests of avoiding unnecessary connections between one ground point and another, avoid the type of patchbay where the socket grounds are all linked together along the length of the patchbay, or you're just creating a whole load more ground loops.

Also, if your patchbay provides the option of removing the ground link between upper and lower socket pairs, then do so wherever a patchbay is being used in a non-normalised application, such as for feeding console line inputs, aux sends/aux returns, or for bringing the inputs and outputs of effects and processors to the patchbay.

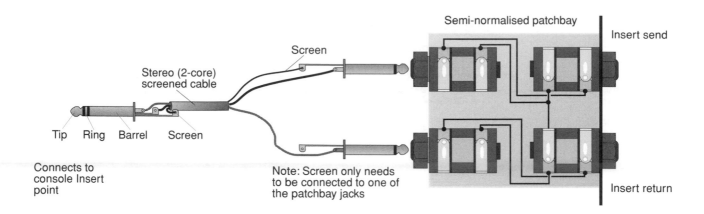

Figure 8.9: Insert-to-patchbay wiring

Normalised patch sockets are usually fed from console insert points, and as long as the distance between the console and patchbay is less than ten feet or so, you can get away with using a stereo cable to carry both the insert send and return connections, as shown in Figure 8.9. The fact that both signals share a common screen means that there can't be a ground loop between the insert point and the patchbay, even if the upper and lower patchbay socket pairs are ground-linked. However, with very long cable runs, sending both signals down the same cable runs the risk of introducing crosstalk, which may lead to instability. If the patchbay is a long way from the mixer, using separate send and return cables is safer.

Usually, the console can be connected directly to the patchbay using conventional cables with no problem; any precautionary measures (such as fitting series resistors) are applied to the cables joining the effects, processors, tape machines and instruments to the patchbay. People pontificate over which end of the cable the resistor ought to be, but in practice I've found that it makes little or no difference, so you may as well put it wherever you find most convenient.

Finding Ground Loops

Even armed with this knowledge, it's virtually impossible to track down ground-loop problems in a complete system, because what you're really dealing with is a large number of separate ground loops, all of which interact with each other. You could fix one loop only to find that the hum gets louder, as may happen where one ground loop is in antiphase with another! Unwelcome though the reality is, the only way to do the job properly is to unplug everything and then start wiring the system from scratch, checking for hum as each new piece of equipment is connected.

You should start with the mixer and the monitor amplifier plus speakers, and if the monitor amp has balanced inputs, use them. Most multitrack mixers have balanced monitor outputs, but even if yours doesn't, you can still use the balanced-to-unbalanced connection technique outlined earlier.

Once you're happy that the system doesn't hum, you can connect the two-track recorder and try again. Because you have four cables (left and right, in and out) going to the two-track, you have the potential for introducing a ground loop, so if hum does appear, use cables with series screen resistors, as shown in Figure 8.7. If the two-track is designed to have no mains earth (ie two-core cable), you'll still need to put resistors in three of the four cables in order to ensure that there's only one ground signal path to the machine. If it is earthed, you may need to treat all four cables. However, try conventional cables first, because if the internal grounding of your mixer has been designed properly, the level of hum may be so low as to be inaudible. Some hiss and hum will always be evident if you turn the monitoring system up far enough, but as long as the hum is at a lower level than the natural background hiss of the mixer with all faders down, it's probably as good as you can hope for. At a realistic monitoring level, neither hiss nor hum should be evident, unless you put your ear right against the speaker in a very quiet room.

Multitrack Connections

When connecting the multitrack recorder, the large number of inputs and outputs again increases the risk of running into multiple ground loops. As before, you'll probably find that everything works OK when using conventional cables, but if problems do arise, use the loop-busting cables with series resistors. Of course, those using digital recorders and digital mixers connected by optical cables won't have to contend with this problem.

Only when you're happy with the basic mixer, monitoring and recorder system should you think about connecting the patchbay. Stage 1 is to confirm that all is quiet when no external equipment is plugged into the patchbay. (Refer back to the earlier section for the warning on linked patchbay grounds.) Only when you're satisfied that the system is still running quietly should you try connecting your outboard equipment, and do this a piece at a time to identify problems as they occur. Furthermore, don't confuse ground loops with the digital noise and hum produced by some budget processors. As a rule, ground-loop hum will remain constant in level, even when the master aux send feeding the outboard equipment is turned down, whereas mix-buss noise or other contamination from the console will go up and down as the relevant aux-send level or effect-input level is adjusted. In theory, only the outboard equipment with mains grounds is likely to cause problems, although if you hear a hum when connecting an ungrounded unit, isolate its chassis from any other metalwork and see if the hum goes away. If it does, you'll need to isolate it from the rest of the metalwork by using plastic screws and washers, as described earlier.

Synths, expanders, sampler and drum modules should be checked in the same way, and if problems occur, they should be tackled in exactly the same way as for outboard equipment. Be aware, however, that the screens of MIDI cables can also aggravate the ground-loop situation, and in extreme cases you might need to use a DI box to get rid of the hum completely. I once had a sampler that refused to co-operate until I fed its audio output via a DI box. Then the hum disappeared.

Ground-Loop Overview

Tracking down and solving ground-loop problems can be tedious, but as long as you're methodical and you follow the guidelines given, it shouldn't be too difficult. Unless you're very unlucky in your choice of mixer, you'll probably find that only a few pieces of equipment give you any real trouble, and most if not all of these should respond to the treatments listed here. As long as you test your system as you assemble it, you should have little difficulty in identifying the areas that need attention and the things you can leave alone.

Grounding Checklist

- Don't disconnect the ground leads from pieces of equipment that are designed to be used grounded.

- Build up your system a piece at a time, checking for hum at every stage. Cure any ground-loop problems before connecting any more equipment. If you experience no hum problems when using standard leads, don't feel you have to fit ground-lifted cables; move onto the next piece of equipment.

- Use balanced wiring wherever your equipment supports balanced connections.

- When working with unbalanced equipment, use ground-lifted leads to ensure that each piece of equipment has only one direct ground path, either via a mains ground or via a signal cable screen. In the case of two-pin mains equipment or that running from mains adaptors, treat it as you would ground-lifted equipment.

- Check individual items of equipment with a meter to identify which have built-in ground-lift resistors. Those that are ground-lifted should be grounded both via the mains and via one signal cable.

- Beware of case-to-case contact causing problems. This is common in metal racks and is usually cured by using special nylon mounting hardware.

- Foil-screened cable is best for permanent wiring, as it's reasonably cost-effective, it has good screening properties and it isn't too thick. It also holds its shape well when made into a harness.

- For flexible wiring, cable with a woven copper screen usually performs best, but conductive plastic cables are fine for short patch cables, instrument leads and so on. Although their screening isn't quite as effective as that of woven-screen-type cables, their pliability tends to make them reliable.

- Don't run signal cables alongside mains cable for any distance, as this alignment allows hum to be introduced, although crossing it at right angles is no problem.

- Anything containing a large transformer is liable to radiate a strong hum field, so mount power amps and mixer power supplies away from other processors. Leave a few U of empty rack space if you have to – this will also help to ventilate your gear.

- Ensure that all connections have the lowest possible resistance. Clean mains-plug pins and jacks using a deoxidising solution and avoid using cables that use poorly made crimped connections.

Studio Mains Wiring

As recording equipment gets quieter, problems such as hum and interference become more significant, and the studio mains supply may not be entirely blameless. If you're setting up a serious private studio in a separate room, you need to think carefully about whether the electricity supply is suitable. Simply plugging into the nearest 13A socket might be OK for making bedroom demos, but depending on the way in which your house is wired, you may run the risk of picking up electrical interference from other systems in the house.

Even if the mains supply is OK, a domestic room will have insufficient mains sockets for all the gear used in a typical project studio, but trying to shoehorn all of your equipment into one wall socket using a nest of domestic distribution boards or adaptors also invites trouble. Even if the total load on the socket doesn't exceed the stipulated 13A, using a mixture of cheap distribution boards and adaptors risks intermittent mains connections, which can arc, causing interference.

If you're wondering why this should be so, try looking inside a typical plastic distribution board and you'll see that the socket contacts are actually small pieces of metal crimped onto rigid wire buss bars, and once you've used them a few times, the sockets lose their springs and fail to make good contact with the plugs. Because such faults are likely to be intermittent, any resulting interference may take a lot of tracking down.

The solution is to use professional-grade mains-distribution boards, which can be built from industrial metal-cased sockets, as described later.

The Mains Supply

The chief cause of concern regarding the mains power supply isn't overloading due to attempts to draw excessive current but interference and mains hum caused by inappropriate wiring. Most pieces of studio equipment actually take relatively little current, and the needs of a typical home studio can often be supplied by just one or two 13A sockets – providing the means of connecting to those sockets is sound. Modern houses use a form of wiring known as a *ring main*, where the main electrical cabling forms a complete loop that starts and finishes at the fuse box. Wall sockets are then positioned at intervals on the loop. Some studio-design specialists prefer to use a *spur-wiring system*, although a properly designed ring main should be fine.

If you're planning a new mains wiring system, you should fit a separate consumer unit for your studio area feeding a dedicated studio ring main – and in a larger facility, you should fit two separate ring mains, one for the 'clean' audio/computer supply and a second for 'dirty' power, such as heating, lighting, coffee machines and so on. A consumer unit is the modern equivalent of a fuse box but will be equipped with resettable circuit breakers, not old-fashioned fuses. The installation should also include an earth-leakage trip. Details of these and other safety trip devices should be discussed with a competent electrician.

Mains-Borne Interference

The reason for using a separate consumer unit fed from the building's main fuse box is that it provides a degree of natural interference rejection, helping to minimise clicks and buzzes caused by the likes of fridge thermostats and central-heating systems elsewhere in the building. However, if these continue to break through onto your audio, engage an electrician to fit suppressors to the offending items, and also get him to check the integrity of your mains earth. If it isn't providing a suitably low impedance path, consider getting a longer earth spike fitted.

Other sources of interference include lighting dimmers (conventional dimmers should never be used in a studio), fluorescent lighting and poorly designed mains power adaptors. It may help to keep mains adaptors away from your signal wiring, as they contain transformers which may induce hum.

Spur Systems

If you opt to install a spur rather than ring-main system, you should have the supply put in by a qualified electrician, as there are certain safeguards required for spur systems that don't apply to normal ring mains. In a spur system, each mains socket is connected back to the consumer unit by a single length of cable, and each spur should be protected separately by a fuse or circuit breaker. In theory, this wiring system provides additional isolation between equipment plugged into the different spurs.

It will also help to use the heaviest mains cable practical, and although the electrician might find your request for 30A cooker cable throughout a little odd, it won't add much to the price and will help keep down interference by providing a lower impedance from the consumer unit to the equipment being powered. If the mains-wiring impedance is excessively high, sound quality can suffer when the mains supply to one piece of gear is modulated by the mains current taken by current-hungry equipment, such as power amplifiers connected to the same supply.

Mains impedance doesn't finish with the mains wiring, though; you also have to consider the connection between the power point and your equipment. For this reason, check the connections inside your mains plugs regularly, and clean any corroded plug pins with wire wool. A wipe-over with WD40 or similar silicone-based lubricant may help keep them clean for longer.

Wiring Topography

To minimise the risk of ground loops and radiated hum, all mains wiring should be run together as far as is possible, and it helps if the cabling can be run around the top of the room with drops to the various sockets. The logic behind this is that it keeps the mains as far as possible from your signal cables (these usually run close to the ground), which reduces the risk of hum pickup. Some benefit may be obtained from running the cable in metal rather than plastic conduit and ensuring that the conduit is earthed. Figure 8.10 shows how a typical ring main is set out, whereas Figure 8.11 shows a spur system for studio use. (Non-UK readers should consult their local electricity regulations for details of permissible wiring systems and requirements.)

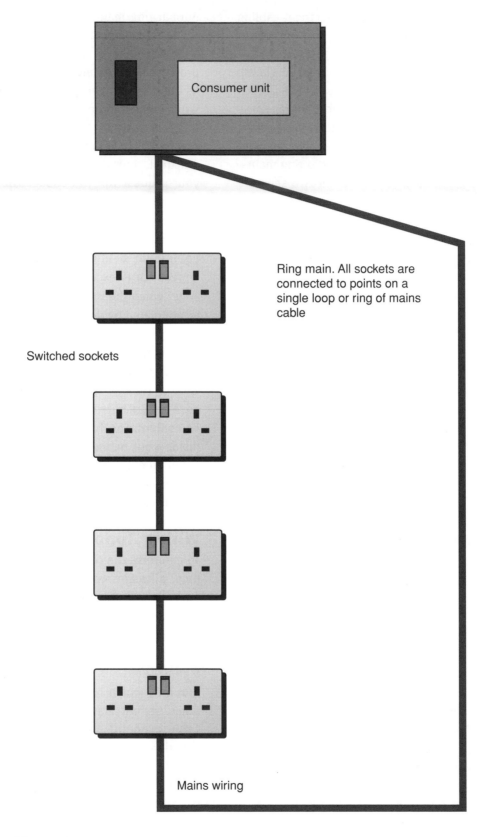

Figure 8.10: Ring wiring system

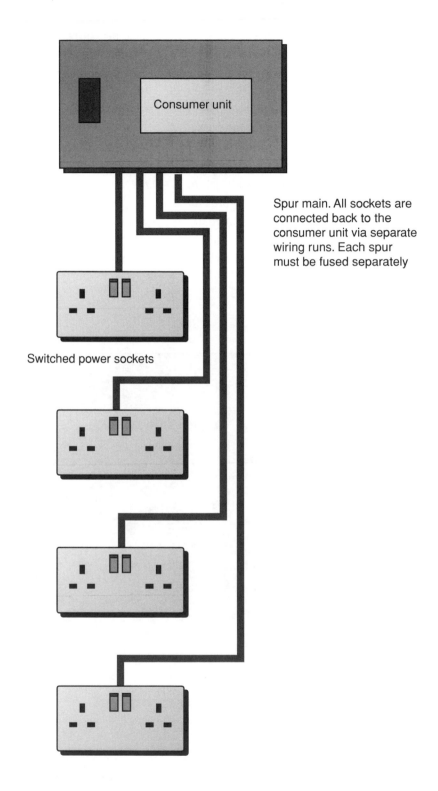

Consumer unit

Spur main. All sockets are
connected back to the
consumer unit via separate
wiring runs. Each spur
must be fused separately

Switched power sockets

Figure 8.11: Spur wiring system

Power Distribution

Plan to fit as many wall sockets in your studio as you can, but also be prepared for the fact that you still won't have enough! To reduce the risk of hum-causing ground loops, all the audio equipment should, if possible, be plugged into the same socket or pair of sockets. If you're not sure about the power consumed by any item of equipment, the power rating is normally quoted in the user handbook or marked on the back of the case. Add the figures for all of your gear together and ensure that you're not connecting more than 3kW to any individual socket. Unless you run a studio with a PA-sized monitoring system, you're unlikely even to come close to this figure; most home studios take well under 1kW. Lighting and heating tends to take much more power than the audio equipment and should, of course, be run on a separate circuit.

In order to split the power from a pair of 13A sockets to drive the studio gear, it's best to make up a distribution board using commercial-grade, metal-cased, switched mains sockets. These may be screwed to a suitably solid piece of wood and then wired spur-wise to a heavy-duty junction box using heavy house-wiring cable. The junction box then terminates in a trailing mains lead made from the heaviest flexible

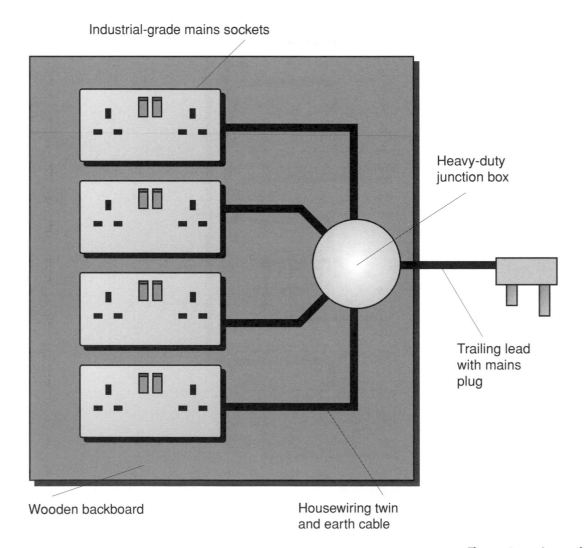

Industrial-grade mains sockets

Heavy-duty
junction box

Trailing lead
with mains
plug

Wooden backboard

Housewiring twin
and earth cable

**Figure 8.12: A practical
mains distribution board**

cable that you can fit into a 13A plug. For a typical studio load, 15A cable is more than adequate, but keep the lengths as short as possible. Also, never coil unused mains cable, especially if it's passing a lot of current – it has been known to melt!

Figure 8.12 shows a practical distribution board, although high-quality commercial alternatives are available, if you're prepared to pay the premium price. By mounting the distribution boards in the back of your equipment racks, the amount of exposed cabling can be kept to a minimum.

For equipment with IEC-type mains connectors, many studio suppliers stock distribution boards with IEC-type sockets, and these boards can help to conserve space. If you use one of these, you'll also need to buy one male-to-female IEC lead for each piece of equipment supplied.

Another useful accessory is the multiple-output IEC lead. This is a straightforward moulded lead with a plug at one end and three or four IEC connectors at the other.

If you decide to risk using cheap consumer distribution boards, snip out the neon indicators, as these can sometimes cause interference. Most importantly, avoid plugging equipment in and out wherever possible. The contacts in these cheap boards are reasonably reliable if left undisturbed, but if you insert or remove plugs a few times, the contact springs will weaken and before you know it you'll have intermittent buzzes and spluttering noises. (Again, non-UK readers should check their local electrical regulations for details of approved wiring systems and of the maximum current that can be drawn from each socket.)

Computer Mains Supply

In a spur-wired installation, computers should be fed from a different spur to the audio, but in any event it's best to plug the computer in via a mains filter that also includes a spike suppressor. Don't plug the computer into a supply handling 'dirty' equipment, such as coffee machines or fridges, as this will increase the risk of crashes. Serious users may also find it worthwhile to fit an uninterruptable power supply that switches the computers over to

power generated by high-capacity batteries if a mains failure occurs. This should provide enough time to shut the computers down properly and to back up any necessary data.

Mains Checklist

- Make sure that mains plugs are wired properly and that fuses of the correct rating are fitted. Aside from being dangerous, loose wires are liable to arc and cause interference.

- Check your plugs carefully, ensuring that the cable grip is clamped firmly on the outer sleeve of the cable. While you're checking the fuse rating, make sure that the fuseholder grips the fuse tightly. If it doesn't, pinch it in a little with a pair of pliers.

- Make sure that the fuseholders on your various pieces of equipment are reasonably tight and that the correct ratings of fuse are fitted.

- Although it's tempting to remove the earth leads from certain pieces of equipment as a quick cure for hum caused by ground loops, this is potentially dangerous – the earth wire is there for your protection in case something else fails. In a correctly designed system, you should be able to cure any ground-loop problems by modifying your signal connections rather than your mains leads.

- Avoid using fluorescent lights or dimmers, as these are known sources of interference problems.

- Use only the correct types of mains power adaptors for your equipment and position them away from signal cabling. If they are a loose fit in the mains socket, consider fixing them to the distribution board using plastic cable ties.

Fuses

Fuses are fitted to equipment in order to protect it, and possibly the user, from further damage in the event of a fault condition. If a fuse blows, especially when you first switch a piece of equipment on, it may simply be the initial surge of current that takes out the fuse, or perhaps the thin wire inside the fuse had become fragile with time. It's also possible that the metal endcaps have come loose, causing the wire inside to fracture. If this happens, you should only ever replace the fuse with the same type and value; if you fit a higher rating and there is a genuine fault, you may cause further damage to the equipment. Quick fixes with pieces of wire or aluminium foil are extremely dangerous and could lead to irreparable damage to the equipment or, worse still, cause it to catch fire.

Equipment that draws a high surge of current at switch-on, such as some power amplifiers, is normally fitted with what are known as *slow-blow fuses*, normally recognisable by a small coiled spring inside one end of the glass fuse casing. Always replace slow-blow fuses with new slow-blow fuses – conventional fuses are likely to fail as soon as the equipment is powered up, as they aren't designed to handle surges of high current.

Always ensure that fuse holders are done up tightly, or they may make a poor contact, resulting in heat and oxidisation of the contacts. If the fuse caps are obviously corroded, clean them with wire wool before refitting them.

Pragmatic Solutions

The next section includes a few problem-solving tips based on using pieces of equipment that you might not normally associate with quality recording. For example, when it seems that you don't have the equipment to do a job, you might find that your hi-fi, combined with a little ingenuity, solves the problem.

Vinyl Challenge

What do you do if you need to record some material from a record deck but your mixer doesn't have a record-deck input? You can't just plug a record deck directly into a line-level mixer, not just because the levels and impedances are all wrong but also because records need to be processed via an RIAA pre-amp. Without getting too technical, records are not recorded 'flat' but instead use a form of pre-emphasis that boosts high frequencies. When played back through a filter with the opposite

characteristics, the original sound is restored and the level of background noise is also reduced, very much like tape noise reduction. All amplifiers with record-deck inputs include RIAA pre-amps, which perform this task, but the only mixers with RIAA pre-amps built in are those designed for DJ or broadcast use.

One simple solution is to plug the recording output of your hi-fi system's amplifier into your mixer to give you a line-level feed from your record deck, complete with RIAA correction. Of course, your hi-fi amp might not have a recording output, but you can still try to take a feed from the headphone socket. Most headphone outputs will match passably well to a mixer's line input, and it's easy to connect up using a 'stereo-to-two-monos' jack adaptor. The quality of the sound ultimately depends on the quality of the headphone amplifier is, but most are adequate.

Cheap Headphone Amps

If you have a spare hi-fi amp, you can use it as the basis for an inexpensive headphone monitoring system. Figure 8.13 shows the wiring arrangement that involves feeding the speaker outlets to a row of stereo headphone jacks via 330-ohm resistors in order to limit the power. Without the resistors, you run the risk of over-driving the headphones. It's also a good idea to include a 33-ohm resistor directly across the speaker outlets, as shown in the diagram, just in case the amplifier in question isn't too happy about running without a speaker load. The 33-ohm resistor should be a 10W wire-wound type, whereas the remaining resistors can be either 1W metal film types or low-wattage wire-wounds.

This system will work with both high- and low-impedance headphones, although the headphone mix will be in mono only. With amplifiers that permit the negative terminals of the left and right speakers to be linked, it's easy enough to create a stereo headphone feed, but because not all amps will operate this way, don't go connecting the output up for stereo unless you've checked with a meter that the left and right speakers' negative terminals are in fact common. The amplifier volume control

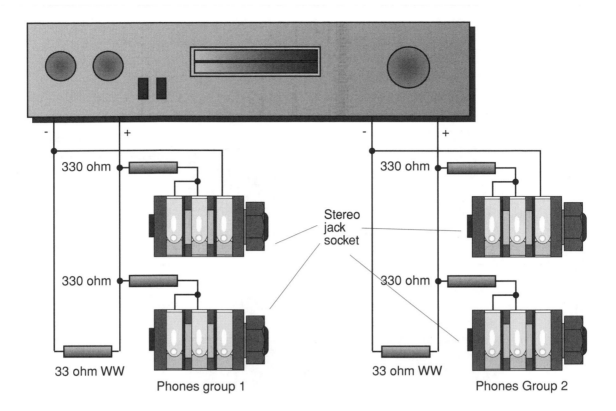

330 ohm

330 ohm

33 ohm WW

Phones group 1

Stereo
jack
socket

330 ohm

330 ohm

33 ohm WW

Phones Group 2

One stereo amplifier provides two sets of mono phones feeds. The relative levels of group 1 and group 2 can be set using the amplifier Balance control. Up to 10 sets of phones may be fed from each amplifier output

Figure 8.13: Using a hi-fi amp to drive studio headphones

will regulate the overall level of the headphone mix, while the balance control sets the relative level of the two headphone groups. The amplifier's Aux, Tuner or CD inputs could be fed from the foldback output of a mixer to provide a cue mix while recording. If you find some of your phones unacceptably louder than others in the same group, you could double (or more) the value of the 330-ohm resistors feeding that particular socket to reduce the power.

Instant Mic Pre-amps

Another way in which your hi-fi can come in handy is to provide a mic input – providing you have a cassette deck with a couple of mic input jacks and not one of those MIDI systems designed with a total

absence of useful orifices. Surprisingly, even relatively cheap cassette decks can have quite good mic amps, so if you're working with a line-level keyboard mixer and want to feed in a mic, just put the cassette deck into Record/Pause mode and feed its output into your mixer. The mic level may then be adjusted using the Record Level control on the cassette deck.

Aside from providing a convenient way of getting a mic input into a line mixer, this trick also helps get around a lack of insert points, if you want to compress or otherwise process a signal as you record it. The mic goes into the cassette deck, the output of the cassette deck feeds the compressor's input and the output of the compressor feeds the mixer's line input as shown in Figure 8.14.

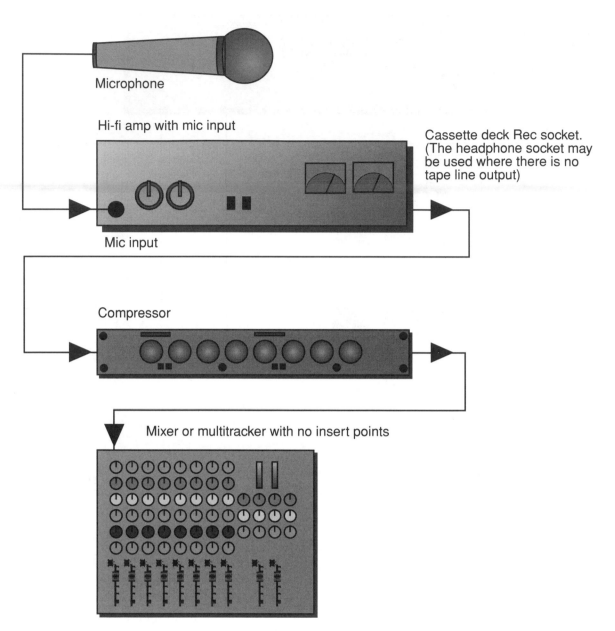

Figure 8.14: Hi-fi amp used as a mic pre-amp

Signal Gremlins

A *gremlin* is a popularly term used to describe anything inexplicable that goes wrong in an audio system and can include (but is by no means limited to) hums, hisses, glitches or mysteriously absent signals. Although gremlins often seem to appear without reason, a little logical thought often reveals the true cause of the problem.

While music is most definitely an art, the studio itself remains rigidly bound by the laws of physics, but even so, signals still disappear, distortions creep in and otherwise-pristine master tapes exhibit inexplicable clicks and pops. The aim of this section is to explore some of the more common gremlins and to provide a few suggestions for keeping them out of your studio.

No Signal?

Perhaps the most common studio gremlin is the one that causes your monitors to remain silent even though you have every reason to believe that music should be pumping through them. The problem is that the signal routing in a typical studio is quite complex, and an error at just one point in the signal chain can lead to complete silence.

Perhaps the most common cause of a disappearing signal is console routing (or being switched to Two-Track Monitor mode when you're hoping to listen to the stereo mix). Before you do anything, however, make sure that everything is switched on and that the power lights are glowing to indicate that the mains fuses are intact. I know this sounds obvious; it's so obvious that nearly everyone – me included – falls for it some time or other. A particular favourite is to have a mixing console that's switched on but a device plugged into the master insert points that's switched off. If you're monitoring via a hi-fi amp, make sure that the source is switched to your desk output, not to your cassette deck or CD player.

Finding The Gremlin

When tracking down a missing signal, first solo the mixer channel to confirm that something is actually getting into the desk, then check your channel routing, including anything that might be plugged into the channel insert point. Getting the inputs and outputs swapped around on a piece of outboard gear is a great way to lose your signal, as is being patched into a processor that's switched off! By using your Solo buttons and by checking any metering along the signal path, it shouldn't be too difficult to identify where the signal stops.

If you suspect a faulty lead, change one lead at a time and check each one with a cable tester. If you don't have a cable tester, I strongly recommend that you buy one – they're not expensive, and they can preserve your sanity! All dubious leads should be labelled clearly as such and put to one side so that, when that elusive spare five minutes finally turns up, you can sit down and fix them.

Always retain a healthy suspicion of insert points or normalised patchbay connections and check that the suspect socket hasn't gone intermittent. You can test this easily by temporarily linking the patchbay send and return points using a patch cable. If you do have a persistently troublesome socket, clean it with isopropyl alcohol or a specialised contact cleaner. If cleaning fails to work, replace the socket.

If the inexplicably silent signal is from a mic, double-check the console mic/line selector switch and make sure that the mic has phantom power, if it's a capacitor model. You might also check that the mic is switched on, if it's fitted with a switch. If you're not sure whether the problem lies with the mic or the wiring, simply plug in a spare mic and check the circuit that way. I once spent several minutes scratching my head at the non-appearance of a drum mic signal only to find that the drummer had knocked the head off the otherwise neat and effective clip-on mic. Fortunately, it was his mic!

In tracking down breaks in circuits, it can also help to have some sort of test signal you can inject into the signal path. I often use the oscillator output from my guitar tuner, but you can also use a synthesiser with a book placed on the keys, a cassette deck playing a continuous music tape or a portable CD player. Take the time to understand the signal flow of your mixing desk and patchbay so that you can follow the signal path a stage at a time until the break is discovered.

Uninvited Signals

Just as frustrating as the missing signal is the presence of unwanted noise, usually traceable to mains hum, circuit hiss or radio-frequency interference, which may be either airborne or carried via the mains supply. Hum is often (but not always) due to ground loops, although it can also be caused by using unscreened cable or cables where the screen has been wired wrongly or has become disconnected. Don't try to cure ground loops by removing mains grounds because this is obviously dangerous; instead, ensure that all of your mains leads are plugged into one distribution board rather than spread around the room, and follow the wiring recommendations that came with your mixer with regard to external connections. Studio equipment takes very little current, so it's unlikely that you'll overload your mains supply, regardless of how many extension boards you have.

RF interference may be due to poor ground connections, poor-quality cables or high contact resistance, either in the mains ground wiring or in the studio's signal wiring.

Ground-Loop Hum

The mechanism of ground loops was described earlier in this chapter, and they're one of the most common causes of unwanted hum in the studio, especially in unbalanced semi-pro systems, but solving them can be tricky and may take persistence.

If a piece of gear runs from an external power supply, the chances are that it's not grounded via the mains, so you should use a connecting cable with the screen connected at both ends – in other words, a conventional instrument lead. However, the casework of the unit might also be grounded via the rack metalwork to another unit, so if you're hearing a background hum, try unbolting it from the rack to see if the hum situation changes. If removing it from the rack cures the hum problem, use plastic screws and washers to isolate the unit from the rack metalwork. Most studio supply companies market kits for this purpose.

Tracking Down Ground Loops

The only sure way to trace ground-loop problems is to disconnect your entire system and then reconnect, starting with just the mixer, the monitor amp and the speakers. If these work without humming, connect your multitrack recorder and listen again. If it's still clear, add the stereo recorders, then the patchbay, then patch in your effects and processors one at a time. As soon as you come across a problem, sort it out before adding any more equipment to the system, or you won't know where to look. You can even get into a situation where two ground loops are causing hum which partially cancels out so that, when you fix one of them, the hum level actually goes up! In reality, some hum will always remain, but this should

be equal to or less than the level of hiss produced by a well-set-up system. If the problem remains persistent, you may have to call in a studio specialist.

Mains Hum

Hum may also be caused by inadequate mains power adaptors, so if you're using a mains PSU that didn't come with the piece of equipment in question, try to eliminate it from your enquires by using a different one. Yet another source of mains hum is electromagnetic radiation from transformers or mains cables, so make sure that mains cables don't run alongside signal cables, and if they must cross, try to arrange it so that they do so at right angles. Keep sensitive equipment, such as mic pre-amps, away from power amplifiers or mixer PSUs, and also be aware that the neon lamps in distribution boards can cause a buzzy kind of hum if brought near sensitive cabling.

Fluorescent lamps, light dimmers and computer monitors all radiate significant amounts of interference. Electronic dimmers should never be used in studios and fluorescent lights should really only be used for maintenance work. The new generation of energy-saving bulbs don't seem to cause any problems, but I can't guarantee them to be safe in all situations. Interference from fluorescent lamps and dimmers can usually be differentiated from ground-loop hum, as their brand of hum contains a large element of buzz due to the high harmonic content of the interference source.

Guitar Hum

For more information on guitar hum, see the section on guitar problems in Chapter 2, 'Vocal And Instrument Recording'. However, it is fair to say that guitars with single-coil pickups pick up hum interference from alternating magnetic fields in surrounding equipment to an almost alarming degree. The only solution is to place as much distance as possible between the guitar and the source of interference and then to move the guitar around to find the angle of least interference. Computer monitors are particularly bad for interfering with guitar pickups, and in some cases they can cause problems at distances up to ten feet or even more. If at all possible, switch off computer monitors when recording the guitar, or explore the possibility of using a laptop computer fitted with an LCD screen.

Crackles And Pops

Crackles and pops are often caused by mains-borne interference such as that caused by thermostats and heating systems switching on or off, although in the case of digital systems, they can also be caused by using the wrong type of cable to carry digital signals from one machine to another. Always buy the proper digital co-axial cable, as its impedance is quite different from that of audio cable.

Running your studio from a separate ring main will help reduce the risk of mains glitches getting onto your recordings, but if the problem is severe, the best answer is to get a qualified electrician to fit suppressor components to the offending devices. It can also help to use mains filters, but in my experience, these seldom offer a complete solution.

Loose Mains Connections

A related source of crackles and bangs can often be traced to loose wires in plugs, loose fuse holders in plugs and cheap extension boards, on which the spring socket contacts have lost their spring. If you're really unlucky, you may also have poor connections in your studio mains wiring, in which case you may need to bring in an electrician.

It's always good practice to check your mains plugs on a regular basis, because wires have a habit of working loose, even if they've never been disturbed. It can also help to clean the contacts of your mains plugs periodically using wire wool, and some hi-fi purists claim that this actually makes things sound better! In any event, keeping mains ground pins clean will help improve your system earth.

Poor Audio Connections

Other areas that may be at fault are poor connections in signal leads and crackly pots or faders. Once a fader has gone crackly, you can clean it with spray cleaner, but in my experience, the only long-term cure is to replace it.

You may experience radio-frequency interference if your ground connections are substandard, but an improperly grounded studio system or poorly designed equipment can also cause similar problems, as can living next door to a radio ham, in which case the laws of both the land and the inverse square are, sadly, on his side. If you live in an environment where there is a high level of airborne RF interference, the only solution may be to enclose the whole studio in a Faraday cage. This sounds drastic, but lining the walls, floor and ceiling with grounded, overlapping aluminium foil can bring about a significant improvement when all else fails.

Hiss

Excessive hiss is nearly always due to a lack of attention to gain structure, and for more information on this, read the 'Gain Structure' section of this chapter. Aside from making sure that the gains are optimised, it's also important to ensure that nothing that isn't needed is being routed into the mix. Unused channels should be de-routed from the mix buss and all unused sends turned down or routed to an unused aux-send output.

In studios where electronic instruments are being recorded, you should also be aware of the amount of noise that's being produced at source. For example, electric-guitar amps tend to be noisy, so gate the track while mixing if you can. Similarly, a lot of synth modules are quite noisy, so in order to make the best of them, work with the MIDI volume set high and use a reasonably high note-velocity level. The loudest notes should come close to the maximum velocity level of 127. If they're not, you're not getting the best possible signal-to-noise ratio.

The other major cause of excessive hiss is using insensitive microphones to capture low-level or distant sounds. There's no cure for this problem, other than either using the right mics for the job or getting the mic closer to the sound source. If you try to record something like remote birdsong or some other low-level sound while using a basic dynamic mic, you'll simply come up against the limits of the equipment.

Equipment Precautions

It's obvious that delicate machinery should be looked after, but what's isn't always evident is just how delicate some pieces of equipment really are.

- Be particularly gentle with tape machines, both digital and analogue, and if you intend to use any of these items in a mobile situation, invest in tough flightcases with resilient shock mounting.

- Never move computer hard drives while they are running.

- Don't move tube equipment while it's on and allow the tubes several minutes to cool after use before moving them. Failure to observe this precaution can result in broken filaments.

- Dust and cigarette smoke can damage electronic equipment, particularly switch contacts, pots and faders. Cover up unused equipment with a cloth and use a vacuum cleaner to remove the dust trapped in air filters.

- Don't handle delicate electronic equipment if there is any danger that you've accumulated a static charge – for example, after having walked over a nylon carpet in dry weather. Discharge yourself to something that is grounded first. This precaution is particularly vital when installing or removing computer soundcards, RAM boards and so on.

- Don't let your equipment overheat. If a particular piece of gear runs hot, leave a space above it in the rack. In extreme cases, install a rack cooling fan, especially if your studio is in a hot climate. Make sure that all air filters are clean.

- Avoid switching on a piece of equipment directly after switching it off; always leave it for 15 seconds or so to allow the power supply's capacitors to discharge. Failure to observe this precaution can generate high voltage surges that can damage power supplies or other parts of the equipment.

- Remove tapes, floppy disks and removable hard disks from your equipment before shutting down. Tapes should be fully rewound and stored in their library cases.

- Hard-disk-based audio recorders don't need to have their heads cleaned or their bias adjusted, but you should defragment the drive periodically using the appropriate software. Although defragmentation shouldn't harm your data, it's safest to back up everything important first.

- When cleaning tape machines, don't allow too much isopropyl alcohol to trickle down the capstan shaft, or it will enter the bearing chamber and dissolve the grease, causing accelerated bearing wear.

- In the event that a microprocessor-controlled piece of equipment malfunctions, switch it off, wait a while and then switch on again. If this doesn't help, check the manual to see if their is a re-initialising procedure. (Note that any user settings or patches are likely to be lost when initialising a machine.) Check also the battery inside the machine, which holds user information when the power is off. These usually need to be replaced every five years or so.

- If all else fails, read the manual!

Tube And Vintage Equipment

There's no doubt whatsoever that properly designed tube equipment possesses a certain sonic quality that is difficult to reproduce using solid-state equipment, and now that so many pieces of studio equipment are becoming digital, it seems that there's renewed interest in tube equipment to help 'warm' up the sound. However, nobody is entirely sure what part of the tube circuitry creates the magic, and I'm not entirely convinced that it's all down to subtle second-harmonic distortion, as some people claim.

The best-sounding tube equipment is nearly always vintage gear that was designed at a time when tubes were all there was to design with. The designers then knew all about tube distortion, and they did their very best to design distortion out of their circuits by using negative feedback and other techniques. True, if you drive a tube too hard, there will be an increase in even harmonic distortion, but what most people fail to realise is that even well-designed loudspeakers produce far more significant levels of even-harmonic distortion than well-designed tube circuits, and reason suggests that the speaker distortion should mask the tube distortion completely. However, tubes also exhibit a very positive transient response, which may account for their ability to interpret detail, and at higher levels their saturation effects tend to introduce an effect not unlike compression, which no doubt helps create a warm sound. Whatever the mechanism, tubes *do* sound different, and whether they are technically superior or inferior to transistors and integrated circuits, on a purely subjective level the human ear generally comes to the conclusion that they sound better.

Some modern tube equipment deliberately 'designs in' distortion with a view to creating a sound that is artificially warm, but in my experience few of the 'deliberately distorting' designs sound as good as those tube designs that aim to deliver a clean sound. Furthermore, some modern circuits run the tubes at a much reduced voltage, and although at least one company has patented a system for making tubes sound the same when run at low voltages, rather than from a proper HT supply, few of these are truly satisfying in the same way as a properly designed circuit. Early tube designs also tended to include matching transformers, and these too introduce a character to the sound that most experienced listeners find pleasant.

Going Vintage

If you're thinking of buying a piece of vintage equipment, be aware that it may require some servicing to get it performing at its best and that, in the case of tubes and other specialist parts, you may

have difficulty in obtaining the correct spares. For example, some of the tubes used in early tube microphones ceased to be produced over 20 years ago. Today, modern tube factories, such as there are, tend to make only the more common tubes, mainly for guitar amplifiers. Furthermore, some early designs had very complex, custom-built switching mechanisms, and some of these may be impossible to replace, except by cannibalising another unit.

Resistors and capacitors should be easier to locate, and in many older pieces of equipment the electrolytic capacitors may have dried out to the point at which they no longer work effectively. Similarly, coupling capacitors may have gone leaky (ie they pass small amounts of DC current), so the need for extensive capacitor replacement isn't at all unusual when refurbishing vintage equipment. Other problems to look out for – other than faulty resistors, capacitors and tubes – include carbonised tube sockets, noisy potentiometers and poor switch contacts.

Modern Tube Equipment

Modern tube equipment is generally based upon readily available tubes, although some microphone manufacturers work from hordes of out-of-production spares of long obsolete tubes, so easy availability of spares isn't always something that you can take for granted. If you are considering something that uses out-of-the-ordinary tubes, get a commitment from the supplier and the manufacturer that spares will be available on a long-term basis.

Other than this, you'll have the benefit of modern capacitors and resistors, readily available switches and controls and probably improved safety features. However, a design doesn't sound good just because there's a tube in it; if you're not sure what to listen for, ask other studio owners to find out what they think sounds good and what doesn't. As mentioned earlier, I usually prefer the sound of tube equipment that runs from a proper HT voltage and that's designed to deliver low distortion. Output transformers also tend to sound warmer than transformerless output stages.

Also, watch out for hybrid equipment which is mainly solid-state but with maybe only one 'marketing' tube in the circuit. Some hybrid devices are very good, as long as the design is sound, but there are also numerous poor designs around on which the tube runs from a very low voltage and introduces massive amounts of distortion to try to emulate the warmth of a properly designed tube device. Don't be seduced by the glow of the tube, though; use your ears, and compare the sound with something you know. Also, allow any tube unit to warm up for at least ten minutes, and ideally more, before doing any critical listening. A well-designed tube circuit has a comfortable yet detailed sound that consolidates and warms the bass end while providing transparency and stereo imaging at the high end. There should also be no cracks, pops, low-level rumblings or whooshings from the valve. Such output noise as there is should be a steady, very low-level hiss.

Alternative Technology

In recent years, FET (Field Effect Transistor) circuits have been used to emulate the behaviour of tubes as their transfer characteristics more closely resemble those of tubes than do conventional transistors. FETs distort in a similar way to tubes when overdriven, and some devices may be driven from a higher voltage than regular ICs, which helps with headroom. Certain compressors may also be designed with optically controlled gain elements comprising a source of illumination and a photocell. Early designs may have used lightbulbs, but modern LED circuits are rather faster and more reliable. Even so, opto gain cells tend to be relatively slow in responding, which is one of the reasons why they produce a characteristic type of compression. Some modern designs based on these principles actually sound very good and are well worth investigating.

Tube-Gear Maintenance

There is little that the owner can do towards maintaining tube equipment, other than looking after it and not moving it during or shortly after use. Sometimes cleaning the tube pins with a hard eraser and then using a deoxidising solution helps reduce spurious noises, but other than that it's mainly a

matter of having the tubes replaced when their performance starts to deteriorate. Gold-plated connections should be cleaned only with a soft eraser. The lifespan of a tube depends very much on the type of tube and the voltage from which it is run. As a rule, pre-amp tubes tend to last rather longer than power-output tubes. Output tubes in class A/B amplifiers should be replaced with matched pairs in order to ensure symmetrical performance for both negative-going and positive-going halves of the waveform.

Soldering

Learning to solder is easy and inexpensive, and it can save you both money and frustration when you need a lead that's a little out of the ordinary. Fortunately, the skill of soldering is quickly picked up, and the necessary equipment costs so little that you'll probably break even after making your first half-dozen leads.

Using The Soldering Iron

It's very tempting to try to heat up a blob of solder on the end of the soldering iron and then carry it to where it's needed, but this is absolutely the wrong approach and will leave you with dry joints (ie those that are both electrically and mechanically dubious). The right way to solder is as follows:

- If the iron has a plain copper bit, it should be filed at an angle of around 45º so as to provide a clean copper surface, especially if the iron has been resting at the bottom of a toolbox for years. However, irons with plated tips should be simply wiped with a piece of cloth once they are hot. Once the iron has been plugged in and has got up to temperature (be careful where you rest it!), melt a little solder on the tip of the iron and wipe off the excess with a piece of rag. This is known as 'tinning the iron'. The end of the iron should now have a nice silvery appearance.

- Strip the wire to be soldered and twist the end. Hold the tip of the soldering iron against the wire and then feed in a little fresh solder between

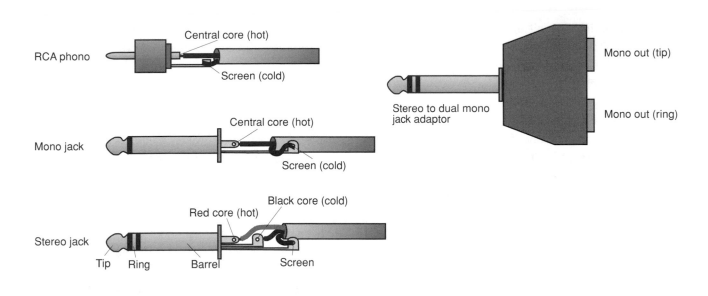

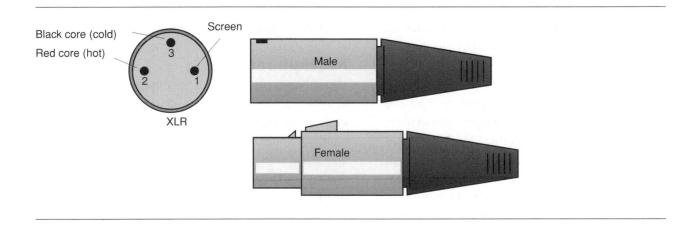

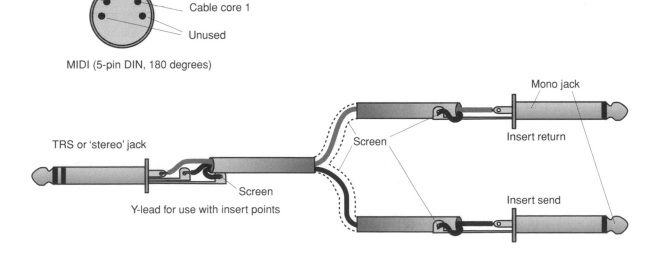

Figure 8.15: Common connector wiring

the soldering-iron bit and the wire. The solder should flow onto the wire and penetrate the spaces between the individual wires, creating a single, stiff conductor.

- Next, tin the tag inside the plug you're wiring in exactly the same way. If the solder blocks the hole in the tag, heat it up again and quickly bang the plug on a hard surface. The excess solder should fall off before it hardens, so don't do this over anything valuable!

- Using small pliers, push the tinned end of the wire through the hole in the tag and then wrap it around the tag once, still using the pliers. Ideally, you should have a reasonable mechanical joint before you solder the two parts together, although with some types of plug you have no choice but to rely on the solder to hold the wire to its destination.

- Place the soldering-iron bit against the joint and feed in a little fresh solder. Keep the iron in place until the solder flows smoothly between the wire and the tag. If it refuses to flow or forms reluctant blobs, heat up the joint again and apply more fresh solder. (The fresh solder is important because it is the chemical flux within it that cleans the joint and makes the solder flow.)

- If the job goes wrong, don't panic – pull the joint apart, strip the wire back a little further, clean the excess solder off the tags and have another go. Within half an hour, you should be soldering like a professional.

Soldering Tools

The ideal soldering iron for wiring small connectors is between 20W and 40W, and they are quite inexpensive. You'll also need a reel of flux-cored solder, a small pair of pliers and a pair of wire cutters. Wire strippers are also useful – if you strip the wire with your cutters, you stand a good chance of cutting right through the conductor by accident. Other than that, all you need is an old file or some wet-and-dry paper to clean up the end of the soldering-iron bit and a piece of rag to wipe off excess solder.

Practical Tips

Most soldering jobs appear to need three hands. Life can be made much easier if you fix an ordinary wooden clothes peg in a vice and use the peg to hold the component you're soldering. Alternatively, in the case of jack plugs, you can simply fit the plug into any convenient jack socket while you work on it. The same is true of most audio connectors, such as DINs, phonos and XLRs. However, make sure that jack-plug covers or XLR shells are threaded onto the cable before you solder the lead to the plug. This sounds so obvious, but we all still forget from time to time! Wiring conventions for the more common audio connectors are shown in Figure 8.15.

Microphone Care

Microphones are designed to convert tiny amounts of acoustic energy into electrical signals – they are precision instruments and don't take kindly to rough handling, no matter how many old Who videos you may have seen! Dynamic mics are designed to be reasonably tough in order to withstand the day-to-day knocks of touring, but avoid dropping them onto hard surfaces. Capacitor mics tend to be less rugged, which is why they're not so widely used on rock tours, but there are considerations other than physical violence! Here are a few tips to help you get a long life from your microphones.

- Don't drop them or pack them where they might sustain physical shocks or knock against other equipment.

- Never plug an unbalanced dynamic microphone into a mic input that has phantom power applied, as there is a possibility of damaging the microphone. It won't sound too good, either! A balanced dynamic mic will sustain no damage.

- Never plug any type of microphone or active DI box into a mic input with the phantom power switched on. Connect everything first, then switch on the phantom power. Modern mics are unlikely to sustain damage if this rule is ignored, but some older mics may be damaged.

- Capacitor microphones can be very susceptible to humidity, resulting in an increase in background noise and a decrease in sensitivity. Don't use a cold capacitor mic without allowing it to get up to room temperature first, and always use a pop shield to prevent the singer's breath from condensing on the capsule.

- Don't blow into microphones to test them, especially delicate capacitor models.

- Tube mics should be left several minutes to warm up before use and should then not be moved until they have been switched off and allowed to cool for ten minutes or more. Moving any tube equipment when hot can shorten the tube life.

- Don't slam the lids of microphone cases as the sudden increase in air pressure could damage the diaphragm or spoil its alignment.

9 COMPUTERS AND AUDIO

Towards the end of the last century, computers were used mainly for MIDI sequencing and stereo-file editing, but today a huge number of project recording studios are based entirely – or almost entirely – around computers. The attraction is obvious insomuch as computer-based systems are relatively cheap, they are immensely powerful and they don't take up too much space, but few things are as frustrating as a computer music system that isn't working properly. The secret of a smoothly running music computer starts with choosing the right system to begin with, then to use that system only for music and not clog it up with games or other non-music-related software. I've lost count of the number of conversations I've had where someone has told me he's decided to go the PC/Windows route so that his children can play games and use the Internet while his wife computerises the accounts. Believe me, this is the road to frustration!

Suitable Computers

Backing up for a moment, I have to answer the question concerning what constitutes a suitable music computer, and in the case of Windows/PC machines I'd say that, unless you really are a PC expert with extensive digital-audio knowledge, it's worth paying a little extra to get a machine that's designed from the ground up to handle music. It's true that you can go to a computer superstore and get an impressively specified machine for less money, but it may well not deliver the performance you expect in a musical context, for a whole host of reasons.

The reason why music places such heavy demands on a computer is because the audio can't be interrupted, ever, or audible glitches and clicks will occur. Video, on the other hand, can suffer missing or delayed frames and still be perfectly watchable. PC music software is generally written to work on Pentium processor chips, as these are the standard for Windows machines, but alternative processor types are available, and while these may work well enough with most music software, you can't guarantee that they'll work with all music software, so the first step you should take if you're considering an alternative to a Pentium processor is to decide what software you want to run and then contact the product-support departments (or website FAQ sections) for the companies concerned and make sure that your choice of processor is suitable. If you buy the computer with the relevant software already installed from a reputable music dealer, this should be taken care of automatically, and if there are problems, you will have right to redress under warranty. However, if you simply buy a PC from a general computer supplier and it doesn't work properly for audio, you may have trouble getting anyone to take your problems seriously; as far as most computer stores are concerned, if your PC runs Microsoft Word and logs onto the Internet OK, it's a working machine.

Other factors that affect audio performance include – but are not limited to – the motherboard chipset, the graphics card and the BIOS settings. Adding PCI graphics cards to Macs or PCs for driving a second monitor can also interfere with other PCI audio devices, so as a rule a double-output AGP card is the best option. Even then, some work better than others in a music context, so it pays to do a little research and ask a few questions before committing yourself. If you're buying a system, I'd advise you to pay the extra and have this fitted at the outset, as modern music software is so sophisticated that trying to run it with a single monitor can be very frustrating.

Some energy-saving settings can also affect audio performance, and the product-support department for the software you're using should be able to provide you with a list of tweaks to optimise your computer's performance in this respect. There are also many useful PC-related FAQs on the *Sound On Sound* website at http://www.sospubs.co.uk. Don't imagine that you can just buy an off-the-shelf computer, load in your music software and immediately get the best possible performance; while you may be lucky enough to get a system that works, it's unlikely to be optimised, and if you're unfortunate in respect of some of the components used inside the box, you may never get satisfactory audio performance.

Power Is Everything

In the early days of computer audio, computers were able to behave as emulations of multitrack tape recorders and mixers, often running alongside MIDI sequencers, but today we have plug-in effects and instruments, all of which use up a share of the processor's resources. To make effective use of all this wonderful software, it is therefore essential to have the most powerful machine you can get your hands on with lots of hard-drive space and plenty of RAM. It's hard to place an exact figure on what's required, as computer technology advances at a spectacular rate, but I'd suggest having a second drive for audio that's no smaller than 80GB, and whatever the normal RAM recommendation is for the machine, double or treble it. Software samplers use the host computer's memory, so if you make extensive use of these, fit as much memory as you can – it's much cheaper than it used to be, so skimping on RAM is really a false economy.

Drives For Audio

There are several reasons why you should fit a second drive for audio. Firstly, it gives you the opportunity to have a swappable drive caddy fitted so that you can change drives between projects. However, it also makes the reading and writing of audio files more efficient and means that you can defragment the drive without disturbing any of your program files. Swappable drive caddies are actually quite inexpensive, and in addition to using them so that you can swap audio drives, it might also be worth using one to house your main system drive. I suggest this for two reasons. The first is so that you can create a duplicate system drive that you can swap over to if anything unfortunate befalls your original system drive. The second is that, in situations where somebody else must use the computer for other purposes, they can have their own system drive with their own settings so that, when the drives are swapped over, you have to all intents and purposes swapped computers. As long as they don't make any BIOS changes, this simple strategy should serve to isolate your audio system from any system-setting changes, although you must ensure that your audio drive is also removed if you demand absolute security against any virus invasion.

Most large hard drives are suitable for audio-recording purposes as the thermal-recalibration problems associated with older, smaller drives (which could cause glitches or breaks in audio transfer) have now been resolved. To obtain the most audio tracks, a high data transfer rate is needed, and as a rule the drives with higher spindle speeds are best in this respect. At one time, it was necessary to use a SCSI drive to get a high track count, but these days you can expect to be able to record in excess of 24 tracks and often double that using a standard IDE drive. It is worth visiting music forums to see what's being said about various drive types, as some are more reliable than others, and – also importantly – some are quieter than others. Where a computer has to be used in the same room in which recording is taking place, it's worth investigating computer-quietening kits, which tend to employ lower-speed fans and acoustically damped drive sleeves. It is also possible to buy silent computer cabinets, although these are fairly expensive and tend to be bulky.

Soundcards

Most computers (other than those designed specifically for music) come fitted with general-purpose soundcards suited for games and multimedia applications, but in my experience these are less than ideal for serious audio work. Even those that are technically capable are burdened by unnecessary complexity, and in some cases the audio passes through a piece of input-routing software that comes with the soundcard, then through your audio program, then back into more mixing and routing software related to the card. This makes setting up very complicated, and as these cards come with so-called entry-level systems it seems ironic that they're the most difficult to get your head around. They may also include on-board synthesiser chips, surround-sound processing and effects, all of which tend to get in the way if all you want is an audio interface.

Is And Os

Your soundcard is the audio gateway to your computer, but the type that you end up buying will depend very much on how you record and mix your music. For example, if you work on your own, overdubbing one audio track at a time, and if you then go on to mix everything inside the computer, adding virtual effects via plug-ins, then a simple stereo-in/stereo-out soundcard is all you need. In most instances, if you do everything inside the computer, there's no need ever to take an audio output from the computer other than to drive your monitor loudspeakers, as the mixed soundfile can be recorded direct to CD-R. This means that the only 'quality bottleneck' is at the analogue-to-digital converters on your soundcard. If these are of a reasonable quality, there's nothing to prevent you from making master-quality recordings.

On the other hand, you may wish to record a group of musicians all playing together, in which case you need to be able to handle several audio inputs at the same time. This requires a multi-input soundcard, with eight inputs being a popular number. More elaborate interfaces may include both analogue and multiple digital inputs (often ADAT format, which can carry eight tracks at a time) as well as stereo S/PDIF and/or AES EBU digital ins and outs. More often than not, a multiple-input audio interface or soundcard will have multiple outputs, but one exception to this is the current crop of USB audio interfaces, on which the bandwidth restrictions of USB means that they're limited to four to six inputs and two outputs running simultaneously, and less if you use high sample rates and 24-bit resolution.

Why Multiple Outputs?

If you mix and process everything within the computer and you're working in stereo, two outputs is fine, but there are occasions where more outputs are necessary. For example, if you're working in 5.1 surround, you'll need five outputs to drive the five main surround speakers plus a further output to feed the LFE (Low-Frequency Effects) sub-bass speaker. Most of the leading multitrack audio software is able to handle surround mixing, so surround files can be created within the computer, but of course the multiple outputs are still necessary for monitoring purposes.

Even if you're working in stereo, as most people still are at the time of writing, you may still benefit from multiple outputs. One reason is so that you can use an external mixer to add different outboard effects or insert different hardware signal processors into the various audio streams before they are mixed. As plug-ins get better, there is less of a need to use external hardware, but in the case of power-hungry effects such as reverb, there is still a benefit to be had from using an external hardware box, as a mid-priced hardware reverb will generally sound noticeably better than a host-powered reverb plug-in. (I'll be covering the ways in which hardware effects can be integrated into software mixing systems later in this chapter.)

Cards or interfaces with ADAT-format outputs are

particularly useful for feeding digital mixers, most of which either have an ADAT interface built in or have one available as a plug-in option. The main advantage of this is that it keeps the signal digital and thus avoids the degradation associated with D-to-A and A-to-D conversion, and it also removes the need to optimise levels.

Cards Or Interfaces?

An audio soundcard is an audio interface, but an audio interface is not necessarily a soundcard – some are external boxes that connect to the computer either via a dedicated PCI interface card or via one of the computer's other data ports. Soundcards tend to plug into the PCI slots in desktop computers or into the PCMCIA slots of laptops, but there are some computers with no PCI or PCMCIA slots, such as the flat-screen iMacs and many laptops. In this case, the only way to get audio in and out of the machine (unless the computer has built-in audio I/O) is to use one of the existing data ports, such as USB or FireWire. As mentioned earlier, USB is practical if you need only a small number of inputs and outputs (at least until the new faster version becomes established), but FireWire is nevertheless a better option where more I/O is needed.

Currently there are FireWire interfaces that offer up to 24 channels of I/O, with 16 or 18 channels being more typical, and in some cases, you can use multiple interfaces to provide even more I/O. These are often a mixture of analogue and digital I/O, and in the case of the ADAT eight-channel digital interface adopted by many manufacturers, this provides a simple means of transferring audio from an audio interface/soundcard to a digital mixer equipped with an ADAT input port or for getting audio from an eight-channel mic pre-amp unit into the audio interface (where the mic pre-amp has an ADAT output option). Not only does the ADAT interface simplify studio wiring by replacing eight balanced cables with a single optical cable but it also eliminates the possibility of setting up any ground loops, as there is no electrical connection between the two pieces of equipment.

Driver Software

The performance of a soundcard is heavily reliant not only on the design of the hardware but also on that of the software driver that comes with it. At the time of writing, the most popular established driver format for both Mac and PC machines is probably ASIO, a Steinberg protocol designed to provide a degree of standardisation between software and soundcard manufacturers. Essentially, if the host software supports ASIO hardware and the soundcard comes with an ASIO driver, you should have no problem in getting them to talk to each other. There are other driver protocols, many of which are manufacturer-specific, but the key point here is that the host software must support the driver protocol used by the interface.

In the case of the Mac, ASIO was necessary because the Mac's own operating system was equipped to handle only stereo audio streams, not multi-channel audio. However, from Mac OSX onwards, multichannel audio is handled within the operating system, so both the audio hardware and host software will communicate via the Core Audio part of OSX. In other words, ASIO won't exist for OSX and beyond. This should eliminate a number of potential compatibility issues and also promotes lower latency. (If you're unfamiliar with the term, latency will be described shortly.) However, the downside of OSX is that VST plug-in effects and instruments that worked under OS9 will have to be rewritten before they can work under OSX. This chapter was written during a time of transition when most of the host software was available in OSX versions as well as OS9, but not all of the hardware drivers necessary to make the soundcards and interfaces work with OSX had been written.

At this time, there was much consternation after Apple's buyout of Emagic was announced, not least because Windows' development of Logic Audio would cease but also because the OSX version of Logic Audio would support only Apple Audio Unit plug-ins and not OSX versions of VST. I'm told that there's little technical difference between the two formats, and most plug-in companies are committed to supporting Core Audio, but some early issues with the graphical user interface delayed widespread Core Audio support until over a year after OSX was being promoted as the Apple OS of choice. It is expected that the majority of plug-ins will have Audio Units support by late 2003. Because the audio industry is in effect riding on the back of the computer market, significant and disruptive changes can occur at any time (such as the aforementioned discontinuation of PC Logic development so soon after Emagic was bought by Apple). For this reason, you should use good music magazines and music Internet sites as references to keep you fully up to speed with current trends.

Mac Or PC?

Other than politics and religion, few topics cause so much self-righteous chest-beating as the Mac-versus-PC debate. Of course, there is no real answer because they are not directly comparable, and even when it comes to something measurable like absolute processing power, Mac hardware and Intel's processors tend to take it in turns to lead. At the moment, the most powerful Windows PC is more powerful than the most powerful Mac, but then new Apple models will be announced in a couple of months that may reverse this situation. There's no doubt that PCs are cheaper than Macs, but whereas you have to have a PC properly configured and designed for music in order to be sure that it will work, the standardisation of Apple hardware means that there's rather less uncertainty when buying a Mac. In fact, when you compare the prices of a properly designed music PC and an off-the-shelf Mac, they're probably not that different.

By saying that you can't compare Macs and PCs directly, I'm saying that PCs require more expertise to configure and maintain, although the advent of Windows XP looks set to improve the situation significantly. Think of it like cars. How do you say which is best between a Mercedes and a fancy sports car? The Mercedes is probably more comfortable but the sports car will be faster. However, the sports car is more likely to be spotted with its hood up by the side of the road while the Mercedes glides by, and so it is with Macs and PCs. If you choose the PC

route, either get the machine set up with all the software installed and ready to run or be prepared to learn a lot about PCs! The Mac will give you smoother ride but probably won't go as fast and may cost you more. At the end of the day, they are both tools to do a job, and used properly they will both do the job well.

Let The Software Decide

Of course, choosing a computer and then finding software to run on it isn't really the best way to go about things, unless all the software you want is available both for Mac and PC. A more logical approach is to find music software that you think you'll feel comfortable with and then pick a computer and an audio interface that will run it. A typical musician will need an audio/MIDI sequencer, a stereo or surround editor, some CD- or DVD-burning software and, of course, a selection of software plug-in processors, effects and virtual instruments. What's more, it's desirable that these will all run under the same OS, as having to restart a Mac to jump between OS9 and OSX or a PC to switch between Windows 98 and Windows XP when you want to switch programs is immensely tedious.

Latency

Latency is a short but unavoidable delay between sound being fed into a computer-based recording system and the same sound emerging via the audio outs. The technical reasons for latency are based on the way in which computers buffer blocks of data, although the software driver for the soundcard also plays a large part in keeping latency low. Latency is particularly significant when doing overdubs, as the sound of your own voice or instruments comes back over the headphones a fraction of a second late, and unless the delay is kept very small, it can affect both your timing and the quality of your performance. The same is true of virtual instruments – having the sound arrive some time after you press a key is clearly distracting.

In the case of a well-designed system, this latency should be only a few milliseconds in length, in which case few people will even notice it's there, but less fortunate combinations of hardware, drivers and host software can throw up delays of more than half a second, and no one can play in time with delays of that magnitude! As a rule, latency is becomes a serious problem only when overdubbing or playing a virtual instrument, as you hear the already recorded tracks with no delay but whatever you're trying to sing or play comes back to you delayed by the system latency.

There are hardware and software approaches to minimising latency, notably ASIO II or other sophisticated audio drivers on the software side and soundcards with 'thru monitoring' on the hardware side. Such hardware automatically passes the audio being overdubbed directly to the soundcard output for monitoring purposes, thus avoiding any delay, but it prevents any software-based plug-in effects from being added to the monitor mix, and of course it doesn't work for virtual instruments, where the computer is generating the sound.

Latency Workarounds

I have to say at the outset that a properly specified modern computer fitted with a suitable soundcard should be able to deliver latencies of only a few milliseconds, which few people are capable of perceiving. However, if you're just starting out on a less optimised system on which latency is an issue, there are workarounds that can be applied, the most effective of which relies on the use of an external mixer.

Unless you have an extremely simple system where you rely on the same soundcard to provide all of your synthesiser sounds as well as audio recording, you're going to need a mixer in order to combine the output from your soundcard with the outputs from your external synths, samplers and drum machines. Furthermore, unless you have a separate microphone pre-amp, you'll need a mixer to provide a mic input with phantom power for your capacitor microphones.

Assuming that you have a mixer, you can set up simple a system where the output from your recording pre-amp is split to feed both the mixer and the soundcard input. At its simplest, this could take the form of a Y-lead (it's always OK to split signals this way, but not to mix them!), but you'll find that many recording pre-amps have two outputs anyway, often one on a jack and the other on an XLR. If this is the case, feed the jack output to the soundcard and then make up a balanced XLR to a balanced quarter-inch jack lead to feed your mixer's line input.

If you don't use a recording pre-amp, you may be able to use one of your mixing channels instead, as long as it has a direct output (or insert send) to feed to the soundcard input. If it doesn't, you can still send a mixer to your soundcard using the channel's pre-fade aux send. This arrangement will allow you to monitor your overdub directly through the mixer when recording, but you'll need to mute the output from the track being recorded within your software – otherwise you'll hear both the direct monitor signal and the delayed signal. Some packages have a Thru Monitoring on/off switch while on others you'll simply have to use the software's virtual mixing facilities to turn down or mute the output from the track being recorded.

After recording, you'll need to unmute the track output before you can hear it (if that's what you did to kill the delayed monitor signal), and you may also want to mute the mixer channel you used for monitoring your recording pre-amp, or your live mic will still be feeding the mix.

A limitation of this system is that, because you're bypassing the computer when monitoring your overdubs, you won't be able to hear the effect of any VST plug-ins until after the track has been recorded. If you need reverb to help you sing better, you can still hook up a regular hardware effects unit to your mixer and so add as much monitor reverb or echo as you like – it won't be recorded. The complete setup is shown in Figure 9.1.

If you're doing a punch-in recording to patch up a mistake, using thru monitoring as described means you won't be able to hear the original track as it will be turned down or muted. A practical workaround is to record the punch-in part on a new track and then to paste it into the original track once you've got it right.

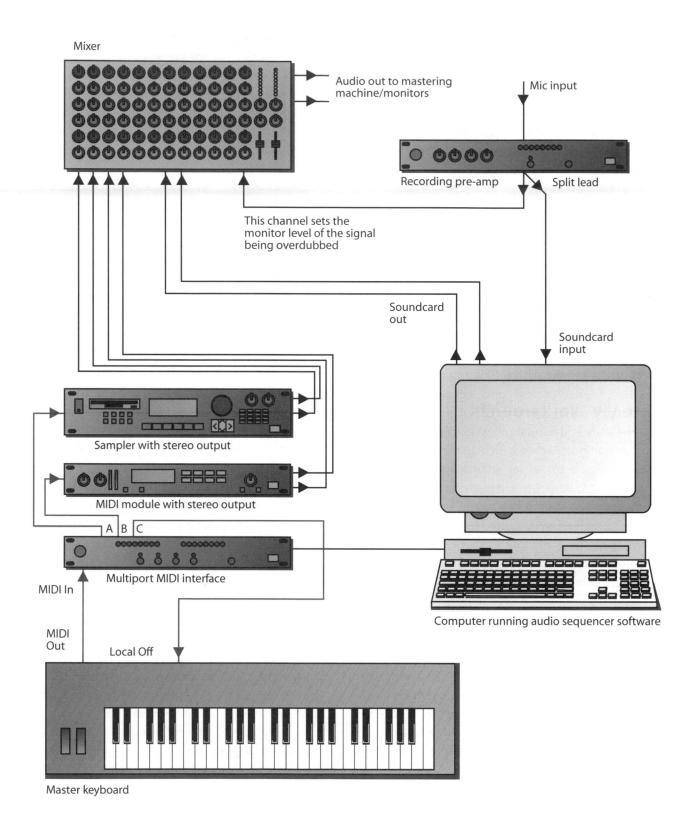

Mixer

Audio out to mastering machine/monitors

Mic input

Recording pre-amp

Split lead

This channel sets the monitor level of the signal being overdubbed

Soundcard out

Soundcard input

Sampler with stereo output

MIDI module with stereo output

A B C

Multiport MIDI interface

Computer running audio sequencer software

MIDI In

MIDI Out

Local Off

Master keyboard

Figure 9.1: Thru monitoring via a mixer

The Voice-Channel Solution

A number of mic pre-amp/voice channels are now built with computer recording in mind and include zero-latency monitoring systems that don't require mixers. Essentially, on these models the soundcard output is fed via a special section of the unit where the pre-amp output is combined with it for monitoring purposes. The principle is basically the same as when using a separate mixer, but here everything is done within the pre-amp unit. The monitor outs from the pre-amp feed the studio monitoring system in the usual way, and many units also include a headphone amplifier for overdubbing purposes. For those recording one track at a time, this is perhaps the best and most elegant solution. I've even tested one such unit that allows an external reverb unit to be connected, so as to provide the monitor mix with reverb, that something a lot of singers need to make them feel comfortable.

Virtual Instruments

I said earlier that none of these latency workarounds apply to virtual instruments, so what's the solution there? The only practical solution is to record the MIDI part using a substitute no-latency sound source, such as a hardware synth or the synth chip on a soundcard. While it may not sound as good, this will at least allow the performer to play in time. Then, once the MIDI data has been recorded, the sequencer track can be switched to play the desired virtual instrument.

As Well As The Computer...

Although it's possible to compose and mix music entirely on a computer, all practical systems must include some external hardware elements, even if only loudspeakers and microphones. For any serious use, you'll need to use a decent microphone, ideally a capacitor model, and because only the more sophisticated audio interfaces come with good-quality microphone pre-amps built in, you'll probably need either a separate mic pre-amp or a small mixer. You also may need to integrate external MIDI instruments and effects boxes into the system, in which case some kind of external mixer becomes essential.

When it comes to systems that use a simple stereo-in/stereo-out audio interface/soundcard, Figure 9.1 shows how a small mixer may be used to combine the soundcard audio outputs with those from external MIDI devices such as synths, samplers and drum machines. The number of inputs you need depends on how much hardware you want to plug into it, but because synths and other MIDI instruments have line-level outputs, you don't need mic inputs on every channel. However, because systems tend to evolve and grow, it's wise to get a mixer that's big enough to leave you with a few spare input channels.

Recording The Mix

The mixer's output carries a stereo, analogue mix of your recording that can be recorded to any mastering machine of your choice – DAT, MiniDisc, CD-R, cassette and so on – or it can be recorded back into your computer as a new audio file via the stereo inputs of your audio interface/soundcard. The latter approach makes sense if you want to do further mastering work on the file after mixing it or if you want to use your computer to your material burn a CD. (Note that the output monitoring level of the stereo track onto which your new file is being recorded should be turned right down so as to avoid electrical feedback.) The system shown in Figure 9.1 uses a conventional hi-fi amp and speakers as a monitoring system, which has the advantage that the signal routing to and from a stereo recorder is handled by the amplifier. You can simply plug your mixer outputs into any spare Aux, CD or Tuner inputs on the back of your hi-fi amp, though don't use the Phono inputs, if provided, as these are designed for turntable cartridges only.

A regular hardware effects box can be used via the post-fade aux sends and aux returns of the mixer in the usual way and will allow you to add different amounts of effect to each sound being mixed. However, what you have to bear in mind when using a soundcard with stereo outs is that all the computer audio tracks (and maybe some MIDI parts too, if you're using your soundcard's synth chip) emerge ready mixed, so there's no way to add hardware

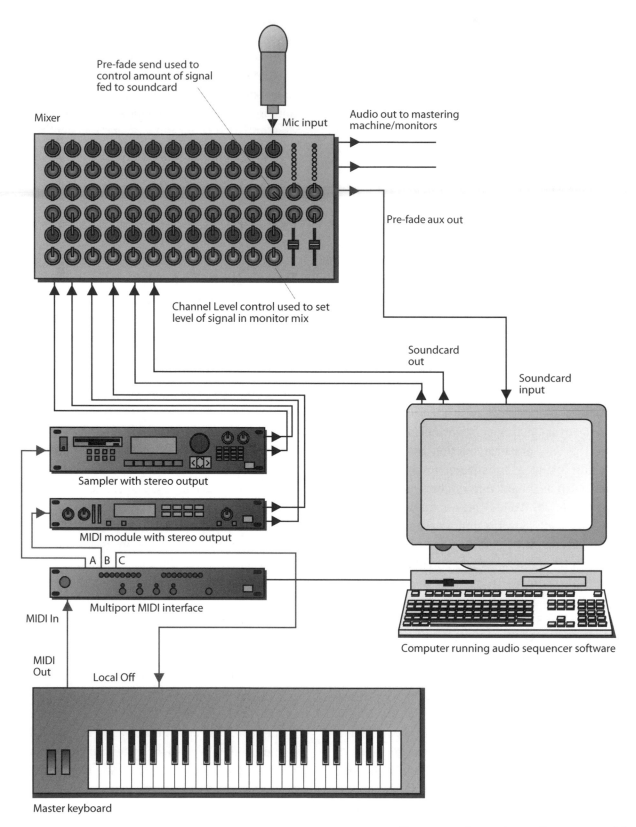

Pre-fade send used to control amount of signal fed to soundcard

Mixer

Mic input

Audio out to mastering machine/monitors

Pre-fade aux out

Channel Level control used to set level of signal in monitor mix

Soundcard out

Soundcard input

Sampler with stereo output

MIDI module with stereo output

A B C

Multiport MIDI interface

MIDI In

MIDI Out

Local Off

Computer running audio sequencer software

Master keyboard

Figure 9.2: Computer audio system with two-in/two-out audio interface

effects to some tracks of your computer audio mix and not to others. Because of this limitation, your computer audio tracks ideally need to be treated using plug-in effects and processors before they are sent out to the mixer. The MIDI tracks may or may not have effects available to them, depending on the design and type of soundcard you're using.

A further option is to mute any tracks to which effects should not be applied and then to create a mix – with effects – of just those tracks that need them. The mix should be recorded back into the computer, where the effected tracks can be used to replace their original uneffected counterparts within the song. Just in case this doesn't work out, it's best to save a copy of the song and work on that rather than risk changing the original.

Connecting A Microphone

As long as you have one spare mixer channel with a mic input, you can use it to feed a signal into the computer for recording, so saving on the expense of a dedicated voice channel or stand-alone mic pre-amp. In many home studios, vocal and instrumental parts are overdubbed one at a time, so one input is often sufficient. On a standard mixer with no multiple busses or other fancy routing options, the easiest way to use a mic channel for feeding a soundcard is to turn its fader fully down and then use the pre-fade send control to send the mic signal to the mixer's pre-fade output jack. This is normally used to set up monitor mixes, but in the smaller studio it can be fed directly into the soundcard input as means of routing the mic signal separately. Essentially, the mic signal goes through the mixer channel, via the pre-fade send and out of the pre-fade send jack, without interacting with anything else the mixer may be doing, almost as though it was a separate piece of hardware. All you have to do is keep its channel fader down when mixing and also ensure that the pre-fade aux send is turned fully down on all channels when recording, except for that being used as a mic input. The diagram in Figure 9.2 shows this routing option.

A further tip here is to turn up the mic channel fader when recording to hear the mic signal in the stereo mix (which you'll need to monitor via headphones while overdubbing). By monitoring the mixer channel in this way, while switching off thru monitoring in the computer, you'll avoid the distracting effects of any system latency, although this means that you'll also lose the ability to monitor the effect of any software plug-ins being applied to the input signal.

Multi-Output Soundcards

Figure 9.3 shows a slightly more flexible solution for users with multi-output audio interfaces/soundcards. If you have eight physical analogue outs, these can feed eight inputs of your analogue mixer, and because these eight signals are independent of each other, effects can be applied to them in different degrees via the mixer's post-fade aux-send system. Furthermore, the mixer insert points may be used to place signal-processing devices, such as compressors or equalisers, into individual signal paths.

If you have more than eight tracks of audio/MIDI on the computer, clearly some mixing must still take place within the computer in order to reduce the number of audio streams to eight, but by mixing sounds in logical groups, this still leaves you plenty of flexibility for adding effects. For example, you might use one output for your lead vocals, a pair of outputs for a stereo mix of your backing vocals, one for bass parts, one for guitar or lead instruments, one for rhythm parts (or subsections thereof) and so on. If you take a little time to think about what effects you're likely to add when mixing, it soon becomes obvious which sounds can be grouped and which need to be kept separate.

One important point to note is that, when you're using an external mixer with a multi-output audio interface, the panning assignments on the computer's internal mixer are more likely to be used for routing rather than actual panning. In the example where the lead vocal is on the first output, this would be achieved by assigning the signal to interface outputs 1/2 and then panning the vocal channel hard left in the computer's Mixer page so that all the signal routes from the odd-numbered

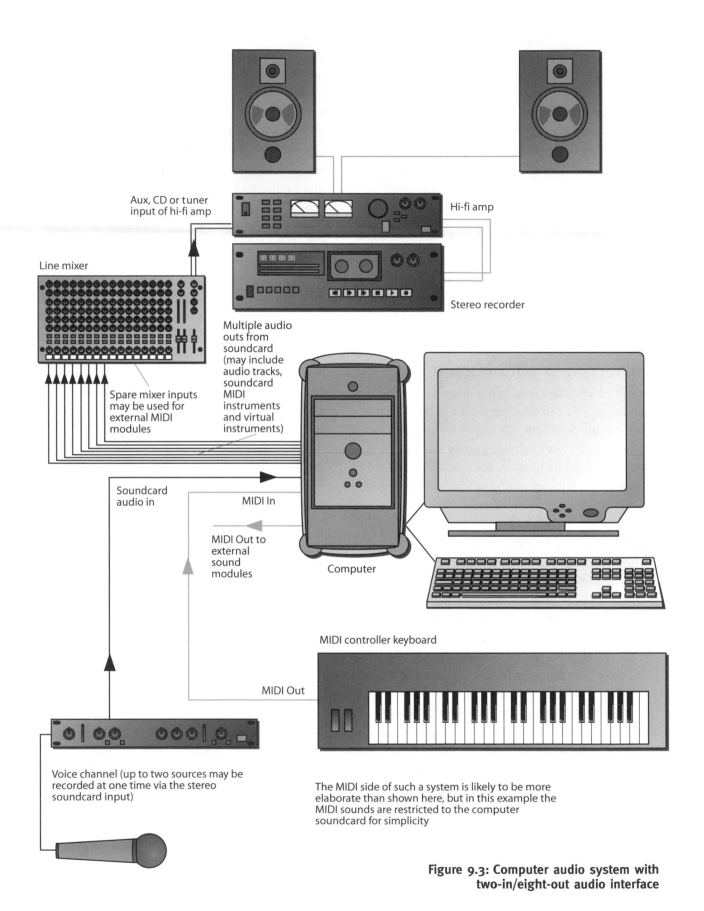

Aux, CD or tuner
input of hi-fi amp

Hi-fi amp

Line mixer

Stereo recorder

Multiple audio
outs from
soundcard
(may include
audio tracks,
soundcard
MIDI
instruments
and virtual
instruments)

Spare mixer inputs
may be used for
external MIDI
modules

Soundcard
audio in

MIDI In

MIDI Out to
external
sound
modules

Computer

MIDI controller keyboard

MIDI Out

Voice channel (up to two sources may be
recorded at one time via the stereo
soundcard input)

The MIDI side of such a system is likely to be more
elaborate than shown here, but in this example the
MIDI sounds are restricted to the computer
soundcard for simplicity

**Figure 9.3: Computer audio system with
two-in/eight-out audio interface**

soundcard output (1). That's because the routing in most software mixers follows the hardware-mixer convention of using the pan control to adjust the balance between odd- and even-numbered output pairs. When the vocal signal reaches your hardware mixer, it is simply a mono source that can be panned anywhere in the mix via the mixer's pan knob. Where stereo mixes have been set up in the computer using an odd/even output pair, the hardware mixer channels into which these are routed need to be panned hard left and right in order to maintain the original stereo perspective.

The pre-fade-send trick used to get a mic signal into a computer soundcard works here exactly the same as described earlier, but if you want to record more mics onto separate tracks at the same time, you'll need either a mixer with more pre-fade sends or you'll have to use the channel direct outputs, where fitted, to send the channel signal directly to the soundcard input. For any larger-scale projects, either a recording mixer with multiple output busses is recommended, or you could use some dedicated mic pre-amps to feed the separate inputs.

Because there are so many good software plug-ins available today, using a two-in/two-out soundcard or interface doesn't impose too many restrictions on how you can mix your tracks, but it does preclude you from using hardware effects and processors to treat individual parts of your mix, other than elements coming from external hardware, such as MIDI modules.

An audio interface with eight outputs offers a good compromise between flexibility and cost as it allows you to separate key sounds for processing with external effects and processors. In all cases where multiple hardware MIDI instruments are used, an external mixer is needed to combine the sound outputs of your computer with the outputs of external MIDI hardware instruments, although this need not be large or expensive. Without a mixer, the only alternative is to record the outputs of the MIDI instruments into the system as audio tracks – one at a time, if you have an interface with a single stereo input. While this is perfectly possible, it is a time-consuming job, but one advantage of

working in this way is that the recorded synth sounds can be further processed using plug-in effects, if required.

Hardware Effects

As you will have discovered by now, using an external hardware effect or processor within your virtual audio software mixer can be tricky to arrange, but sometimes it is necessary. For reasons of CPU power, hardware reverbs still tend to be better than their soft counterparts, but if you have an audio interface with more than two outputs, you can use an external hardware reverb device, with or without an external hardware mixer. I imagine most computer studio users will have at least a small hardware mixer to combine their soundcard outputs with the outputs from any external MIDI synths, in which case all you need is a pair of spare inputs and you can use a hardware effects unit. This works by having the post-fade send in your software's virtual mixer set up as usual, but instead of routing it to an effects plug-in, you send it to one of the spare outputs on the audio interface. This output feeds the input to your reverb unit and the reverb outs go into the hardware mixer panned left and right, as shown in Figure 9.4.

If you have spare audio-interface inputs and your sequencer can add live inputs to the mix (as can the current versions of both Cubase and Logic), you also have the option of feeding the hardware reverb outputs directly back into the mix, which avoids the need for a hardware mixer. In some cases, working this way will add a little delay to the reverb due to the system latency, but as reverb is traditionally pre-delayed by several tens of milliseconds anyway, this is unlikely to cause problems. This arrangement is shown in Figure 9.5.

It's less easy to use external processors as insert effects, especially if you have a limited number of additional audio outputs on your interface card. The usual method is to route the track to be processed to one of the spare audio outputs, then feed it into a hardware mixer channel with the desired processor connected via its insert point. If there is no hardware mixer, you can route the

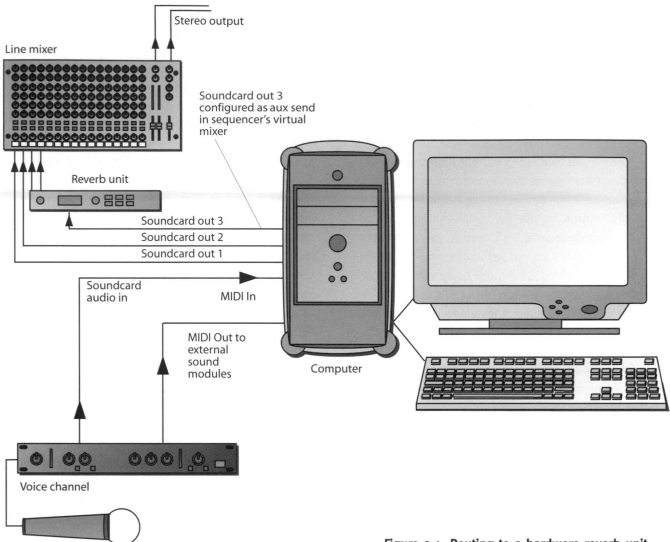

Figure 9.4: Routing to a hardware reverb unit and an external mixer

soundcard output directly to the processor and then feed the processor's output back into a spare soundcard input and add it to the mix this way. If you find that the system latency delays the processed input by any significant degree, you can either record the processed signal as a fresh audio track or apply negative delay to the audio track being processed in order to bring the processed input back into line with the rest of the song. Of course, you can only use as many hardware insert effects as you have spare soundcard/interface inputs and outputs available.

VST Instrument FAQs

Usually, virtual instruments simply install and play without any trouble, but occasionally problems do occur. The following questions and answers are not supposed to be a comprehensive treatise on the subject but are instead a quick reference to some of the more common problems and solutions.

Q: There's an audible delay between pressing a key and hearing any sound.

A: The latency is too high for real-time playing,

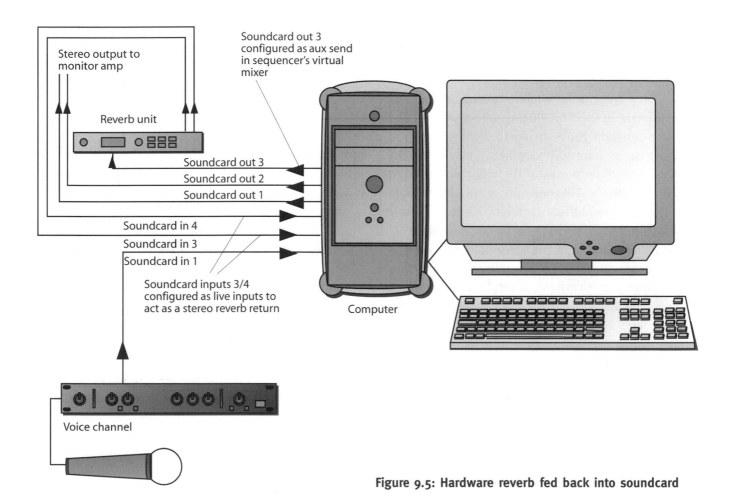

Stereo output to
monitor amp

Soundcard out 3
configured as aux send
in sequencer's virtual
mixer

Reverb unit

Soundcard out 3
Soundcard out 2
Soundcard out 1

Soundcard in 4
Soundcard in 3
Soundcard in 1

Soundcard inputs 3/4
configured as live inputs to
act as a stereo reverb return

Computer

Voice channel

Figure 9.5: Hardware reverb fed back into soundcard

although with a well-written audio driver you should be able to get the figure down to an acceptable value, providing you don't have a slow computer. Check the audio-driver settings, where you should be able to adjust the latency. Depending on your computer and soundcard driver, there will be a minimum value you can set, and it's also quite possible that, if you select the minimum value, the audio side of the program will become unstable or subject to glitching. Through experimentation, choose the setting that gives you the lowest latency with reliable performance. If this results in a latency

of less than 10ms, you'll probably be comfortable playing virtual instruments in real time. You may even find that you get the best results by using a low latency setting that's near the system's limit for recording and then switch back to a higher latency setting for reliable playback when mixing.

Q: What if the minimum latency is still too high to be able to play in real time?

A: You can use a hardware sound source, such as your soundcard or a synth module, to provide the sound when you're recording, then switch the track to the desired virtual instrument for playback. Latency is compensated for on playback, so your track will play in time.

Q: I've installed a new VST instrument but it doesn't appear in the VST instrument list within my program.

A: Check that the installation has placed the VST instrument in the 'VSTPlugins' folder used by the audio program you're trying to work with. If you have two or more VST programs, you can usually put shortcuts or aliases of the original plug-ins in the respective VSTPlugins folders, and they should still work. Alternatively (and less messily), simply create a single VSTPlugins folder and place an alias/shortcut of it in the same folder as each of your VST audio programs. Then restart your computer (just in case this particular VST instrument also includes system files) and then try again. Procedures may be different under Mac OSX, but no OSX-compatible VST plug-ins were available at the time of writing.

Q: The VST instrument appears but none of its factory preset sounds are available.

A: Often the factory presets come in separate folders which have to be located as specified in the installation instructions. Usually the installation procedure will do this for you, but occasionally you may have to move things manually, especially if you're running two or more 'VSTPlugins' folders. Again, you should be able to use aliases and shortcuts to simplify access to your plug-ins by all your VST audio programs.

Q: How can I minimise the CPU drain cause by VST instruments?

A: Some instruments allow you to choose the sample rate at which they run, so choose the lowest that still sounds good. This won't affect the sample rate of your final audio output. You'll also find that most VST instruments allow you to specify the maximum

polyphony (number of notes that can sound at the same time), and the lower the value that this is set to, the less CPU drain there will be, especially when the playing gets busy. Long release times also eat up polyphony due to the large numbers of overlapping notes that can occur.

Q: I've bought some plug-in instruments to use within Logic Audio, but they aren't accessible from within my other VST programs.

A: Although they may appear to work the same way as VST plug-ins, many of the Logic VST instruments are dedicated to running only within Emagic programs, although some, such as the EXS-24, are also available as true VST plug-ins. Because Logic instruments (and processors) are not actually VST instruments, there is no way to use them from within another program.

Q: Can I use regular VST effects to process the output from VST instruments?

A: Normally, you can use any VST plug-in effect or processor after a VST instrument. In effect, the VST instrument behaves much like any other audio track, although the way in which subsequent plug-ins may be deployed depends on the design of the host software.

Q: Will adding more RAM allow me to run more VST instruments at the same time?

A: If your computer is short on memory, you'll run into trouble, but the only benefit of adding more than you need is that any sample-based VST instruments (such as samplers) will be able to load more or longer samples. Most VST instruments overtax the computer's CPU before its RAM. If you have a virtual sampler, you should add at least an extra 256MB of RAM, as this will give your sampler considerably more capacity, especially when used multitimbrally or where a lot of long multisamples are involved. Mac OS9 users should follow the manufacturer's guidelines concerning how much

RAM to assign to the host program when running VST instruments.

Q: I know that virtual instruments can use a lot of processing power, so even a powerful computer may not be able to run all the instruments I wish to use in a song. However, I don't want to compromise my arrangement by leaving instruments out, so what can I do to get around this problem?

A: The simplest option is to record the virtual-instrument part and any plug-ins used to process it as a regular audio track. Methods of doing this vary a little from one software package to another, but there is invariably some system for bouncing one or more tracks to a new audio file (something you might also do when mixing a song using all virtual instruments and no external MIDI sources). From version 6, Logic Audio has implemented a Freeze Track function, which does this for you automatically but also allows you to unfreeze the track and go back to the original virtual instrument/plug-in combination to allow subsequent editing. This is such an obvious and useful feature that it seems almost certain that the other major sequencers will add something similar in the near future.

Some Strategies For Computer Audio

When working with any kind of computer audio system, the first thing to establish once you get the system up and running is a viable backup regime. It has often been said that digital data isn't actually real until it exists in at least two different places, and that's something I'd go along with 100 per cent. There are various options, the most obvious being copying your files to a second hard drive, but in an ideal world you also need to save important work in a form you can archive.

When it comes to sequencer projects, the first stage is to compile a folder containing everything you need to restore your project, which generally means the song file plus any associated audio files. If you're using a plug-in soft sampler, you may also wish to back up any samples used within that song.

Whether you store all associated audio files, including alternative takes, or just the ones used in the song is up to you. The project folder may then be copied to another drive for increases security, but CD-R and DVD-R also provide a very practical means of backing up that is easy to archive. However, you should only use the best-quality media for important work as budget media may not have as long a shelf life and may be more prone to errors. Because projects are backed up as data files and not as CD audio tracks, the data error correction is very robust and there are no problems with timing jitter or other forms of digital audio degradation, but you still need to choose a media that will retain its data intact for many years. A standard CD-R will hold around 70 minutes of two-track audio along with the song file and a small number of samples, which equates to approximately one five-minute song comprising 24 busy audio tracks and a few alternative takes. A typical complete album project may be stored on one or two DVDs, depending on your track usage, although working at esoteric 96kHz or even 192kHz sample rates will reduce the storage time accordingly, as will surround mixes, which comprise six discrete audio tracks rather than the two needed for stereo.

When archiving stereo mixes, backing up you final audio CD is fine, but it's also wise to back up your original mixes as data files, ideally in 24-bit format. Some CD-burning software insists on trying to burn an audio CD if it sees audio files, but in most instances, if you put your audio files into a folder and then load up a copy of the folder, this will force it to burn your files as data, which is a more robust format than CD audio.

Be aware that, when you come to restore a project from a data backup disk, the song may initially be confused as to where to find the audio files, so the first time you work on the song, you may have to direct your computer to look in the project folder that you've copied from the CD-R or DVD-R back onto your hard drive. Once this has been done and the song resaved, the files should be located automatically the next time you access the song.

Computer Multitrack Strategies

It isn't the place of this book to offer an introduction MIDI or to sequencing, so I'm assuming you have a basic knowledge of these matters. A modern sequencer is an incredibly sophisticated software tool and most users spend most of their time working with only a small percentage of the available functions. If this allows you to get the job done, that's fine, but where the facility is available to allow you to define your own key commands, you'll find that your work regime will become much more efficient if you make use of it. Similarly, using screen sets to bring up pre-designated screens or combinations of screens can save a lot of dragging and clicking.

All serious sequencers now offer both MIDI and audio recording with full dynamic automation and plug-in effects and instruments. It is possible to automate plug-in parameters, but for many routine recording tasks, this isn't necessary. For example, if you have a vocal part that has a very different character in the choruses to the verses, perhaps because the singer shifts up a gear in the choruses, you could automate both EQ and compression to even out any excessive differences, or you could simply use the scissors tool to divide the vocal track into verse and chorus sections, then move the choruses to a different audio track. Once you've done this, you can set up the necessary EQ and compressor plug-ins in the two tracks and use static plug-in settings to deal with the differences.

When setting up mix automation, it is of course possible to do everything using a mouse and keyboard, but a hardware moving fader controller makes mixing more of a hands-on experience. I've used both manual and motorised fader controllers and have come to the conclusion that manual units make more work than they save, owing to the fact that the physical fader positions seldom relate to the actual stored values. This is a particular issue if the unit includes bank-switching to allow it to address extra channels or other functions, such as aux send levels, because whenever you switch banks, you have to null the faders you wish to use with their stored values before proceeding. Moving faders, on the other hand, automatically take up their new positions whenever you change between banks or select a different fader function, so no time is wasted.

Timing Is Everything

Sequencers make it easy for us to force MIDI events into time by invoking quantising, but audio tracks aren't always so precise. A very common fault when working with inexperienced musicians is that the bass guitar and drum parts aren't adequately tight. Providing you have a little patience, you can usually fix this by slicing up the bass-guitar track into one-bar segments and then sliding these bars back or forward in time slightly until they are in time with the drums. The easiest way to do this is to set up the two parts on adjacent tracks and then expand the display until you can see the kick-drum and bass-guitar waveforms next to each other. This makes it easy to slide errant bars into time, and if the timing drifts within a bar, you can slice again and drag the offending note or notes into place. A tenuously related but useful tip when working with drums is to use a sub-bass synthesiser plug-in to fatten up kick drums that are lacking in depth. These often succeed where EQ fails.

Tuning

How did we manage before Auto-Tune came along? Automatic pitch correction is now pretty routine stuff, but too often people end up compromising the audio quality by setting the pitch-correction speed to fast. At very fast settings, you end up with the familiar vocoder-like pitch-quantised vocal sound, but even at medium settings you may still hear slightly artificial artifacts creeping in. The trick is to set the correction speed as slow as you can while still getting the job done, and if you're able to automate the parameters, you can change the correction speed throughout the song to optimise performance. Where a song involves key changes, splitting the vocals over several tracks and setting up a different version of your pitch-correction plug-in for each one is often the simplest way of getting the job done.

Although automatic pitch correction was originally designed for vocals, it works well on many monophonic instruments and I find it particularly useful on fretless bass guitar and on lead-guitar solos. Even though these sounds aren't always strictly monophonic, you'll find that the software generally refuses to do anything until it recognises a single note, so in the case of lead guitar or fretless bass, setting a slow correction speed will help pull sustained bent notes into pitch without affecting the natural vibrato of the instrument.

Tempo Delays

One of the most common plug-ins is the digital delay, and the facility for synchronising to the song's tempo is also a common and useful feature, but you can come unstuck when the song you're working on includes one or more tempo changes. If you've ever turned the Delay Time control on a hardware delay unit when sound is passing through it, you'll probably have noticed that the delays shift in pitch while you're moving the control, and this is exactly what happens when a tempo change is encountered. What's more, where the feature exists to smoothe the tempo change applied to the delay, this just seems to prolong the agony, so you'll either need to reduce the delay output at the point where the tempo changes or pick a delay that isn't locked to tempo.

Mastering

There's a big difference between what goes on in a really good professional mastering suite and what the average home studio owner can do at home, but as more computer-based mastering tools become available, it's easily possible to achieve very impressive results in the project studio using relatively inexpensive equipment. However, there's a lot more to mastering than simply compressing everything to make it as loud as possible, although compression does play an important role in mastering. Arguably the most important tool, however, is the ear of the mastering engineer, because successful mastering is about treating each mix individually; there is no standard mastering treatment that can be applied simply like a coat of paint, even though hardware mastering boxes filled with presets might seem to suggest otherwise.

To make any sense of mastering, you need a benign monitoring environment and accurate speakers that have a reasonable bass extension. Any computer audio program that permits basic cut-and-paste editing and that can run plug-ins can be used for mastering, although a dedicated mastering program such as Wavelab, Bias Peak or TC Spark might be better.

A professional may want to start off with a 20- or 24-bit master tape or to work from a half-inch analogue master, but in the home studio most recording is still done to 16-bit DAT or CD-R. This shouldn't be a problem for most pop music, as long as you proceed carefully, but if you can save your mixes in 24-bit format, you can preserve more of the original sound quality when you finally reduce to 16 bits for transfer to an audio CD.

Most mastering mistakes are due to over-processing, particularly over-compression so don't feel that you have to process a piece of music just because you can.

Useful Mastering Guidelines

Where possible, handle fade-out endings in the computer editor rather than using a mix that was faded while mixing. Not only does the computer provide more control but it will also fade out any background noise along with the music so that the songs ends in perfect silence. Ideally, you should do your fades after processing but before dithering down to 16 bits (if you are editing a 24-bit file), as this will preserve the best audio quality.

Once you've transferred your mixes into the editing program, you should clean up the starts of songs using the Silence function. Note, however, that, if you intend to use a 'fingerprint' noise-removal program, you should avoid cleaning up the starts until you've done the de-noising, as most of these programs require a short sample of noise to analyse in order to optimise their filter settings.

• Use the waveform display to make sure that you silence right up to the start of the song without clipping it. As a rule, endings should be faded out rather than silenced, as most instruments end with a natural decay. When the last note or beat has decayed to around five percent of its maximum level, start your fade and make it around one second long so that the song finishes in complete silence without the natural decay of the last note being compromised. You can still try this if the song already has a fade-out, although you may want to set a slightly longer fade time. Listen carefully to make sure you aren't shortening any long reverb tails or making an existing fade sound unnatural. Being pedantic, the fade should be done after any EQ, compression or limiting, but in the context of pop music, where the dynamic range is limited, you're unlikely to hear any difference if you do the fades first.

- Once you've decided on a running order for the tracks on the album, you'll need to get the levels to match, but don't attempt to do this until all other processing has been carried out, as compression in particular can change both the actual and subjective loudness of a mix.

  Adjusting levels doesn't simply mean settin everything to the same peak level, though, as this will make any ballads seem very loud compared to those songs that are supposed to sound loud. The vocals often give you the best idea of how well matched songs are, but ultimately your ears are the best judges. Use the computer's ability to access any part of the album at random to compare the subjective levels of different songs after processing is complete and pay particular attention to the levels of the songs on either side of the one you're working on. It's in the transition of one song to the next that poor level matching shows up most.

- If the tracks were recorded at different times or in different studios, they may not sound consistent enough to sit together comfortably on the album without further processing. Often a little careful EQ will improve matters, but you

need a good parametric equaliser (either hardware or software) if you're not to make matters worse. Listen to the bass end of each song to hear how that differs and use the EQ to try to even things out. For example, one song might have all the bass energy bunched up at around 80Hz or 90Hz while another might have an extended deep bass that goes right down to 40Hz or below. By rolling off the sub-bass and peaking up the 80Hz area slightly, you might be able to bring the bass end back into focus. Similarly, the track with the bunched-up bass could be treated by adding a gentle 40Hz boost combined with a little cut at around 120Hz. All equalisers behave differently, so there are no hard-and-fast figures – you'll need to experiment.

At the mid and high end, use gentle boost at between 6kHz and 15kHz to add air and presence to a mix while cutting at between 1kHz and 3kHz to reduce harshness. Boxiness tends to occur between 150Hz and 400Hz. If you need to add top to a track that doesn't have enough natural high-frequency content, try a harmonic enhancer such as an Aphex Exciter or one of the many harmonic-enhancer plug-ins currently available.

Multiband Compression

Most compressors are so-called full-band types, which means that the entire audio signal is processed via a single gain-control element. When gain reduction occurs, the whole signal level is reduced, so whenever a loud peak occurs, whatever its frequency content, the level of the whole signal is reduced until the loud event has passed. A common problem arising from full-band compression is that a loud kick drum or other powerful low-frequency event will trigger the compressor and consequently pull down the gain of everything else that happens to be passing through the compressor at the same time, even though those other sounds might not need compressing. If the compressor is acting on a solo kick-drum track, clearly this isn't a problem, but it's different when you're compressing a whole mix, because the low-frequency sounds in the mix

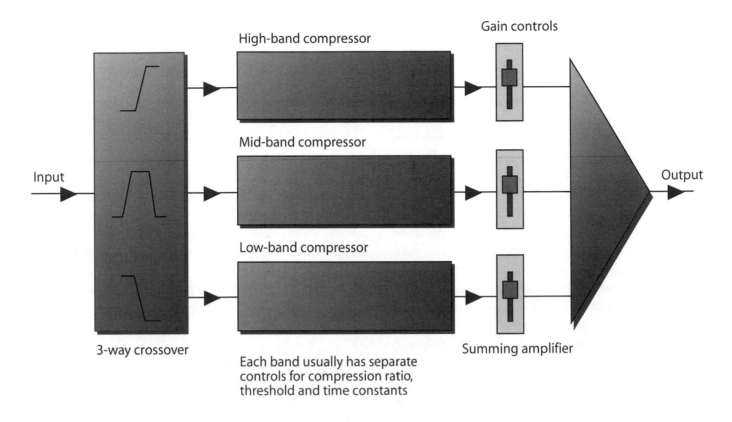

Gain controls

High-band compressor

Mid-band compressor

Low-band compressor

Input

Output

3-way crossover

Summing amplifier

Each band usually has separate
controls for compression ratio,
threshold and time constants

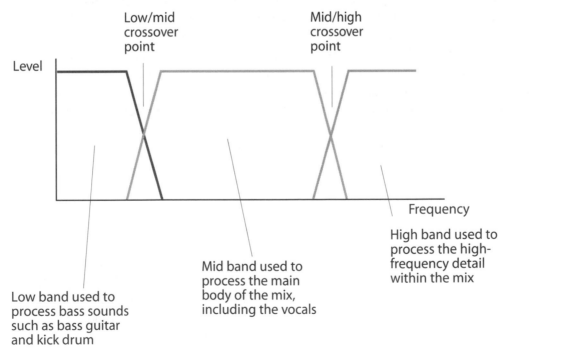

Low/mid
crossover
point

Mid/high
crossover
point

Level

Frequency

High band used to
process the high-
frequency detail
within the mix

Mid band used to
process the main
body of the mix,
including the vocals

Low band used to
process bass sounds
such as bass guitar
and kick drum

**Figure 9.6: Operation of a
multiband compressor**

determine the compression applied to everything else. What tends to happen is that the kick drum and bass line dictate how the mix will be compressed.

One way to disguise this aspect of full-band compression is to set a slightly longer attack time so that transients can pass through cleanly before the gain reduction takes place, but for mastering and other critical applications multiband compressors can offer advantages, not least that high-energy bass events don't dominate the way in which the compressor reacts across the entire audio spectrum.

How Multiband Works

A multiband compressor comprises a set of crossover filters that splits the audio signal into two or more frequency bands. Three or four band compressors are perhaps the best compromise between versatility and ease of setting up. After passing through the filters, each frequency band is fed into its own compressor, after which the signals are recombined, as shown in Figure 9.6. Now, when that loud kick drum comes along, instead of pulling the whole mix down with it, only the low-frequency sounds (ie those in the low-frequency band as defined by the crossover filter) will be compressed, leaving the mid range and high frequencies unchanged. Similarly, a loud event in the mid range won't affect the extreme high or low frequencies for the same reason.

Using a multiband compressor also allows you to apply different compressor settings in each band if necessary, so if you need more density at the bass end, you can use a higher ratio or different threshold setting in that band without affecting the mid and high sections of your mix. Furthermore, if the effects of compression change the overall tonal balance unfavourably, you can restore it by changing the levels of the individual compressor bands relative to each other. For example, if the mix needs to sound brighter, you can increase the level of the high-frequency band's compressor output.

Stereo

Conventional full-band compressors designed to be used in stereo invariably have two audio channels plus a stereo-link control. The link control sums the two side-chain signals and then uses that to control both compressor channels so that the same amount of gain reduction is always applied to both channels. With hardware compressors, control of the compressor parameters is usually handed over to just one set of the front-panel controls in order to avoid having to set up two channels identically. Without linking, there could be audible image shift triggered by signals that are louder on one channel than on another. A multiband compressor works in a similar way, except that each band has its own side chain, so a three-band, stereo compressor would have three stereo-linked sections, comprising high frequencies, mid frequencies and low frequencies. The good news is that, when it comes to plug-ins, most multiband compressors are available in both mono and stereo versions, where the linking is looked after automatically when you choose the stereo version.

Fingerprint EQ

Another powerful tool in matching the sounds of tracks is the so-called fingerprint equaliser. This uses hundreds or even thousands of separate frequency bands and works by analysing the overall spectral response of one piece of music (the reference) and then analysing the target mix that you want to adjust. Having done this, it computes an EQ-correction curve that will make the overall response of the target mix the same as that of the source mix. Providing the mixes use similar instrumentation and are in similar styles, this technique can be very useful, but often some manual adjustment is needed to fine-tune the result. It's also possible to use a commercial track as a reference and use this to modify your own target mixes, but again this depends on picking a track that has similar characteristics – trying to make a ballad conform to the spectrum of a heavy dance track makes no sense at all. The better fingerprint-EQ plug-ins allow you to adjust the degree to which the target mix is modified and should also allow you to determine parts of the spectrum that should be left untreated. For example, if you need to match only the bass end, confining the processing to under 500Hz might be wise.

Mastering And Dynamics

One of the objectives of mastering is to make the best use of the available dynamic range of a CD and also to ensure that your mix sounds as loud as other commercial mixes. To make a track sound even louder when it's already peaking close to digital full scale, you need to use a limiter to pull down the levels of any short peaks, such as those that occur at the starts of snare-drum beats. In many cases, you can increase the overall level by up to 6dB or even more before your ears notice that the peaks have been processed in any way, and many plug-in limiters can effectively limit and normalise in one operation. It's always good practice to normalise the loudest track on an album to peak at around −0.5dB and then balance the others to that one, but if you're using a limiter that also handles dithering from 24-bit to 16-bit resolution, leave this process until everything else – including level changes – has been completed. Normalising or other level-matching changes should always be the last thing you do prior to limiting and dithering, as all EQ, dynamics or enhancement involves some degree of level changing. Dithering is not required if you're recording the result to an analogue machine, but these days this tends to be done only in specialist situations where the analogue tape is being used because of its 'warming' influence on the sound.

- When mastering, always keep a CD player and some reference recordings to hand so that you can compare what you're doing with known good commercial recordings. Not only does this help you keep a sense of perspective regarding the tonality of your mixes but it will also give you a final loudness level to aim for, providing you calibrate your system to play back material at the same level from the computer and from CD. You can do this by recording a CD (digitally) into your computer editor and then switching back and forth between the original CD played on your CD player and the computer audio while adjusting the playback levels so that they sound the same.

- Overall compression can add energy to a mix and help to even out a performance, but it isn't mandatory. Music needs some light and shade to provide dynamics. Often a compressor will change the apparent balance of a mic slightly, so you may need to use it in combination with EQ. Putting the EQ before the compressor results in any boosted frequencies being compressed most, while putting it after the compressor allows you to equalise the compressed sound without affecting the compressor operation. The best method depends on the material being treated, so try both.

- A split-band compressor or dynamic equaliser will give you more scope to change the spectral balance of a mix, but these devices take a little practice before you feel that you're controlling them and not vice versa. Many professional mastering engineers still use full-band compression, so don't assume that you have to use a multi-band compressor.

- One way to homogenise a mix that doesn't quite gel, or one that sounds too dry, is to add reverb to the entire mix. This has to be done very carefully, however, as excess reverb tends to make things sound washy or cluttered, but small-room or ambience programs work well for giving a mix a sense of space and identity without adding an obvious reverb sound.

- If you want to add a stereo-width-enhancing effect to a mix that's already completed, there are two main areas that you have to consider: the balance of the mix and the mono-compatibility of the end result. Most width enhancers tend to increase the level of panned or stereo sounds while suppressing centre sounds slightly. Sometimes this can be compensated for by EQ, but be aware that the balance may change slightly when you listen in mono, so always listen to your mastered work in both stereo and monitoring modes before decreeing that it's OK.

Other than the simple phase-inversion width-enhancement system used in many plug-ins and hardware boxes, where some out-of-phase left channel signal is fed to the right hand speaker and vice versa, and which is completely mono-compatible, width enhancement tends to compromise mono compatibility. While most serious listening equipment is stereo these days, a lot of TVs and portable radios are still mono, so mono compatibility is still important.

- Always listen to your finished album master all the way through, preferably over headphones, as these have the ability to show up small glitches and noises that loudspeakers may mask. Digital clicks can appear in even the best systems, although using good-quality digital interconnects that are no longer than necessary helps to reduce this risk. If you're mastering to CD-R, you can help to reduce errors by buying a can of compressed air spray from a photographic suppliers to remove any dust particles from the CD-R surface prior to recording. Audio recordings are also generally best made at low speeds using media specifically designed for low-speed writing.

- Try to work from a 44.1kHz master tape if the end product is going to be a CD master. If you have to work from a 48kHz file or one with different tracks recorded at a different sample rates, you can either use a stand-alone sample-rate converter as you transfer the material into the computer or use a software sample-rate converter. Most editor software has sample-rate conversion capability.

  When you're working with a software sample-rate converter, make sure that you enter the sample rate of the source material correctly if this isn't recognised automatically. If you don't have a sample-rate converter, you can record material into the computer in the analogue domain. As long as you're careful with your recording levels, you probably won't notice any loss of quality.

- When transferring digital material into a computer, make sure that the computer hardware is set to External Digital Sync mode when you're recording and Internal Sync when you play back. Also, double-check that your record sample rate matches the source sample rate – I've had clients bring along DAT tapes either at the wrong sample rate or even with different tracks at different sample rates. Often this is overlooked until the client realises that some of their songs are now playing back around ten percent too slow!

- When deciding on the space between tracks on an album, listen to how the first track ends and the second one starts. Gaps are rarely shorter than two seconds, but if the starts and ends are very abrupt, you may need to leave up to four seconds between tracks. Use the pre-roll feature of your digital editor to listen to the transition so that you can get a feel for when the next track should start. There is no absolute right gap length; it depends entirely on what feels right.

- If you're using a digital de-noising program, don't expect it to work miracles if your source material is unduly noisy, as there may be some audible side-effects, but where the noise level is low to moderate, de-noising software can be incredibly effective. Digital de-noisers are effectively multi-band expanders with hundreds or thousands of separate frequency bands. The expander threshold for each band is set automatically by allowing the program to sample a short section of noise, usually from before the start of the song – which is why it's good practice not to try to clean up the starts of your original masters prior to editing. If the software is poorly designed, or if the noise contamination is severe, the background noise is modulated in a way that can only be described as 'chirping', an artifact caused by individual frequency bands being switched on and off by their expanders. The more noise reduction you try to achieve, the worse the chirping, so it's best to use as little noise reduction as you can get away with. A good rule of thumb is to monitor a quiet section at a loud level and then adjust the amount of noise reduction so that the remaining hiss still masks any unnatural side-effects.

- When editing individual tracks – for example, when compiling a version from all the best sections of several mixes or recordings – try to make your edits just before or just after a drum beat. This makes it easy to identify the correct edit point and also helps to ensure any minor discontinuities are masked by the beat. However, if you have to use a long crossfade edit to smoothe over a transition, try to avoid including a drum beat in the crossfade zone or you may hear a phasing or doubling effect where the two beats overlap. As a rule, crossfades should be as short as you can get away with, where as little as between 10ms and 30ms is enough to avoid producing a click. Longer times are usually necessary only when you're trying to smoothe over a small music discontinuity.

- Always run off two or more copies of the final master and where the master is a DAT tape or similar format, write the sample rate on the box along with all other relevant data. If you include test tones, document their level and include a list of all the track start times and running lengths for the benefit of the CD manufacturer. If for any reason you have produced a 48kHz sample rate master, mark this clearly on the production DAT master so that the CD manufacturer can sample rate convert it for you.

- It is always a good idea to avoid recording audio during the first minute or so of a new DAT tape in order to avoid the large number of dropouts commonly caused by the leader-tape clip in the tape spool hub. However, you can use this section to record test tones, which will also demonstrate to the person playing your tape that it isn't blank! If you put DAT start IDs on each track, check them carefully to make sure that there are no spurious ones, and don't use skip

IDs. It's also a good idea to manually replace the track IDs so that they start around half a second before each track so that, when these are transferred to CD, the player won't miss the start of any track.

CD-R Masters

When using CD-R to produce a master that will itself be used for commercial CD production, the disk must be written in Disk At Once mode rather than a track at a time, and the software must support PQ encoding to Red Book standard. Check with your CD manufacturer to confirm that they can work from CD-R as a master and take note of any special requirements they may have. Be very careful how you handle blank CD-Rs – there are commercial CDs on the market with beautiful fingerprints embodied in the digital data! As mentioned earlier, record masters at low speed, ideally single speed, using suitable mastering-grade media and make sure that the media is absolutely clean before recording. Occasionally a pressing plant will come back and say that a CD-R has too high an error rate to be used as a master, even though it sounds perfectly OK. Some brands of CD-R recorder produce better block error rates (BLERs) than others, but also using high-quality, clean media makes a big difference. When mastering, any Burn Proof feature should be switched off to avoid the risk of producing a master that wasn't recorded in a single pass.

Be aware that many stand-alone audio CD recorders have an automatic shut-off function that activates if gaps in the audio exceeds a preset number of seconds, usually between 6 and 20. This may be a problem if you need to put large gaps between tracks for any reason, and just occasionally classical music with very low-level passages can be interpreted as a gap. Also, note that these recorders will continue to record for that same preset number of seconds after the last track, so you'll need to stop recording manually if you don't want a section of silence tacked onto the end of the album. As a rule, a computer CD burner provides the most flexibility for producing masters, but if you have a hardware-based studio or have no access to computer editing, a hardware CD recorder is a viable option.

Mastering Using Plug-Ins

Although there is no standard mastering setting, there is a fairly standard set of mastering processors, which normally comprises at least a compressor, an equaliser and a limiter, in that order. The compressor may be either of the full-band or split-band variety (many commercial mastering hardware boxes use three- or four-band compression) and the EQ should be a good-sounding parametric type. A software harmonic enhancer may also be useful for adding crispness to a mix.

You can buy either separate plug-ins or invest in a mastering bundle, but in many instances the plug-ins supplied with your editor or sequencer will get you off to a good start. At least try them before deciding to spend money on something you may not need.

Perhaps the most important element in any mastering processor is the compressor, which goes right at the start of my own processing chain. Where using a multiband compressor, I feel that three bands are enough, but if you have only a single-band compressor, try that first, as you'll often find that it's perfectly OK.

For mastering applications, I like to set the crossovers within the multiband compressor so that the majority of the mid range sits within a single band – a low crossover point at around 150Hz and a high crossover point at around 3-5kHz works for most material. This way, the low band influences mainly bass and kick-drum sounds while the high band covers that area of the spectrum that conveys sizzle and detail. The vulnerable mid range is contained within a single band, where the processing is least likely to damage it.

As an initial default, I set the compression ratios to between 1.1:1 and 1.2:1 and this applied both to full and multiband compressors. The more density you need, the higher you have to set the ratio in that particular band, but it's unwise to go much above 1.2:1 in combination with the low threshold values used in mastering, which in this case usually end up being between –30dB and –35dB. I usually adjust

the threshold while watching the compressor gain-reduction meters, and because such a low ratio is being used, by the time you've achieved the necessary 4–6dB of gain reduction, the threshold is very low, which means that more of the dynamic range is being compressed rather than just the peaks. The whole dynamic range of the signal is squeezed gently to produce a smoother, more dense overall sound, and a fast attack (around 5ms) combined with a release time of around 150ms usually works well. As a rule, the release time should be as short as possible without causing audible gain pumping.

Although the gain-reduction meters may show as little as 3dB or 4dB of gain reduction, that's usually enough to homogenise the mix and to add density. In a multiband compressor, you can also change the levels of the individual bands to effect a tonal change, but again it's best to stick to small changes of no more than 2–3dB. If you need more than that, use EQ.

Mastering EQ

A typical plug-in parametric EQ comprises five or more bands, the middle three of which are often bandpass filters and the outer two shelving (although they may be switchable between bandpass and shelving). To add air and detail, set the highest parametric band to between 12kHz and 16kHz with a Q of approximately 0.5 and then use just one or two decibels of boost. Because the EQ is applied high up with a wide bandwidth, it has the effect of enhancing detail without adding harshness.

At the bass end, a little 80Hz boost may be used to lift the kick-drum sound or to fatten bass instruments, but a useful technique is to balance this using a gentle dip at around 250Hz, which helps prevent the low-frequency EQ from clouding the lower mid range. Of course, the precise setting depends on what your mix needs to make it sound properly balanced, but it is worth noting that most mastering EQ boost settings are quite gentle. EQ cut can be more drastic, as the human ear is less sensitive to missing or attenuated frequencies than to peaks, but as a rule any problems that require serious EQ should be dealt with at the individual track stage wherever possible.

If you decide to use an enhancer, it should come after the EQ and before the limiter. I treat enhancers as an extension of EQ, although, unlike EQ, a typical enhancer generates new harmonics based on existing information. This makes it useful for synthesising high-end detail where it is lacking in the original mix, but it's an effect you have to use with care, as it can end up sounding harsh. Combining more gentle high-end EQ with a very moderate amount of high-frequency enhancement can add a very professional sizzle to a track, but be careful not to set the enhancer's Frequency control too low or you may end up with a harsh, aggressive quality being added to the sound. I'd recommend setting the enhancer's filter to no less than 2.5–3kHz, but, as ever, you have to rely on your ears to tell you what's needed.

Take It To The Limiter

The last process is limiting, and it's most convenient to use the type of limiter where you set a maximum output level and then adjust the input gain until the desired amount of gain reduction is achieved, as this limits and normalises at the same time. I usually set the target output level at −0.5dB to leave just a little safety headroom and then push the gain until the gain-reduction meter shows between 3dB and 6dB of gain reduction on the peaks. This simple strategy increases the overall loudness of the track significantly but won't generally make the track sound as though it has been processed heavily. If there's any sign of the mix sounding squashed or harsh, back off the amount of limiting – unless that's the effect you're after.

Although the chain of mastering processors described here uses plug-ins of the type provided with most serious audio editors and sequencers, you can achieve extremely good results providing the material being processed doesn't need radical adjustment. Subtle adjustments invariably lead to the most natural sound and double-checking your settings over your headphones is a good way to identify distortions, clicks, glitches, gain pumping and just about any other unwanted artifact. Individual plug-ins can always be bypassed to check their contribution to the process, and don't forget to keep referring back to commercial recordings, as it's very easy to lose perspective when

you're processing a mix, especially if you've been working on it for any length of time without a break.

The Bits And Pieces Of Digital

Today we can record digital audio at 16 bits or 24 bits and with sample rates of 44.1kHz, 48kHz, 88.2kHz, 96kHz and even 192kHz. The more bits you record at, the greater the dynamic range you have at your disposal, where multiplying the number of bits used by 6dB gives you the theoretically best dynamic range you can achieve. From this, it follows that a 16-bit recording can have a dynamic-range of 96dB, whereas a theoretically perfect 24-bit system has a 144dB dynamic range. In reality, the results are usually a few decibels short of perfection, but what you have to keep in mind is that these figures only mean anything if your signal is fully recorded. For example, if you leave a safely margin of 12dB between your peak signals and the maximum recording level, the best you can do with a 16-bit system is 84dB.

In reality, even 84dB is extremely good and far better than the dynamic range of most of the sources that we record when making pop music. The real disadvantage of recording at too low a level isn't noise but resolution. Digital bits are used to measure audio waveforms in finite steps, and while a fully recorded signal might comprise thousands of steps, a very low-level signal uses fewer bits and is therefore measured in fewer steps. Unlike analogue, therefore, where signals get more distorted at higher recording levels, digital signals are cleanest when fully recorded and most distorted at very low levels. If this seems counter-intuitive to you, imagine a sine wave 1,000 feet high built out of regular house bricks. Because it is so big, the fact that the bricks are rectangular will have little effect on the accuracy of the overall shape, so the amount of distortion (the difference between the original waveform and the digital representation) is small. Now, if we use those same bricks to build a sine wave only a foot high, it's going to look pretty rough to the point of being almost unrecognisable because the bricks are large compared to the shape we're trying to represent. This is a close analogy to what happens with low-level digital signals, where distortion is consequently very high.

Whenever we change the level of a digital signal, mix it with another signal or process it in some other way, the multiplication and division processes used to achieve this result end up rounding off some of the calculations, which results in the overall resolution getting slightly worse every time a process is applied. In a modern system using floating-point arithmetic, the loss of resolution through processing is very small compared to what we expect when processing analogue signals, but some degradation still takes place.

Bit Reduction

In order to produce a 16-bit CD with the best possible resolution, we should ideally record, mix and process at 24-bit resolution so that we retain better than 16-bit quality throughout the project, even taking into account losses caused by under-recording, processing and so on. At the end of the mastering stage, we can then reduce the finished work to 16 bits ready for CD production and know that as much quality has been preserved as possible. Whether you'd notice any difference when working with pop music is a difficult question, as most pop music has a fairly narrow dynamic range and quiet passages are rare. However, in classical and other forms of acoustic music, where there's a lot of light and shade in the playing, low-level sounds might sounds smoother and more natural if recorded at 24-bit resolution.

Dither

The next question involves how 24-bit files can best be converted to 16-bit files for CD production. You could simply throw away the six least significant bits (a process known as *truncation*) and it wouldn't sound bad, at least not for music with a restricted dynamic range, but you may notice a loss of smoothness during low-level passages or at the ends of reverb tails. A better system is to use dither, a mathematical process that adds tiny amounts of pseudo-noise to the signal so that, instead of the least significant bit fizzling into extinction when the signal level falls below −90dB, the added noise keeps it active. The audible result is akin to what happens with analogue tape, where the signal appears to disappear smoothly into the noise

floor, except with digital the noise floor is very much lower. More important still is the fact that these low-level signals sound smooth and clear when dither is added rather than sounding grainy and distorted.

Noise Shaping

Even so, adding a few decibels of audible noise isn't something we'd normally wish to do, so most dither noise is modified so that it has most of its energy in the parts of the audio spectrum to which our ears are least sensitive, usually above 15kHz. This spectral tailoring is known as *noise-shaping dithering*, and various types of noise-shaped dither are available to suit different musical styles. I must stress that dither noise is extremely low level, so you're unlikely to hear any hiss unless you select a very quiet passage and then turn up the monitoring to very loud. What you should notice when doing this test is that properly dithered audio sounds far smoother and less distorted during quiet passages than audio initially recorded at 16 bits or 24-bit recordings that have been simply truncated to 16 bits.

The most important thing to note about dither, however, is that it is only beneficial if dithering from 24 bits to 16 bits is the very last thing that happens to a piece of audio. Any subsequent changes – even altering levels – will re-introduce rounding-up and -down errors, and the benefits of low-level smoothness will be lost.

Sample Rates

Even though we can hear only up to 20kHz or less, listening tests indicate that recording audio at sample rates higher than 44.1kHz or 48kHz can improve the sense of stereo imaging, which is why some specialised listening formats use recordings made at these high sample rates. However, you need to be using top-class equipment in an extremely quiet acoustic environment to make anything like the best use of these sample rates, so for pop music that is destined to be released on a 44.1kHz/16-bit CD, the benefits are dubious, especially when you consider that doubling the sample rate halves the amount of audio you can fit onto a hard drive, halves the track count in your audio software and halves the number of plug-ins you can run on any given system. What's more, if you do record at one of these high sample rates, you'll still have to convert the sample rate down to 44.1kHz for CD production, and unless the sample-rate converter is very good, you may lose more quality in the conversion than if you'd worked at 44.1kHz all along. My own personal view is that it's only worth working at these high sample rates if your final release medium supports them, although others may put forward different arguments. As computers become more powerful and storage gets even cheaper, the penalties of working at such sample rates will become less significant.

Clocking Issues

There's a common assumption that, because a digital signal comprises nothing more than a string of ones and zeroes, there will be no quality loss when transferring it from one system to another or from one recording medium to another. This turns out to be quite untrue, because in order to get an accurate reproduction of a digital audio signal, two things are needed: the original string of numbers and the original timing relationships between those numbers. If the right numbers turn up at slightly the wrong time, the result is an increase in noise and distortion. It's just the same as if you sampled the waveform at the right time but stored numerical values that were slightly inaccurate.

Digital timing errors of this type come under the heading of *jitter*, and even connecting one digital device to another via an AES/EBU or S/PDIF cable can introduce jitter if the cable is of poor quality or the wrong type. The reason for this is because, at the high frequencies used for digital data transfer, cables of a very precise impedance are needed to prevent some of the energy from reflecting back into the cable from a mismatched termination. Even low-level reflections can cause problems, as they in effect add to the real signal, making the rising and falling edges of the digital ones and zeroes less distinct. Once these edges lose their definition, the circuit that detects them may do so slightly later or earlier than it should, thus introducing a tiny timing error – jitter. If you think about it, digital

signals travelling down cables are actually analogue waveforms (and high-frequency ones at that) and are thus susceptible to analogue distortions, ground-loop hum contamination, loss of harmonics due to cable capacitance and everything else that affects analogue waveforms, so it pays to look after them to the best of your ability by using only appropriate connecting cables.

To minimise jitter, runs of digital cable should be kept as short as possible and cable of the correct impedance should be used. S/PDIF and word clock use 75-ohm cables while AES/EBU cable is 110 ohms, balanced. Consumer audio cables may appear to work, but at best you'll lose quality through jitter and at worst you may even experience clicks and glitches.

Word Clock

Digital equipment can be connected directly only if their sample-rate clocks are synchronised, as this is the only way to pass on the right numbers and get them into the right time slots. In semi-pro and consumer digital systems, the device sending the signal generally provides the clock reference needed by the receiving device, but as this clock is embedded in the normal digital signal, no extra cables are needed. All you need to do is set the receiving device to External Digital Sync mode and everything should work. However, in larger or more complex signals, this type of daisy-chain clocking can introduce serious jitter when three or more pieces of equipment are connected in series, so a far better solution is to have one master clock for the whole system and to feed each individual piece of gear directly from this master clock. To permit this, many pieces of professional audio equipment have word clock inputs, usually on BNC connectors, and unlike semi-pro connections this clock travels separately to the audio. Each piece of digital gear is linked star-fashion back to the central clock and its sync mode switched to Word Clock. A typical commercial word clock generator will have multiple outputs to facilitate this type of connection, and in a mixed audio-and-video environment, the word clock generator may itself have the facility to lock to a master video clock generator or other high-quality clock source,

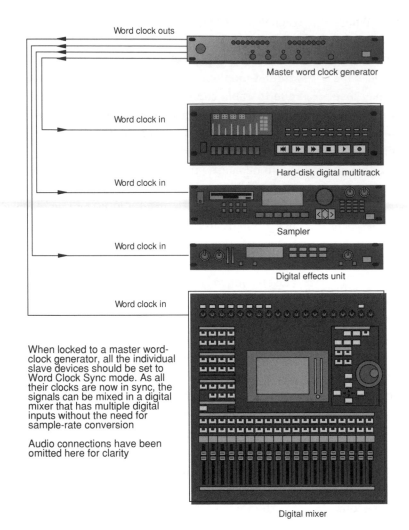

Word clock outs

Master word clock generator

Word clock in

Hard-disk digital multitrack

Word clock in

Sampler

Word clock in

Digital effects unit

Word clock in

Figure 9.7: Connections of a basic system incorporating a master clock

When locked to a master word-clock generator, all the individual slave devices should be set to Word Clock Sync mode. As all their clocks are now in sync, the signals can be mixed in a digital mixer that has multiple digital inputs without the need for sample-rate conversion

Audio connections have been omitted here for clarity

Digital mixer

Aside from the convenience aspect (you don't have to keep switching from Internal to External Sync mode), a high-quality clock will reduce jitter throughout the entire system, improving the audio quality, and some pieces of semi-pro equipment sound noticeably better when locked to a high-quality external clock than when running from their own jittery internal clocks.

However, a potential problem arises when you want to introduce some pieces of equipment that don't have word-clock inputs, as these can't always be locked to the master source. Some are able to lock via an AES/EBU or S/PDIF signal carrying clock only (know as *audio black*), and many clock generators include audio-black outputs for this purpose. However, where even this facility isn't available, it is possible to run the outputs of the consumer equipment through sample-rate converters synced to the master clock. Better still is to use a master clock generator that also includes a few channels of sample-rate conversion that are locked to its own high-quality internal master clock. To my knowledge, the relatively inexpensive Drawmer M-Clock is the only unit to offer all of these facilities in one affordable unit. Figure 9.7 shows how a basic system incorporating a master clock is connected.

GLOSSARY

AC

Abbreviation of *alternating current*.

Active

Describes a circuit containing transistors, ICs, tubes and other devices that require power to operate and are capable of amplification. In the context of monitor loudspeakers, *active* means that the speaker also incorporates amplifiers and electronic crossover units.

Active Sensing

System used to verify that a MIDI connection is working. Operates via a process that involves the sending device sending frequent short messages to the receiving device to reassure it that all is well. If these active-sensing messages stop, the receiving device will recognise a fault condition and switch off all notes. Not all MIDI devices support active sensing.

A/D Converter

Circuit for converting analogue waveforms into a series of values represented by binary numbers. The more 'bits' a converter has, the greater the resolution of the sampling process. Current effects units are generally 16 bits or more with most units being 24-bit models.

Additive Synthesis

A system for generating waveforms or sounds by combining basic waveforms or sampled sounds prior to further processing with filters and envelope shapers.

ADSR

Envelope generator with Attack, Sustain, Decay and Release parameters. This is a simple type of envelope generator and was first used on early analogue synthesisers. This form of envelope generator continues to be popular on modern instruments. (See *Decay* for more details.)

AES/EBU

Digital-interface protocol designed to accommodate stereo audio signals at sample rates up to 48kHz using balanced cable, normally connected via a standard three-pin XLR connector. There are systems that deliver audio at sample rates of up to 96kHz comprising of a pair of AES/EBU cables. Certain consumer 'flags' are not recognised by AES/EBU, including SCMS copy-protection data and DAT track-start IDs.

AFL

Abbreviation of *after-fade listen*, a system used within mixing consoles to allow specific signals to be monitored at the level set by their fader of level control knob. Aux sends are generally monitored AFL rather than PFL. (See *PFL*.)

Aftertouch

A means of generating a control signal based on how much pressure is applied to the keys of a MIDI keyboard. Most instruments that support this do not have independent pressure sensing for all keys but instead detect the overall pressure by means of a sensing strip running beneath the keys. Aftertouch may be used to control such functions as vibrato depth, filter brightness, loudness and so on.

Algorithm

A computer program designed to perform a specific task. In the context of effects units, algorithms usually describe a software building block designed to create a specific effect or combination of effects.

Aliasing

When an analogue signal is sampled for conversion into a digital data stream, the sampling frequency must be at least twice that of the highest frequency component of the input signal. If this rule is disobeyed, the sampling process becomes ambiguous, as there are insufficient points to define each cycle of the waveform, resulting in enharmonic frequencies being added to the audible signal.

Ambience

The result of sound reflections in a confined space being added to the original sound. Ambience may also be created electronically by some digital reverb units. The main difference between ambience and reverberation is that ambience doesn't have the characteristic long delay time of reverberation – the reflections mainly give the sound a sense of space.

Amp

Abbreviation of *ampère*, the SI unit of electrical current.

Amplifier

Device that increases the level of an electrical signal.

Amplitude

Another word for *level*. Can refer to sound levels or electrical signal levels.

Analogue

Circuitry that uses a continually changing voltage or current to represent a signal. The origin of the term is that the electrical signal can be thought of as being analogous to the original signal.

Analogue Synthesis

A system for synthesising sounds by means of analogue circuitry, usually by filtering simple repeating waveforms.

Anti-Aliasing Filter

Filter used to limit the frequency range of an analogue signal prior to A/D conversion so that the maximum frequency does not exceed half the sampling rate.

Application

Alternative term for computer program.

Arpeggiator

Hardware or software device that allows a MIDI instrument to sequence around any notes currently being played. Most arpeggiators also allows the sound to be sequenced over several octaves so that holding down a simple chord can result in an impressive repeating sequence of notes.

ASCII

Abbreviation of *American Standard Code for Information Interchange*, a standard code for representing computer keyboard characters by binary data.

ASIO

Software driver standard developed by Steinberg to allow compatible soundcards/audio interfaces and software to work together effectively and with low latency. ASIO II also provides the option for source monitoring with compatible hardware to avoid the effects of latency when recording or overdubbing.

ATRAC

Data-compression system used in commercial MiniDisc recorders.

Attack

The time it takes for a sound to achieve maximum amplitude. Drums have a fast attack, whereas bowed strings have a slow attack. In compressors and gates, the attack time equates to how quickly the processor can change its gain.

Attenuate

To make lower in level.

Audio Frequency

Signals in the human audio range, nominally 20Hz–20kHz.

Audio Unit

Audio plug-in format supported by Apple's OSX software and above.

Autolocator

Feature of a tape machine or some other recording device that enables specific locations to be stored. At some later time, these locations within the recording may then be recalled. For example, you may store the start of a verse as a locate point so that you can get the tape machine to wind back the start of the verse after you've recorded an overdub.

Auto-Tune

Software or hardware designed by Antares to correct vocal pitching problems by forcing notes to the nearest correct note in a selected musical scale.

Aux

Control on a mixing console designed to route a proportion of the channel signal to the effects or cue mix outputs (aux send).

Aux Return

Mixer inputs used to add effects to a mix.

Aux Send

Physical output from a mixer aux-send buss.

Azimuth

Alignment co-ordinate of a tape head which references the head gap to the true vertical relative to the tape path.

Backup

A safety copy of software or other digital data.

Balance

This word has several meanings in recording. It may refer to the relative levels of the left and right channels of a stereo recording, or it may be used to describe the relative levels of the various instruments and voices within a mix.

Balanced Wiring

Wiring system which uses two out-of-phase conductors and a common screen to reduce the effect of interference. For balancing to be effective, both the sending and receiving device must have balanced output and input stages respectively.

Bandpass Filter

Filter that removes or attenuates frequencies above and below the frequency at which it is set. Frequencies within the band are emphasised. Bandpass filters are often used in synthesisers as tone-shaping elements.

Bandwidth

A means of specifying the range of frequencies passed by an electronic circuit such as an amplifier, mixer or filter. The frequency range is usually measured at the points where the level drops by 3dB relative to the maximum.

Bass Trap

Acoustic absorber designed to absorb low frequencies, often positioned in the corner of a room.

Beta Version

Software which is not fully tested and may include bugs.

Bias

High-frequency signal used in analogue recording to improve the accuracy of the recorded signal and to drive the erase head. Bias is generated by a bias oscillator.

Binary

Counting system based on two states: one and zero.

BIOS

Part of a computer operating system held on ROM rather than on disk. This handles basic routines such as accessing the disk drive.

Bit

Abbreviation of *binary digit*, which may represent either one or zero.

Boost/Cut Control

A single control which allows the range of frequencies passing through a filter to be either amplified or attenuated. The centre position is usually the 'flat' or 'no effect' position.

Bouncing

The process of mixing two or more recorded tracks together and re-recording these onto another, separate track.

BPM

Abbreviation of *beats per minute*.

Breath Controller

Device that converts breath pressure into MIDI controller data.

Buffer

Circuit designed to isolate the output of a source device from loading effects due to the input impedance of the destination device.

Buffer Memory

Temporary RAM used in some computer operations, sometimes to prevent a break in the data stream when the computer is interrupted to perform another task. All audio software employs buffer memory to ensure a continuous stream of audio. The greater the buffer size, the less likely it is that glitches or other problems will occur, but at the same time, a larger buffer size increases the system latency.

Bug

Slang term for software fault or equipment design problem.

Burner

Drive mechanism capable of recording CD-R and/or DVD-R discs.

Buss

Common electrical signal path along which signals may travel. In a mixer, there are several busses carrying the stereo mix, the groups, the PFL signal, the aux sends and so on. Power supplies are also fed along busses.

Byte

A piece of digital data comprising eight bits.

Capacitance

Property of an electrical component able to store electrostatic charge.

Capacitor

Electrical component exhibiting capacitance. Capacitor microphones are often abbreviated to *capacitors*.

Capacitor Microphone

Microphone that operates on the principle of measuring the change in electrical charge across a capacitor, where one of the electrodes is a thin conductive membrane that flexes in response to changes in sound pressure.

Cardioid

Literally 'heart-shaped'. Describes the polar response of a unidirectional microphone.

CD-R

Recordable type of compact disc that can be recorded on only once – it cannot be erased and reused.

CD-R burner

Device capable of recording data onto blank CD-R discs.

Channel

A single strip of controls in a mixing console relating to either a single input or a pair of main/monitor inputs.

Channel

In the context of MIDI, *channel* refers to one of 16

possible data channels over which MIDI data may be sent. The organisation of data by channels means that up to 16 different MIDI instruments or parts may be addressed using a single cable.

Channel
In the context of mixing consoles, a channel is a single strip of controls relating to one input.

Chase
Term describing the process whereby a slave device attempts to synchronise itself with a master device. In the context of a MIDI sequence, *chase* may also involve chasing events – ie looking back to earlier positions in the song to see if there are any program changes or other events that need to be acted upon.

Chip
Integrated circuit.

Chord
Three or more different musical notes played at the same time.

Chorus
Effect created by doubling a signal and adding delay and pitch modulation.

Chromatic
Term used to describe a scale of pitches rising in semitone steps.

Click Track
Metronomic pulse that helps musicians to play in time.

Clipping
Severe form of distortion which occurs when a signal attempts to exceed the maximum level that a piece of equipment can handle.

Clone
Exact duplicate. Often refers to digital copies of digital tapes.

Common-Mode Rejection
A measure of how well a balanced circuit rejects a signal that is common to both inputs.

Compander
Encode/decode device that compresses a signal while encoding it, then expands it when decoding it.

Compressor
Device designed to reduce the dynamic range of audio signals by reducing the levels of high signals or by increasing the levels of low signals.

Computer
Device used to store and process sequences of digital data.

Conductor
Material that provides a low resistance path for electrical current.

Console
Alternative term for mixer.

Contact Enhancer
Compound designed to increase the electrical conductivity of electrical contacts such as plugs, sockets and edge connectors.

Continuous Controller
Type of MIDI message used to translate continuous change, such as from a pedal, wheel or breath-control device.

Control Voltage
Used to control the pitch of an oscillator or filter frequency in an analogue synthesiser. Most analogue synthesisers follow a one-volt-per-octave convention, although there are exceptions. To use a pre-MIDI analogue synthesiser under MIDI control, a MIDI-to-CV converter is required.

Copy Protection
Protocol used by software manufacturers to prevent unauthorised copying.

Crash

Slang term relating to the malfunctioning of a program.

Cut-And-Paste Editing

The copying or moving of sections of a recording to new locations.

Cut-Off Frequency

The frequency above or below which attenuation begins in a filter circuit.

Cycle

One complete vibration of a sound source or its electrical equivalent. One cycle per second is expressed as 1Hz (Hertz).

Daisy Chain

Term used to describe a serial electrical connection between devices or modules.

Damping

In the context of reverberation, damping refers to the rate (usually frequency dependent) at which the reverberant energy is absorbed by the various surfaces in the environment.

DAT

Abbreviation of *digital audio tape*. The commonly used DAT machines are more correctly known as R-DATs because they use a rotating head similar to that in a video recorder. Digital recorders using fixed or stationary heads (such as DCC) are known as S-DAT machines. Most DAT recorders work at 44.1kHz or 48kHz sampling rates with a 16-bit resolution, although some 24-bit models have been developed.

Data

Information that is stored and used by a computer.

Data Compression

System used to reduce the amount of data needed to represent an audio signal, usually by discarding audio information that is being masked by more prominent sounds. Data-compression algorithms are based on psychoacoustic principles designed to ensure that only components which cannot be heard are lost, although in practice heavy compression does compromise the subjective audio quality. Both MiniDisc (ATRAC) and MP3 files use a type of data compression.

dB

Abbreviation of *decibel*, a unit used to express the relative levels of two electrical voltages, powers or sounds.

dBm

Variation on dB referenced to 0dB = 1mW into 600 ohms.

dB/octave

A means of measuring the slope of a filter. The more decibels per octave, the sharper the filter slope.

dBv

Variation on dB referenced to 0dB = 0.775 volts.

dBV

Variation on dB referenced to 0dB = 1 volt.

dbx

Commercial encode/decode tape-noise-reduction system that compresses the signal during recording and expands it by an identical amount on playback.

DC

Abbreviation of *direct current*.

DCC

Stationary-head digital recorder format developed by Phillips that uses a data-compression system to reduce the amount of data that needs to be stored. DCC is now obsolete, although some machines are still in circulation.

DCO

Abbreviation of *digitally controlled oscillator*.

DDL

Abbreviation of *digital delay line*.

Decay

Progressive reduction in amplitude of a sound or electrical signal over time. In the context of an ADSR envelope shaper, the Decay phase starts as soon as the Attack phase has reached its maximum level. In the Decay phase, the signal level drops until it reaches the Sustain level, set by the user. The signal then remains at this level until the key is released, at which point the Release phase is entered.

De-Esser

Device for reducing the effect of sibilance in vocal signals.

Defragmentation

Process of rearranging the files on a hard disk so that all the files are as contiguous as possible and that the remaining free space is also contiguous.

Deoxidising Compound

Substance formulated to remove oxides from electrical contacts.

Detent

Physical click-stop in the centre of a control such as a pan or EQ cut/boost knob.

DI

Abbreviation of *direct injection*, where a signal is plugged directly into an audio chain without the aid of a microphone, often via an impedance-matching device called a *DI box*.

DI Box

Device for matching the signal level impedance of a source to a tape machine or mixer input.

Digital

Term used to describe an electronic system that represents data and signals in the form of codes comprising ones and zeros.

Digital Delay

Digital processor that generates delay and echo effects.

Digital Reverb

Digital processor that simulates reverberation.

DIN Connector

Consumer multipin signal connection format, also used for MIDI cabling. Various pin configurations are available.

Direct Coupling

Means of connecting two electrical circuits so that both AC and DC signals may be passed between them.

Dithering

System of adding low-level noise to a digitised audio signal in such a way as to extend the low-level resolution at the expense of a slight deterioration in noise performance. Special 'noise shaped' dither algorithms are used to minimise the subjective effects of the added noise by adding it in those areas of the spectrum where the human hearing system is least sensitive.

Disc

Term used to describe vinyl discs, CDs and MiniDiscs.

Disk

Abbreviation of *diskette* but now used to describe computer floppy, hard and removable disks.

DMA

Abbreviation of *direct memory access*, part of a computer operating system that allows peripheral devices to communicate directly with the computer memory without going via the central processor or CPU.

Dolby

An encode/decode tape-noise-reduction system that amplifies low-level, high-frequency signals during recording and then reverses this process during playback. There are several different Dolby systems in use: types B, C and S for domestic and semi-professional machines, and types A and SR for professional machines. Recordings made using one of these systems must also be replayed via the same system.

Dolby Digital

Means of digitally encoding a surround audio soundtrack so that discrete signals can be fed to each of the surround speakers and to a separate sub-bass (LFE) speaker. AC3 compression is used to enable a movie and its soundtrack to fit onto a DVD.

Dolby Surround

Means of encoding an analogue two-channel signal so that information can be extracted to drive rear speakers as well as stereo front speakers. This system drives the rear speakers from a mono source and has limited channel separation due to the matrixing process employed.

DOS

Abbreviation of *disk operating system*, part of the operating system of PC and other IBM-compatible computers.

Driver

Piece of software that handles communications between the main program and a hardware peripheral, such as a soundcard, printer or scanner.

Drum Pad

Synthetic playing surface that produces electronic trigger signals in response to being hit with drum sticks.

Dry

Term used to describe a signal that has had no effects added.

DSP

Abbreviation of *digital signal processor*, a powerful microchip used to process digital signals.

Dubbing

The process of adding further material to an existing recording. This process is also known as *overdubbing*.

Ducking

System for controlling the level of one audio signal with another. For example, background music can be made to 'duck' whenever you need a voice-over to be heard.

Dumping

Transferring digital data from one device to another. A sysex dump is a means of transmitting information about a particular instrument or module over MIDI, and may be used to store sound patches, parameter settings and so on.

DVD

Abbreviation of *digital versatile disc*, used for consumer playback of video, for computer data storage and for specialised surround audio playback formats, such as DVD-A.

Dynamic Microphone

Type of microphone that operates on the same principle as electric generators, where an internal diaphragm moves a coil of wire within a magnetic field.

Dynamic Range

The range in decibels between the highest signal that can be handled by a piece of equipment and the level at which small signals disappear into the noise floor.

Dynamics

Way of describing the relative levels within a piece of music.

Early Reflections

Initial sound reflections from walls, floors and ceilings following a sound created in an acoustically reflective environment.

Effect

Device for treating an audio signal in order to change it in some creative way. Effects often involve the use of delay circuits and include such treatments as reverb and echo.

Effects Loop

Connection system that allows an external signal processor to be connected into the audio chain.

Effects Return

Additional mixer input designed to accommodate the output from an effects unit.

Electret Microphone

Type of capacitor microphone utilising a permanently charged capsule.

Encode/Decode

Term used to describe a system that requires a signal to be processed prior to recording. The process is then reversed during playback.

Enhancer

Device designed to brighten audio material using techniques such as dynamic equalisation, phase shifting and harmonic generation.

Envelope

Term used to describe the way in which the level of a sound or signal varies over time.

Envelope Generator

Circuit capable of generating a control signal which represents the envelope of the sound you want to recreate. This may be used to control the level of an oscillator or other sound source, although envelopes may also be used to control filter/modulation settings. The most common example is the ADSR generator.

E-PROM

Similar to ROM, but the information on the chip can be erased and replaced using special equipment.

Equaliser

Device for selectively cutting or boosting selected parts of the audio spectrum.

Erase

To remove recorded material from an analogue tape or remove digital data from any storage medium.

Event

In MIDI terms, an event is a single unit of MIDI data, such as a note being turned on or off, a piece of controller information, a program change message, and so on.

Exciter

Enhancer that works by synthesising new high-frequency harmonics.

Expander

Device designed to decrease the levels of low-level signals and increase the levels of high-level signals, thus increasing the dynamic range of the signal.

Expander Module

Synthesiser with no keyboard, often rack mountable or in some other compact format.

Fader

Sliding potentiometer control used in mixers and other processors.

Ferric

Variety of magnetic tape coating that uses iron oxide.

FET

Abbreviation of *field-effect transistor*.

Figure-Of-Eight

Term used to describe the polar response of a microphone that is equally sensitive to sounds coming from both front and rear, yet rejects sounds coming from the sides.

File

Meaningful list of data stored in digital form. A Standard MIDI File is a specific type of file designed to allow sequence information to be interchanged between different types of sequencer.

Filter

Electronic circuit designed to emphasise or attenuate a specific range of frequencies.

FireWire

Also known as IEEE 1394, FireWire is a high-speed data-transfer format used with computers, often to connect hard drives, digital video cameras or other peripherals. It has the capacity to carry multiple channels of audio, MIDI and sync data. A number of FireWire-connected audio interfaces are available for computer audio use. Yamaha have built a dedicated audio protocol using FireWire which they call mLAN and which is supported by dedicated chip sets.

Flanging

Modulated delay effect using feedback to create a dramatic, sweeping sound.

Floppy Disk

Computer disk that uses a flexible, magnetic medium encased in a protective plastic sleeve. The maximum capacity of a standard high-density disk is 1.44MB. Earlier double-density disks held only around half that amount of data.

Flutter Echo

Resonant echo that occurs when sound reflects back and forth between two parallel, reflective surfaces.

Foldback

System for feeding one or more separate mixes to the performers for use while recording and overdubbing. Also known as a *cue mix*.

Formant

Frequency component or resonance of an instrument or voice sound that doesn't change with the pitch of the note being played or sung. For example, the body resonance of an acoustic guitar remains constant, regardless of the note being played.

Format

Procedure required to ready a computer disk for use. Formatting organises the disk's surface into a series of electronic pigeonholes into which data can be stored. Different computers often use different formatting systems.

Fragmentation

Process by which the available space on a disk drive gets split up into small sections due to the storing and erasing of files. (See *Defragmentation*.)

Frequency

Indication of how many cycles of a repetitive waveform occur in one second. A waveform which has a repetition cycle of once per second has a frequency of 1Hz.

Frequency Response

Measurement of the frequency range that can be handled by a specific piece of electrical equipment or loudspeaker.

FSK

Abbreviation of *frequency shift keying*, a method of recording a sync clock signal onto tape by representing it as two alternating tones.

Fundamental

All sounds comprise a fundamental or basic frequency plus harmonics and partials at higher frequencies.

FX

Abbreviation of *effects*.

Gain

Amount by which a circuit amplifies a signal.

Gate

Electrical signal that is generated whenever a key is depressed on an electronic keyboard, used to trigger envelope generators and other events that need to be synchronised to key action.

Gate

Electronic device designed to mute low-level signals so as to improve noise performance during pauses in the wanted material.

General MIDI

Addition to the basic MIDI specification to assure a

minimum level of compatibility when playing back GM-format song files. The specification covers type and program number of sounds, minimum levels of polyphony and multitimbrality, response to controller information and so on.

Glitch

Unwanted short-term corruption of a signal, or the unexplained short-term malfunction of a piece of equipment. For example, an inexplicable click on a DAT tape would be termed a glitch.

GM Reset

Universal sysex command that activates the General MIDI mode on a GM instrument. The same command also sets all controllers to their default values and switches off any notes still playing by means of an All Notes Off message.

Graphic Equaliser

Equaliser that controls several narrow segments of the audio spectrum with individual cut/boost faders. The name comes about because the fader positions provide a graphic representation of the EQ curve.

Ground

Electrical earth, or oV. In mains wiring, the ground cable is physically connected to the ground via a long, conductive metal spike.

Ground Loop

Wiring problem where multiple ground connections are causing audible mains hum to be picked up. Also known as *earth loop*.

Group

Collection of signals within a mixer that are mixed and then routed through a separate fader to provide overall control. In a multitrack mixer, several groups are provided to feed the various recorder track inputs.

GS

Roland's own extension of the General MIDI protocol.

Hard Disk

High-capacity computer storage device based on a rotating rigid disk with a magnetic coating onto which data may be recorded.

Harmonic

High-frequency component of a complex waveform, being a direct multiple of the fundamental frequency.

Harmonic Distortion

Addition of harmonics that were not present in an original signal.

Head

Part of a tape machine or disk drive that reads and/or writes data to and from the storage media.

Headroom

Safety margin in decibels between the highest peak signal being passed by a piece of equipment and the absolute maximum level the equipment can handle.

High-Pass Filter

Filter that attenuates frequencies below its cut-off frequency.

Hiss

Noise caused on tape by random electrical fluctuations.

Hum

Signal contamination caused by the addition of low frequencies, usually related to the mains power frequency.

Hz

Abbreviation of *Hertz*, the unit of frequency.

IC

Abbreviation of *integrated circuit*.

Impedance

Can be visualised as the 'AC resistance' of a circuit that contains both resistive and reactive components.

Inductor

Reactive component that presents an increasing impedance with frequency.

Initialise

To restore a piece of equipment to its factory default settings automatically.

Insert Point

Connector that allows an external processor to be patched into a signal path so that the signal flows through the external processor.

Insulator

Material that does not conduct electricity.

Interface

Device that acts as an intermediary between two or more other pieces of equipment. For example, a MIDI interface enables a computer to communicate with MIDI instruments and keyboards.

Intermittent

Term usually used to describe a fault that appears only occasionally.

Intermodulation Distortion

Form of distortion that introduces frequencies not present in an original signal, invariably based on the sum and difference products of the original frequencies.

I/O

The part of a system that handles inputs and outputs, usually in the digital domain.

IPS

Abbreviation of *inches per second*, used to describe tape speed.

IRQ

Abbreviation of *interrupt request*, part of the operating system of a computer that allows a connected device to request attention from the processor in order to transfer data to it or from it.

Isopropyl Alcohol

Type of alcohol commonly used for cleaning and degreasing tape-machine heads and guides.

Jack

Common audio connector. May be mono or stereo.

Jargon

Specialised words associated with a specialist subject.

Jitter

Timing errors in digital data caused by poor clock timing at the A-to-D or D-to-A conversion stages. Jitter translates into a loss of audio quality, especially stereo imaging, and in extreme cases can manifest itself as an increase in background noise. Daisy-chaining clocks can increase the risk of jitter, which is why running a studio from a central, high-accuracy master word-clock generator is desirable.

Joystick

Controlling device able to input data in three dimensions. Often used for controlling surround audio panning, both left/right and front/rear.

k

Abbreviation for 1,000 (*kilo*). Used as a prefix to other values to indicate magnitude.

LCD

Abbreviation of *liquid-crystal display*.

LED

Abbreviation of *light-emitting diode*, a solid-state lamp.

LFO

Abbreviation of *low-frequency oscillator*, used as a modulation source, usually below 20Hz. The most common LFO waveshape is the sine wave, although there is often a choice of sine, square, triangular and sawtooth waveforms.

Limiter

Device that controls the gain of a signal so as to prevent it from ever exceeding a preset level. A limiter is essentially a fast-acting compressor with an infinite compression ratio.

Linear

Term used to describe a device on which the output is a direct multiple of the input.

Line Level

Nominal signal level which is around −10dBV for semi-pro equipment and +4dBu for professional equipment.

Load

Electrical circuit that draws power from another circuit or power supply. Also describes the reading of data into a computer.

Local On/Off

Function that allows the keyboard and sound-generating section of a keyboard synthesiser to be used independently of each other.

Logic

Type of electronic circuitry used for processing binary signals, comprising two discrete voltage levels.

Loop

Circuit where the output is connected back to the input.

Low-Pass Filter

Filter that attenuates frequencies above its cut-off frequency.

LSB

Abbreviation of *least-significant byte*. If a piece of data has to be conveyed as two bytes, one byte represents high-value numbers and the other low-value numbers, much in the same way as tens and units function in the decimal system. The high value, or most significant part of the message, is called the MSB (Most Significant Byte).

Machine Head

The tuning heads of a guitar.

MDM

Abbreviation of *modular digital multitrack*, a digital recorder that can be used in multiples to provide a greater number of synchronised tracks than a single machine.

Memory

Computer's RAM, used to store programs and data. This data is lost when the computer is switched off and so must be stored to disk or other suitable media.

Menu

List of choices presented by a computer program or a device with a display window.

Mic Level

Low-level signal generated by a microphone. This must be amplified many times to increase it to line level.

Microprocessor

Specialised microchip at the heart of a computer. It is here that instructions are read and acted upon.

MIDI

Abbreviation of *musical instrument digital interface*.

MIDI Analyser

Device that gives a visual readout of MIDI activity when connected between two pieces of MIDI equipment.

MIDI Bank Change

Type of controller message used to select alternate banks of MIDI programs where access to more than 128 programs is required.

MIDI Control Change

Also known as *MIDI controllers* or *controller data*, these messages convey positional information relating to performance controls such as wheels, pedals and switches. This information can be used to control functions such as vibrato depth, brightness, portamento, effects levels and many other parameters.

MIDI Controller

Term used to describe the physical interface by means of which the musician plays the MIDI synthesiser or other sound generator. Examples of controllers include keyboards, drum pads and wind synths.

(Standard) MIDI File

Standard file format for storing song data recorded on a MIDI sequencer in such as way as to allow it to be read by other makes or model of MIDI sequencer.

MIDI Implementation Chart

Chart usually found in MIDI product manuals providing information as to which MIDI features are supported. Supported features are marked with a o while unsupported feature are marked with a X. Additional information may be provided, such as the exact form of the bank-change message.

MIDI In

Socket used to receive information from a master controller or from the MIDI Thru socket of a slave unit.

MIDI Merge

Device or sequencer function that enables two or more streams of MIDI data to be combined.

MIDI Module

Sound-generating device with no integral keyboard.

MIDI Mode

MIDI information can be interpreted by the receiving MIDI instrument in a number of ways, the most common being polyphonically on a single MIDI channel (Poly/Omni Off mode). Omni mode allows a MIDI instrument to play all incoming data regardless of channel.

MIDI Note Number

Each key on a MIDI keyboard has its own note number, ranging from 0–127, where 60 represents middle C. Some systems use C3 as middle C while some use C4.

MIDI Note Off

Message sent when key is released.

MIDI Note On

MIDI message sent when note is played (key pressed).

MIDI Out

MIDI connector used to send data from a master device to the MIDI In of a connected slave device.

MIDI Port

MIDI connections of a MIDI-compatible device. In the context of a MIDI interface, a multiport is a device with multiple MIDI output sockets, each capable of carrying data relating to a different set of 16 MIDI channels. Multiports are the only means of exceeding the limitations imposed by 16 MIDI channels.

MIDI Program Change

MIDI message used to change sound patches on a remote module or effects patch on a MIDI effects unit.

MIDI Splitter

Alternative term for MIDI Thru box.

MIDI Sync

Description of the synchronisation systems available to MIDI users – MIDI clock and MIDI time code.

MIDI Thru

Socket on a slave unit used to feed the MIDI In socket of the next unit in line.

MIDI Thru Box

Device that splits the MIDI Out signal of a master instrument or sequencer in order to avoid daisy chaining. Powered circuitry is used to 'buffer' the outputs so as to prevent problems when many pieces of equipment are driven from a single MIDI output.

Mixer

Device for combining two or more audio signals.

mLAN

See *FireWire*.

Monitor

Reference loudspeaker used for mixing.

Monitor

To listen to a mix or a specific audio signal.

Monitor

VDU display for a computer.

Monophonic

One note at a time.

Motherboard

Main circuit board within a computer into which all the other components plug or connect.

MP3

Form of data compression used to minimise the sizes of mono or stereo audio files so that they can be transmitted over the Internet or used in a portable MP3 player. Various levels of compression are available depending on how much quality can be sacrificed for the sake of small file size, but a typical MP3 file takes up around ten per cent of the size of an uncompressed 16-bit/44.1kHz file.

MTC

Abbreviation of *MIDI time code*, a MIDI sync implementation based on SMPTE time code.

Multisampling

Creation of several samples, each covering a limited musical range, the idea being to produce a more natural range of sounds across the range of the instrument being sampled. For example, a piano may need to be sampled every two or three semitones in order to sound convincing.

Multitimbral

Term used to describe a synthesiser, sampler or module that can play several parts at the same time, each under the control of a different MIDI channel.

Multitimbral Module

MIDI sound source capable of producing several different sounds at the same time and controlled on different MIDI channels.

Multitrack

Recording device capable of recording several 'parallel' parts or tracks , which may then be mixed or re-recorded independently.

Near Field

Some people prefer the term *close field*, used to describe a loudspeaker system designed to be used close to the listener. The advantage is that the listener hears more of the direct sound from the speakers and less of the reflected sound from the room.

Noise Reduction

System used to reduce analogue tape noise or to reduce the level of hiss present in a recording. Noise-reduction systems generally employ a coding process while recording and an inverse decoding process during playback. Examples are Dolby A, B, C, S and SR as well as dbx type I and type II.

Noise Shaping

System used to create digital dither such that any added noise is shifted into those parts of the audio spectrum where the human ear is least sensitive.

Non-Linear Recording

Term used to describe the process carried out by digital recording systems that allows any parts of the recording to be played back in any order with no gaps. Conventional tape is referred to as *linear*, because the material can play back only in the order in which it was recorded.

Non-Registered Parameter Number

Addition to the basic MIDI specification that allows Controllers 98 and 99 to be used to control non-standard parameters relating to particular models of synthesiser. This is an alternative to using system-exclusive data to achieve the same ends, although NRPNs tend to be used mainly by Yamaha and Roland instruments.

Normalising

A socket is said to be normalised when it is wired

so that the original signal path is maintained unless a plug is inserted into the socket. The most common examples of normalised connectors are the insert points on a mixing console.

Normalising

The process of increasing the level of an audio file so that its loudest peak reaches exactly digital full scale.

Nut

Slotted plastic or bone component at the headstock end of a guitar neck used to guide the strings over the fingerboard and space the strings above the frets.

Nyquist Theorem

Rule which states that a digital sampling system must have a sample rate at least twice as high as that of the highest frequency being sampled in order to avoid aliasing. Because anti-aliasing filters aren't perfect, the sampling frequency has usually to be made more than twice that of the maximum input frequency.

Octave

When a frequency or pitch is transposed up by one octave, its frequency is doubled.

Offline

Term used to describe a process carried out while a recording is not playing. For example, some computer-based processes have to be carried out offline as the computer isn't fast enough to carry out the process in real time.

Ohm

Unit of electrical resistance.

Omni

Literally 'all', omni refers to a microphone that is equally sensitive in all directions or to the MIDI mode where data on all channels is recognised.

Open Circuit

Break in an electrical circuit that prevents current from flowing.

Open Reel

Tape machine on which the tape is wound on spools rather than sealed in a cassette.

Operating System

Basic software that enables a computer to load and run other programs.

Opto-Electronic Device

Device on which some electrical parameters change in response to a variation in light intensity. Variable photo-resistors are sometimes used as gain-controlling elements in compressors, where the side-chain signal modulates the light intensity.

Oscillator

Circuit designed to generate a periodic electrical waveform.

Overdub

To add another part to a multitrack recording or to replace one of the existing parts.

Overload

To exceed the operating capacity of an electronic or electrical circuit.

Pad

Resistive circuit used for reducing the level of a signal.

Pan Pot

Control enabling the user of a mixer to move the signal to any point in the stereo soundstage by varying the relative levels fed to the left and right stereo outputs.

Parallel

Means of connecting two or more circuits together so that their inputs are connected together and their outputs are all connected together.

Parameter

Variable value that affects some aspect of a device's performance.

Parametric EQ

Equaliser with separate controls for frequency, bandwidth and cut/boost.

Passive

Term used to describe a circuit with no active elements.

Patch

Alternative term for *program*, referring to a single programmed sound within a synthesiser that can be called up using program-change commands. MIDI effects units and samplers also have patches.

Patch Bay

System of panel-mounted connectors used to bring inputs and outputs to a central point from which they can be routed using plug-in patch cords.

Patch Cord

Short cable used with patch bays.

Peak

Maximum instantaneous level of a signal.

Phase

Timing difference between two electrical waveforms expressed in degrees, where 360º corresponds to a delay of exactly one cycle.

Phaser

Effect that combines a signal with a phase-shifted version of itself to produce creative filtering effects. Most phasers are controlled by means of an LFO.

PFL

Abbreviation of pre-fade listen, a system used within a mixing console to allow the operator to listen in on a selected signal, regardless of the position of the fader controlling that signal.

Phantom Power

48V DC supply for capacitor microphones, transmitted along the signal cores of a balanced mic cable.

Phono Plug

Hi-fi connector developed by RCA and used extensively on semi-pro, unbalanced recording equipment.

Pickup

Part of a guitar that converts the string vibrations to electrical signals.

Pitch

Musical interpretation of an audio frequency.

Pitch Bend

Special control message designed specifically to produce a change in pitch in response to the movement of a pitch-bend wheel or lever. Pitch-bend data can be recorded and edited, just like any other MIDI controller data, even though it isn't part of the controller message group.

Pitch Shifter

Device used to change the pitch of an audio signal without changing it's duration.

Plug-in

Modular software program that adds functionality to a host program – for example, musical instruments or audio effects. Common audio plug-in formats are VST, Audio Units, MAS (Digital Performer) and ProTools TDM.

Poly Mode

Most common MIDI mode, allowing and instrument to respond to multiple simultaneous notes transmitted on a single MIDI channel.

Polyphony

Ability of an instrument to play two or more notes simultaneously. An instrument that can play only one note at a time is described as *monophonic*.

Port

Connection for the input or output of data.

Portamento

Gliding effect that allows a sound to change pitch

at a gradual rate, rather than abruptly, when a new key is pressed or MIDI note sent.

Post-Fade

Aux signal taken from after the channel fader so that the aux-send level follows any channel fader changes. Normally used for feeding effects devices.

Post-Production

Work done to a stereo recording after mixing is complete.

Power Supply

Unit designed to convert mains electricity to the voltages necessary to power an electronic circuit or device.

PPM

Abbreviation of *peak programme meter*, designed to register signal peaks rather than the average level.

PPQN

Abbreviation of *pulses per quarter note*. Used in the context of MIDI-clock-derived sync signals.

PQ Coding

Process for adding pause, cue and other subcode information to a digital master tape in preparation for CD manufacture. A master properly prepared for commercial production is sometimes said to be 'Red Book' compatible.

Pre-Emphasis

System for applying high-frequency boost to a sound before processing so as to reduce the effect of noise. A corresponding de-emphasis process is required on playback so as to restore the original signal and to attenuate any high-frequency noise contributed by the recording process.

Pre-Fade

Aux signal taken from before the channel fader so that the channel fader has no effect on the aux send level. Normally used for creating foldback or cue mixes.

Preset

Effects unit or synth patch that cannot be altered by the user.

Print-Through

Undesirable process that causes some magnetic information from a recorded analogue tape to become imprinted onto an adjacent layer. This can produce low-level pre or post echoes.

Processor

Device designed to treat an audio signal by changing its dynamics or frequency content. Examples of processors include compressors, gates and equalisers.

Pulse Wave

Similar to a square wave but non-symmetrical. Pulse waves sound brighter and thinner than square waves, making them useful in the synthesis of reed instruments. The timbre changes according to the mark/space ratio of the waveform.

Pulse-Width Modulation

Means of modulating the duty cycle (mark/space ratio) of a pulse wave. This changes the timbre of the basic tone. LFO modulation of pulse width can be used to produce a pseudo-chorus effect.

Punching In

Action of placing an already recorded track into record at the correct time during playback so that the existing material may be extended or replaced.

Punching Out

The action of switching a tape machine (or other recording device) out of record after executing a punch-in. With most multitrack machines, both punching in and punching out can be accomplished without stopping the tape.

PZM

Abbreviation of *pressure-zone microphone*, a type of boundary microphone designed to reject out-of-phase sounds reflected from surfaces within the recording environment.

Q

Measure of the resonant properties of a filter. The higher the Q, the more resonant the filter and the narrower the range of frequencies that are allowed to pass.

Quantising

Means of moving notes recorded in a MIDI sequencer so that they line up with user defined subdivisions of a musical bar – for example, 16th notes. The facility may be used to correct timing errors, but over-quantisation can remove the human feel from a performance.

RAM

Abbreviation of *random-access memory*, a type of memory used by computers for the temporary storage of programs and data. All data is lost when the power is turned off, and for this reason work needs to be saved to disk if it is not to be lost.

R-DAT

Digital tape machine using a rotating-head system.

Real Time

Term used to describe an audio process that can be carried out as the signal is being recorded or played back. Conversely, offline describes a situation where the signal is processed in non-real time.

Release

Time it takes for a level or gain to return to normal, often used to describe the rate at which a synthesised sound reduces in level after a key has been released.

Resistance

Opposition to the flow of electrical current, measured in ohms.

Resolution

Accuracy with which an analogue signal is represented by a digitising system. The more bits that are used, the more accurately the amplitude of each sample can be measured, but there are other elements of converter design that also affect accuracy. High-conversion accuracy is known as *high resolution*.

Resonance

Same as Q.

Reverb

Acoustic ambience created by multiple reflections in a confined space.

RF Interference

Radio-frequency interference significantly above the range of human hearing.

Ribbon Microphone

Microphone where the sound capturing element is a thin metal ribbon suspended in a magnetic filed. When sound causes the ribbon to vibrate, a small electrical current is generated within the ribbon.

Ring Modulator

Device that accepts and processes two input signals in a particular way. The output signal does not contain any of the original input signal but instead comprises new frequencies based on the sum and difference of the input signals' frequency components. The best known application of ring modulation is in the creation of Dalek voices, but it may also be used to create dramatic instrumental textures. Depending on the relationships between the input signals, the results may be either of a musical nature or extremely dissonant – for example, ring modulation can be used to create bell-like tones. (The term *ring* is used here because the original circuit which produced the effect used a ring of diodes.)

RMS

Abbreviation of *root mean square*, a method of measuring the voltage of a complex audio waveform.

Roll-Off

Rate at which a filter attenuates a signal once it has passed the filter cut-off point.

ROM

Abbreviation of *read-only memory*, a permanent, non-volatile type of memory containing data that can't be changed. Operating systems are often stored on ROM, as it remains intact when the power is removed.

Safety Copy

Copy or clone of an original tape for use in case of loss of or damage to the original.

Sample

Digitised sound used as a musical sound source in a sampler or additive synthesiser.

Sample And Hold

Usually refers to a feature whereby random values are generated at regular intervals and then used to control another function such as pitch or filter frequency. Sample-and-hold circuits were also used in old analogue synthesisers to 'remember' the note being played after a key had been released.

Sample Rate

Number of times an A/D converter samples an incoming waveform each second.

Sampling

Process carried out by an A/D converter where the instantaneous amplitude of a signal is measured many times per second (44.1kHz in the case of CD).

Sawtooth Wave

So called because it resembles the teeth of a saw, this waveform contains only even harmonics.

SCSI

Abbreviation of *small-computer system interface*, an interfacing system for using hard drives, scanners, CD-ROM drives and similar peripherals with a computer. Each SCSI device has its own ID number and no two SCSI devices in the same chain must be set to the same number. The last SCSI device in the chain should be terminated, either via an internal terminator, where provided, or via a plug-in terminator fitted to a free SCSI socket.

Session Tape

Original tape made during a recording session.

Sequencer

Device for recording and replaying MIDI data, usually in a multitrack format, allowing complex compositions to be built up a part at a time.

Short Circuit

Low resistance path that allows electrical current to flow. The term is usually used to describe a current path that exists through a fault condition.

Sibilance

High-frequency whistling or lisping sound that affects vocal recordings, due either to poor mic technique or excessive equalisation.

Side Chain

Part of a circuit that splits off a proportion of the main signal to be processed in some way. Compressors use side-chain signals to derive their control signals.

Signal

Electrical representation of input such as sound.

Signal Chain

Route taken by a signal from the input to a system to the output.

Signal-To-Noise Ratio

Ratio of maximum signal level to residual noise, expressed in decibels.

Sine Wave

Waveform of a pure tone with no harmonics.

Single-Ended Noise Reduction

The use of a device that removes or attenuates the noise component of a signal but doesn't require previous coding, as in the case of Dolby or dbx.

Slave

Device that operates under the control of a master device.

SMPTE

Time code developed for the film industry but now extensively used in music and recording. SMPTE is a real-time code and is related to hours, minutes, seconds and film or video frames rather than to musical tempo.

Soundfield

A British four-capsule microphone designed for surround recording applications. Its output is in the so-called B format, which can be decoded to provide any desirable surround audio format, in both horizontal and vertical space.

SPL

Abbreviation of *sound-pressure level*, measured in decibels.

SPP

Abbreviation of *song-position pointer* (MIDI).

Square Wave

Symmetrical, rectangular waveform containing a series of odd harmonics.

SRC

Abbreviation of *sample-rate conversion*, a system used to convert the sample rate of a piece of digital audio from one standard to another – for example, from 48kHz to 44.1kHz. Both hardware and software SRCs are available.

Standard MIDI File

See *MIDI File*.

Step Time

System for programming a sequencer in non-real time.

Stereo

Term used to describe a two-channel system that feeds both left and right loudspeakers.

Sticky-Shed Syndrome

Problem affecting some brands of analogue audio tape after prolonged periods of storage and caused by the breakdown of the chemical binder holding the oxide onto the tape's backing film. In extreme cases, the tape sheds large amounts of oxide and may even stick to the heads during playback. In most cases, the tape can be rendered playable for a few days by baking it at approximately 50ºC for 24–48 hours. Once it has been allowed to cool naturally, it should be copied to a suitable medium before the problem returns.

Square Wave

Symmetrical rectangular waveform. Square waves contain a series of odd harmonics.

Stripe

To record time code onto one track of a multitrack tape machine.

Sub-Bass

Frequencies below the range of typical monitor loudspeakers. Some define sub-bass as frequencies that can be felt rather than heard.

Subcode

Hidden data within CD/DAT format that includes such information as the absolute time location, number of tracks, total running time and so on.

Subtractive Synthesis

Process of creating a new sound by filtering and shaping a raw, harmonically complex waveform.

Subwoofer

Loudspeaker that handles only very low frequencies. In a surround system, the subwoofer carries the LFE (Low Frequency Effects) channel.

Surge

Sudden increase in mains voltage.

Surround

Audio playback format for film soundtracks or music employing more than two speakers to carry different information in order to recreate the effect of sounds arriving at the listener from different directions. The current commercial standard is 5.1 surround, where the 5 refers to left, centre, right, left surround and rear surround speakers and the .1 refers to the subwoofer.

Sustain
Part of the ADSR envelope that determines the level to which the sound will settle if a key is held down. Once the key is released, the sound decays at a rate set by the Release parameter. Also refers to a guitar's ability to hold notes that decay very slowly.

Sweet Spot
Optimum position for a microphone or for a listener relative to monitor loudspeakers.

Switching Power Supply
Type of power supply that uses a high-frequency oscillator prior to the transformer so that a smaller, lighter transformer may be used. These power supplies are commonly used in computers and some synthesiser modules.

Sync
Abbreviation of *synchronisation*, a system for making two or more pieces of equipment run together.

Synthesiser
Electronic musical instrument that is designed to create a wide range of sounds, both imitative and abstract.

Tape Head
Part of a tape machine that transfers magnetic energy to the tape during recording or reads it during playback.

Tempo
Rate of the 'beat' of a piece of music, measured in beats per minute.

Test Tone
Steady, fixed-level tone recorded onto a multitrack or stereo recording to act as a reference when matching levels.

TFT
Abbrevitation of *thin-film transistor*, referring to the transistor technology used in flat-screen, solid-state monitor displays.

THD
Abbreviation of *total harmonic distortion*.

Thru
MIDI connector which passes on the signal received at the MIDI In socket.

Timbre
Tonal colour of a sound.

TOSLINK
Standard optical interface used by the S/PDIF and ADAT interfaces.

Track
Term that dates back to the days of using multitrack tape, where the tracks are physical stripes of recorded material located side by side along the tape's length.

Tracking
System whereby one device follows another. Tracking is often discussed in the context of MIDI guitar synthesisers or controllers, where the MIDI output attempts to track the pitch of the guitar strings.

Transducer
Device used to convert one form of energy to another. A microphone is a good example of a transducer as it converts mechanical energy to electrical energy.

Transparent
Subjective term used to describe audio quality where the high-frequency detail is clear and individual sounds are easy to identify and separate.

Transpose
To shift a musical signal by a number of semitones.

Tremolo
Modulation of a sound's amplitude using an LFO.

Triangle Wave

Symmetrical wave containing odd harmonics only, but with a lower harmonic content than a square wave.

TRS Jack

Stereo-type jack plug with tip, ring and sleeve connections.

Truss Rod

Metal bar within a guitar neck that is tensioned in order to counteract the tendency for the neck to bend under the tension of the strings.

Unbalanced

Term used to describe a two-wire electrical signal connection where the inner (or hot, or positive) conductor is usually surrounded by the cold (or negative) conductor, which forms a screen against interference.

Unison

Term used to describe the playing of a melody using two or more different instruments or voices simultaneously.

USB

Abbreviation of *universal serial buss*, a computer interfacing standard used to connect printers, scanners and modest audio interfaces. USB II is much faster and is comparable in performance with FireWire, enabling it to be used for multichannel audio and video applications.

Valve

Vacuum-tube amplification component, also known as a *tube*.

Velocity

Rate at which a key is depressed. This may be used to control loudness (to simulate the response of instruments such as pianos) or other parameters on later synthesisers.

Vibrato

Pitch modulation using an LFO to modulate a VCO.

Vocoder

Signal processor that imposes a changing spectral filter on a sound based on the frequency characteristics of a second sound. By taking the spectral content of a human voice and imposing it on a musical instrument, talking-instrument effects can be created.

Voice

Term used to indicate the capacity of a synthesiser to play a single musical note. An instrument capable of playing 16 simultaneous notes is said to be a 16-voice instrument.

VST

Abbreviation of *virtual studio system*, a Steinberg-originated standard for plug-in design to be used with their Cubase VST software. VST is now supported by other leading sequencers, although Emagic's Logic supports only Audio Units from OSX onwards. Other Apple systems that do support the VST protocol require special versions when used with OSX or later.

VST Effect

Plug-in effect or processor written to the VST standard that may be used within any VST-compliant music software package. Both Mac and PC versions are available for many VST products. VST II-compliant plug-ins can receive MIDI data, which makes automation possible.

VST Instrument

Plug-in MIDI instrument, such as a synth, sampler or drum machine, written to the VST standard and which may be used within any VST-compliant music software package. Both Mac and PC versions are available for many VST products. VST instruments are played like any other MIDI instrument, and most have comprehensive parameter automation.

VU Meter

Meter designed to interpret signal levels in roughly the same way as the human ear, which responds more closely to the average levels of sounds than to the peak levels.

Wah-Wah Pedal

Guitar effects device where a bandpass filter is varied in frequency by means of a pedal control.

Warmth

Subjective term used to describe sound where the bass and low-mid frequencies have depth and where the high frequencies are smooth-sounding rather than aggressive or fatiguing. Warm-sounding tube equipment may also exhibit some aspects of compression.

Watt

SI unit of electrical power.

Waveform

Graphic representation of the way in which a sound wave or electrical wave varies with time.

White Noise

Random signal with an energy distribution that produces the same amount of noise power per Hz.

Word-Clock Generator

Hardware device capable of generating an accurate digital word-clock signal for distribution to multiple digital audio devices within a studio. All the slave devices are then synced to this master clock, which simplifies operation and reduces jitter.

Wrapper

Software program that allows one type of plug-in to emulate another format. For example, there are wrappers that allow VST programs compiled for Mac OSX to run as Audio Units in programs that don't support VST directly.

Write

To save data to a digital storage medium, such as a hard drive.

XG

Yamaha's alternative to Roland's GS system for enhancing the General MIDI protocol to provide extra banks of patches and further editing facilities.

XLR

Variety of connector commonly used to carry balanced audio signals, including the feeds from microphones.

Y-Lead

Lead split so that one source can feed two destinations. Y-leads may also be used in console insert points, in which case a stereo jack plug at one end of the lead is split into two monos at the other.

Zenith

Parameter of tape-head alignment relating to whether or not the head is perpendicular to the tape path and aligned so as to be in the same plane.

Zero-Crossing Point

Point at which a signal waveform crosses over from being positive to negative, or vice versa.

Zipper Noise

Audible steps that occur when a parameter is being varied in a digital audio processor.

NOTES

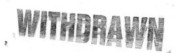

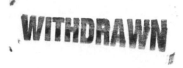

Also available from SANCTUARY PUBLISHING

CREATIVE RECORDING 1 - EFFECTS AND PROCESSORS (SECOND EDITION)
Paul White | £11.95 | $17.95 | 1-86074-456-7

MIDI FOR THE TECHNOPHOBE (SECOND EDITION)
Paul White | £11.95 | $19.95 | 1-86074-444-3

RECORDING AND PRODUCTION TECHNIQUES (SECOND EDITION)
Paul White | £11.95 | $19.95 | 1-86074-443-5

HOME RECORDING MADE EASY (SECOND EDITION)
Paul White | £11.95 | $19.95 | 1-86074-350-1

DESKTOP DIGITAL STUDIO
Paul White | £11.95 | $20 | 1-86074-324-2

BASIC SAMPLING
Paul White | £5 | $7.95 | 1-86074-477-X

BASIC KIT REPAIR
Robbie Gladwell | £5 | $7.95 | 1-86074-384-6

GIANTS OF ROCK
Jamie Humphries | £19.99 | $24.95 | 1-86074-509-1

GIANTS OF BLUES
Neville Marten | £19.99 | $24.95 | 1-86074-211-4

HOW TO GET THE SOUND YOU WANT
Michael and Tim Prochak | £11.95 | $19.95 | 1-86074-348-X

RHYTHM PROGRAMMING
Mark Roberts | £11.95 | $19.95 | 1-86074-412-5

CUBASE SX - THE OFFICIAL GUIDE
Michael Prochak | £11.95 | $17.95 | 1-86074-470-2

MACWORLD MUSIC HANDBOOK
Michael Prochak | £20 | $28 | 1-86074-319-6

FOR MORE INFORMATION on titles from Sanctuary Publishing visit our website at www.sanctuarypublishing.com or contact us at: Sanctuary House, 45-53 Sinclair Road, London W14 ONS. Tel: +44 (0)20 7602 6351

To order a title direct call our sales department or write to the above address. You can also order from our website at www.sanctuarypublishing.com